# THE ULTIMATE
# BMAT GUIDE

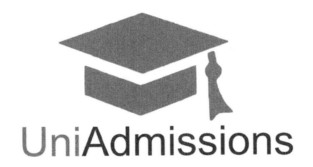

ISBN 978-1-915091-00-0

Published by *RAR Medical Services Limited*
www.uniadmissions.co.uk
info@uniadmissions.co.uk
Tel: +44 (0) 208 068 0438

# THE ULTIMATE BMAT GUIDE

DR. ROHAN AGARWAL

MATTHEW WILLIAMS

EDITED BY DR. CHLOE GAMLIN

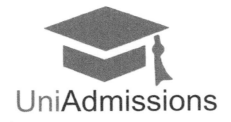

UniAdmissions

# ABOUT THE AUTHORS

**Rohan** is the **Director of Operations** at *UniAdmissions* and is responsible for its technical and commercial arms. He graduated from Gonville and Caius College, Cambridge and is a fully qualified doctor. Over the last five years, he has tutored hundreds of successful Oxbridge and Medical applicants. He has also authored ten books on admissions tests and interviews.

Rohan has taught physiology to undergraduates and interviewed medical school applicants for Cambridge. He has published research on bone physiology and writes education articles for the Independent and Huffington Post. In his spare time, Rohan enjoys playing the piano and table tennis.

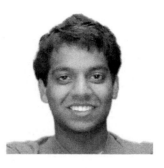

**Matthew** is **Resources Editor** at *UniAdmissions* and a 5th year medical student at St Catherine's College, Oxford. As the first student from Barry Comprehensive School in South Wales to receive a place on the Oxford medicine course he embraced all aspects of university life, both social and academic. Matt Scored in the **top 5% for his UCAT and BMAT** to secure his offer at the University of Oxford.

Matt has worked with UniAdmissions since 2014 – tutoring several applicants successfully into Oxbridge and Russell group universities. His work has been published in international scientific journals and he has presented his research at conferences across the globe. In his spare time, Matt enjoys playing rugby and golf.

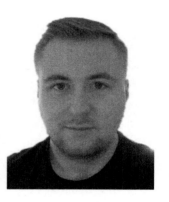

# CONTENTS

# THE ULTIMATE BMAT GUIDE

## THE BASICS

### What is the BMAT?

The BioMedical Admissions Test (BMAT) is a 2-hour written exam for medical and veterinary students who are applying for competitive universities.

### What does the BMAT consist of?

| Section | SKILLS TESTED | Questions | Timing |
|---|---|---|---|
| ONE | Problem-solving skills, including numerical and spatial reasoning. Critical thinking skills, including understanding argument and reasoning using everyday language. | 32 MCQs | 60 minutes |
| TWO | Ability to recall, understand and apply GCSE level principles of biology, chemistry, physics and maths. Usually the section that students find the hardest. | 27 MCQs | 30 minutes |
| THREE | Ability to organise ideas in a clear and concise manner, and communicate them effectively in writing. Questions are usually but not necessarily medical. | One essay from three | 30 minutes |

### Why is the BMAT used?

Medical and veterinary applicants tend to be a bright bunch and therefore usually have excellent grades. For example, in 2013 over 65% of students who applied to Cambridge for Medicine had UMS greater than 90% in all of their A level subjects. This means that competition is fierce, so universities must use the BMAT to help differentiate between applicants.

### When can I sit BMAT?

There are two sittings for the BMAT – the second week of September and the first week of November (normally Wednesday mornings). You can generally sit the BMAT on either date. Be aware, however that some universities will ask that you sit the test on a specific date e.g. Oxford, Lee Kong Chian and Chulalongkorn University will only accept results from the November BMAT sitting. You're highly advised to check which date you should sit the BMAT depending on your university choices. This information is available online, on the official BMAT page of the Cambridge Assessment admissions testing site, as well as on individual university websites.

### When should I sit the BMAT?

The difficulty and content of both sittings is the same so the answer will depend on how much time you have over the summer and how important it is for you to know your BMAT result before you submit your UCAS application. In general, if you're applying for two or more BMAT universities, it's a good idea to sit the BMAT in September if circumstances allow.

|  | **SEPTEMBER** | **NOVEMBER** |
|---|---|---|
| **Positive** | Get BMAT Results before UCAS Deadline Can use the summer to prepare thoroughly | More time to prepare overall Will have covered more science topics in school |
| **Negative** | Less time to prepare overall May conflict with UCAT, Personal Statement etc | Hard to balance school-work with BMAT revision Won't get BMAT results until after UCAS Deadline |

### Who has to sit the BMAT?

Applicants to the following universities must sit the BMAT:

| University | Course |
|---|---|
| **University of Cambridge** | Medicine and Veterinary Medicine |
| **University of Oxford** | Medicine, Graduate Medicine, Biomedical Sciences |
| **University College London** | Medicine |
| **Imperial College London** | Medicine, Graduate Medicine, Biomedical Science |
| **Brighton and Sussex** | Medicine |
| **University of Leeds** | Medicine, Gateway Year to Medicine, Dentistry |
| **Lancaster University** | Medicine |
| **Keele University** | Medicine (International Applicants) |
| **Royal Veterinary College** | Veterinary Medicine |
| **Lee Kong Chian (Singapore)** | Medicine |
| **Thammasat University** | 642901( Medicine) and 642902 (Dental Surgery) |
| **Universidad de Navarra** | Medicine |
| **Mahidol University** | Medicine |

### How is the BMAT Scored?

**Section 1 and Section 2** are marked on a scale of 0 to 9. Generally, 5 is an average score, 6 is good, and 7 is excellent. Very few people (<5%) get more than 8.

The marks for sections 1 + 2 show a normal distribution with a large range. The important thing to note is that the difference between a score of 5.0 and 6.5+ is often only 3-4 questions. Thus, you can see that even small improvements in your raw score will lead to massive improvements when they are scaled.

**Section 3** is marked on 2 scales: A-E for Quality of English and 0-5 for Strength of Argument

The marks for section 3 show a normal distribution for the strength of argument; the average mark for the strength of argument is between 3 – 3.5. The distribution of quality of English marks is negatively skewed. In other words, the vast majority of students will score A or B for quality of English. The ones that don't tend to be students who are not fluent in English.

This effectively means that the letter score (A-E) is used to flag students who have a comparatively weaker grasp of English- i.e. it is a test of competence rather than excellence like the rest of the BMAT. In practice this means that essays scoring a C or below are therefore likely to be more heavily scrutinised by admissions tutors than essays graded A or B.

Finally, section 3 is marked by two different examiners. If there is a large discrepancy between their marks, it is marked by a third examiner.

### Can I resit the BMAT if I'm unhappy with my score?

No, you can only sit the BMAT once per admissions cycle. You can resit the BMAT if you apply for medicine again in the future.

### Do I have to resit the BMAT if I reapply?

You must resit the BMAT with each admissions cycle, if you applying to a university that requires it. You cannot use your score from any previous attempts.

### Where do I sit the BMAT?

For the September sitting, you will need to register yourself and sit the test at one of 20 authorised centres. In November, your school will normally register you and you can usually sit the BMAT at your school or college (ask your school exams officer for more information). Alternatively, if your school isn't a registered test centre or you're not attending a school or college, you can sit the BMAT at an authorised test centre.

### When do I get my results?

For the September sitting, you will get your results by the end of September online. You are then responsible for informing the University of your BMAT score. For the November sitting, the BMAT results are usually released to universities in mid-late November and then to students in late November.

### How is the BMAT used?

**Cambridge:** Cambridge interviews more than 90% of students who apply so the BMAT score isn't vital for making the interview shortlist. However, it can play a huge role in the final decision – for example, 50% of overall marks for your application may be allocated to the BMAT. Thus, it's essential you find out as much information about the college you're applying to, as each college places a slightly different weighting on each part of your application.

**Oxford:** Oxford typically receives thousands of applications each year and they use the BMAT to shortlist students for interview. Typically, 450 students are invited for interview for 150 places. Thus, if you get offered an interview- you are doing very well! Oxford centralise their short listing process and use an algorithm that uses your % A*s at GCSE along with your BMAT score to rank all their applicants of which the top are invited to interview. BMAT sections 1 + 2 count for 40% each of your BMAT score whilst section 3 counts for 20% [the strength of argument (number) contributes to 13.3% and the quality of English (letter) makes up the remaining 6.7%].

**UCL:** UCL make offers based on all components of the application and whilst the BMAT is important there is no magic threshold that you need to meet in order to guarantee an interview. Applicants with higher BMAT scores tend to be interviewed earlier in the year.

**Imperial:** Imperial employs a BMAT threshold to shortlist for interview. This exact threshold changes every year but in the past has been approximately 4.5-5.0 for sections 1 + 2 and 2.5 B for section 3.

**Leeds:** The BMAT contributes to 15% of your academic score at Leeds. You will be allocated marks based on your rank in the BMAT. Thus, applicants in the top 20% of the BMAT will get the full quota of marks for their application and the bottom 20% will get the lowest possible mark for their application. Thus, you can still get an interview if you perform poorly in the BMAT (it's just much harder!). Leeds will calculate your BMAT score by attributing 40% to section 1, 40% to section 2 and 20% to section 3 (lower weighting as it can come up during the interview).

**Brighton & Sussex:** BSMS recently started using the BMAT as part of the shortlisting process to decide which students to interview. They assign a total score of 28 to the BMAT (9 marks for Section 1, 9 marks for Section 2 and 5 marks for each component of Section 3 – letter and number grade). An example score at BSMS for a BMAT score of 5.0 in Section 1, 4.0 in Section 2 and 3.5A in Section 3 would be 17.5/28. The medical school rank all applicants based on their total score out of 28 and work down the rankings until all interview spots are filled. There is no specific cut off score, so it will vary each year depending on applicants' BMAT scores. In addition, they state on their website that it "may also be used as a final discriminator if needed after interview."

**Royal Veterinary College:** It is unclear how the RVC use the BMAT- it has influenced applications both before and after interview and it's likely that they use it on a case-by-case basis rather than as an arbitrary cut-off.

# GENERAL ADVICE

### Start Early

It is much easier to prepare and do well if you practice little and often. Start your preparation well in advance; ideally by mid September but at the latest by early October for the November sitting, or 8-12 weeks prior to the earlier sitting. This way you will have plenty of time to complete as many papers as you wish to feel comfortable with the exam content and style and won't have to panic and cram just before the test, which is a much less effective and more stressful way to learn. In general, an early start will give you the opportunity to identify the complex issues and work at your own pace to better your understanding of the material.

### Prioritise

Some questions in sections 1 + 2 can be long and complex — and given the intense time pressure in the BMAT you need to know your limits. It is essential that you don't get stuck and waste valuable time on very difficult questions. If a question looks particularly long or complex, mark it for review and move on. You don't want to be caught 5 questions short at the end just because you took more than 3 minutes in answering a challenging multi-step physics question. If a question is taking too long, choose a sensible answer, mark for review if you have time later, and move on. Remember that each question carries equal weighting and therefore, you should adjust your timing accordingly. With some disciplined practice under timed conditions, you can get very good at this and learn to maximise your efficiency. In short, exam technique is a crucial part of the BMAT, and matters almost as much as learning the content, so it is wise to spend your preparation time developing a consistent approach to the exam.

### Positive Marking

There are no penalties for incorrect answers in the BMAT; you will gain one mark for each right answer and will not lose a mark for a wrong or unanswered question. This affords you the luxury of being able to guess if you are completely unable to figure out the right answer to a question or find yourself running out of time. Since each question provides you with 4 to 6 possible answers, you have a 16-25% chance of guessing correctly. Therefore, if you aren't sure (and are running short of time), you can make an educated guess and move on without risking being penalised for an incorrect answer. Before 'guessing' you should try to eliminate a couple of answers to increase your chances of getting the question correct. For example, if a question has 5 options and you manage to eliminate 2 options, your chances of getting the question correct increase from 20% to 33%!

It is important also to try to avoid losing easy marks on other questions because of poor exam technique. The BMAT is very time pressured, so you must attempt to get through as many questions as you can by doing plenty of practice under timed conditions well in advance of the exam. If you have failed to finish the exam on the day, take the last 10 seconds to guess the remaining questions to at least give yourself a chance of getting them right.

## Practice

This is the best way to familiarise yourself with the style of questions and the timing for BMAT. Although the BMAT tests only GCSE level knowledge, you are unlikely to be familiar with the style of questions in all 3 sections when you first encounter them. Although you will have previously encountered all of the scientific ideas in the BMAT specification, often the questions use a different approach to questions on the school exams syllabus. This means you will be required to apply principles rather than knowledge acquired from rote-learning, so it is important to ensure you fully understand the material on the test specification.

Practising questions will put you at ease and make you more comfortable with the exam. The more comfortable you are, the less you will panic on the test day when confronted with tricky questions, and the more likely you are to score highly. Initially, work through the questions at your own pace, and spend time carefully reading the questions and looking at any additional data provided on the test paper. As you get closer to the test, **make sure you practice the questions under exam conditions**.

## Past Papers

Official past papers and answers from 2003 onwards are freely available online and once you've worked your way through the questions in this book, it's a good idea to attempt as many of them as you can. You should aim to complete at least 5 full BMAT papers from the most recent specification under timed conditions prior to taking your test. Keep in mind that the specification was changed in 2009 so some things asked in earlier papers may not be representative of the content that is currently examinable in the BMAT. If a topic has been removed from the BMAT specification, this is usually made clear on the older past papers, so they are still a useful resource for practice. In general, **it is worth doing at least all the papers from 2009 onwards**. If time permits, you could work backwards from 2009 for additional Section 1 & 2 practice, although there is little point doing the section 3 essays pre-2009 as they are significantly different to the current style of essay questions.

## Scoring Tables

Use these to keep a record of your scores – you can then easily see which paper you should attempt next to build on your syllabus knowledge and exam technique (always the one with the lowest score).

| SECTION 1 | 1st Attempt | 2nd Attempt | SECTION 2 | 1st Attempt | 2nd Attempt |
|---|---|---|---|---|---|
| 2003 | | | | | |
| 2004 | | | | | |
| 2005 | | | | | |
| 2006 | | | | | |
| 2007 | | | | | |
| 2008 | | | | | |
| 2009 | | | | | |
| 2010 | | | | | |
| 2011 | | | | | |
| 2012 | | | | | |
| 2013 | | | | | |
| 2014 | | | | | |
| 2015 | | | | | |
| 2016 | | | | | |
| 2017 | | | | | |
| 2018 | | | | | |
| 2019 | | | | | |
| 2020 | | | | | |

## Repeat Questions

When checking through your answers to practice papers, pay particular attention to questions you have got wrong. If there is a worked solution, look through that carefully until you feel confident that you understand the reasoning, and then repeat the question without help to check that you can do it. If only the answer is given, have another look at the question and try to work out why that answer is correct. You can refer to worked solutions for similar types of questions for some pointers if the answer doesn't seem obvious. This is the best way to learn from your mistakes, and means you are less likely to make similar mistakes when it comes to the real BMAT. The same applies for questions which you were unsure of and made an educated guess which was correct, even if you got it right. When working through this book, **make sure you highlight any questions you are unsure of**, to ensure you know to spend more time looking over them once marked.

### No Calculators

You aren't permitted to use a calculator in the BMAT – thus, it is essential that you have strong numerical skills and feel confident manipulating figures with pen and paper. For instance, you should be able to rapidly convert between percentages, decimals and fractions. You will seldom get questions that would require calculators but you would be expected to be able to arrive at a sensible estimate. Consider for example:

Estimate $3.962 \times 2.322$;

$3.962$ is approximately 4 and $2.323$ is approximately $2.33 = 7/3$.

Thus, $3.962 \times 2.322 \approx 4 \times \frac{7}{3} = \frac{28}{3} = 9.33$

It is an important part of exam technique to know that in the BMAT you will rarely be asked to perform difficult calculations. In fact, you can use this as a marker of whether you are tackling a question correctly.

For example, when solving a physics question, if you end up having to divide values such as 8,079 by 357- this should raise alarm bells as calculations in the BMAT are rarely this difficult.

### A word on timing...

> "If you had all day to do your BMAT, you would get 100%. But you don't."

Whilst this isn't completely true, it illustrates a very important point. Once you've practiced and know how to answer the questions, the clock is your biggest enemy. This seemingly obvious statement has one very important consequence. The way to improve your BMAT score is to improve your speed. There is no magic bullet. But there are a great number of techniques that, with practice, will give you significant time gains, allowing you to answer more questions and score more marks.

Timing is tight throughout the BMAT – mastering the timing of each section is the first key to success. Some candidates choose to work as quickly as possible through every question to save up time at the end to check their answers, but this is generally not the best approach.

BMAT questions can have a lot of information in them – each time you start answering a question it takes time to get familiar with the instructions and information given. By splitting the question into two sessions (the first run-through and the return-to-check) you double the amount of time you spend familiarising yourself with the data, as you have to do it twice instead of only once. This costs valuable time. In addition, candidates who do check back may spend 2–3 minutes doing so and yet not make any actual changes.

> **Top tip!** In general, students tend to improve the fastest in Section 2 and slowest in Section 1; Section 3 usually falls somewhere in the middle. Thus, if you have very little time left to prepare for the BMAT, it's best to prioritise Section 2 in order to maximise your overall score.

While this can feel reassuring in a high-stakes exam, it is actuallly false reassurance as this approach is unlikely to have a significant impact on your actual score. Therefore, it is usually best to pace yourself very steadily, aiming to spend the same amount of time on each question and finish the final question in a section just as time runs out. This reduces the time spent on re-familiarising yourself with the content of the questions and maximises the time spent arriving at the answer. This approach is the most efficient way to gain the maximum marks you are capable of.

It is essential that you don't get stuck with the hardest questions – no doubt there will be some tough ones scattered through each section of the BMAT. In the time you might spend attempting to answer only one of these questions you could miss out on answering three easier questions, worth three times as many marks! If a question is taking too long, choose a sensible answer (through educated guesswork) and move on. Never see this as giving up or in any way failing – rather, it is the smart way to approach a high stakes test with a tight time limit. With practice and discipline, you can get very good at this and learn to maximise your efficiency. It is not about being a hero and aiming for full marks – this is almost impossible and very much unnecessary (even Oxbridge will regard any score higher than 7 as exceptional). It is about maximising your efficiency and gaining the maximum possible number of marks within the time you have. In summary, perfecting your exam timing and technique is an important way for you to give yourself the best chance of achieving a score that will secure you an interview at medical school.

*Top tip!* Ensure that you take a watch that can show you the time in seconds into the exam. This will allow you have a much more accurate idea of the time you're spending on a question. In general, if you've spent >150 seconds on a section 1 question or >90 seconds on a section 2 questions – move on regardless of how close you think you are to solving it, to ensure you have enough time to answer all the other questions too.

### *Use the Options:*

Some questions may try to overload you with information. You could see this as a distraction technique designed to intimidate candidates, so knowing what to do in this situation is critical.

When presented with large tables and data, it's essential that you look at the answer options so you can focus your mind. This can allow you to reach the correct answer a lot more quickly. Consider the example below:

The table below shows the results of a study investigating antibiotic resistance in staphylococcus populations. A single staphylococcus bacterium is chosen at random from a similar population. Resistance to any one antibiotic is independent of resistance to others.

Calculate the probability that the bacterium selected will be resistant to all four drugs.

A. 1 in $10^6$
B. 1 in $10^{12}$
C. 1 in $10^{20}$
D. 1 in $10^{25}$
E. 1 in $10^{30}$
F. 1 in $10^{35}$

| Antibiotic | Number of Bacteria tested | Number of Resistant Bacteria |
|---|---|---|
| Benzyl-penicillin | $10^{11}$ | 98 |
| Chloramphenicol | $10^9$ | 1200 |
| Metronidazole | $10^8$ | 256 |
| Erythromycin | $10^5$ | 2 |

Looking at the answer options first makes it obvious that there is **no need to calculate exact values**- only in powers of 10. This makes your life a lot easier. If you hadn't noticed this, you might have spent well over 90 seconds trying to calculate the exact value when it wasn't even being asked for.

In other cases, you may actually be able to use the answer options to arrive at the solution quicker than if you had tried to solve the question from scratch as you normally would. Consider the example below:

A region is defined by the two inequalities: $x - y^2 > 1$ and $xy > 1$. Which of the following points is in the defined region?

A.  (10,3)          B.  (10,2)          C.  (-10,3)          D.  (-10,2)          E.  (-10,-3)

Whilst it's possible to solve this question both algebraically or graphically by manipulating the identities, by far **the quickest way is to simply use the options given to you in the question**.

Note that options C, D and E violate the second inequality, narrowing down to answer to either A or B. For A: $10 - 3^2 = 1$ and thus this point is on the boundary of the defined region and not actually in the region. Thus, the answer is B (as $10 - 4 = 6 > 1$)

In general, it pays dividends to look at the answer options briefly to see if they can help you arrive at the solution more quickly. Get into this habit early on in your BMAT preparation – it may feel unnatural at first, but it's guaranteed to save you time in the long run.

### Key Words

If you're stuck on a question; pay particular attention to the options that contain key modifiers like "**always**", "**only**", "**all**" as examiners like using them to test if there are any gaps in your knowledge. For example, the statement "arteries carry oxygenated blood" would normally be true. However, the statement "**all** arteries carry oxygenated blood" would be false because there is an exception: the pulmonary artery carries deoxygenated blood.

# SECTION 1

This is the first section of the BMAT and as you walk in, it is inevitable that you will feel nervous. Make sure that you have been to the toilet prior to the exam because once it starts you cannot simply pause and go due to the time pressure. Take a few deep breaths and calm yourself down. Remember that panicking will not help and may negatively affect your marks - so try and avoid this as much as possible.

You have one hour to answer 32 questions in section 1. The questions fall into two categories:
- Problem solving (16 questions)
- Critical thinking (16 questions)

Whilst this section of the BMAT is renowned for being difficult to prepare for, there are a number of powerful shortcuts and techniques that you can use. Learning specific exam techniques and practising plenty of example questions will train you to work efficiently and make the best of the time available for Section 1.

You have approximately 100 seconds per question. Although this may initially sound like plenty of time the questions in Section 1 often require you to read and analyse passages or graphs to find the correct answer, meaning it is important to work as quickly and efficiently as possible.

Nevertheless, this part of the BMAT is not as time pressured as Section 2 so most students usually finish the majority of questions in time. However, some questions in Section 1 are very tricky and can be a big drain on your limited time. **The people who fail to complete section 1 are those who get bogged down on a particular question**.

Therefore, it is vital that you start to get a feel for which questions are going to be easy and quick to do and which ones should be left until the end. The best way to do this is through practice and the questions in this book will offer extensive opportunities for you to do so.

# SECTION 1: CRITICAL THINKING

BMAT critical thinking questions require you to understand the components of a good argument and be able to pick them apart. The majority of BMAT critical thinking questions tend to fall into 3 major categories:
1.  Identifying Conclusions
2.  Identifying Assumptions + Flaws
3.  Strengthening and Weakening arguments

> ***Top tip!*** Though it might initially sound counter-intuitive, it is often best to read the question **before** reading the passage.  Then you'll have a much better idea of what you're looking for in the text and are therefore likely to pick out the relevant information quickly.

Having a good grasp of language and being able to filter unnecessary information quickly and efficiently is a vital skill in medical school – you simply do not have the time to sit and read vast numbers of textbooks cover to cover. Instead, you will need to be able to filter the information to quickly identify the key points. Ultimately this skill will contribute to your success in your studies, which is why it forms part of the BMAT.

Selecting the most relevant pieces of information from a larger passage is also a key skill for qualified doctors, who simply do not have the time to read pages and pages of notes on the wards to make important healthcare decisions. As such, it is important not to underestimate the importance of getting to grips with verbal reasoning skills at this stage and throughout university.

### Key Tips & Tricks for Section 1

### 1. Only Use the Passage
Your answer must only be based on the information available in the passage provided by the question. Do not try and guess the answer based on your general knowledge as this can be a trap. For example, if the passage says that spring is followed by winter, then take this as true even though you know that spring is followed by summer.

### 2. Take your time
Unlike the problem solving questions, critical thinking questions are less time pressured. Most of the passages are well below 300 words and therefore don't take long to read and process (unlike the UCAT in which you should skim read passages). Thus, your aim should be to understand the intricacies of the passage and identify key information so that you don't lose easy marks.

**Section 1 Question Types**

**Identifying Conclusions**

Students often struggle with these types of questions because they confuse a premise for a conclusion.

Let's start by defining the differences between the two:

- A **conclusion** is a summary of the arguments being made and is usually explicitly stated or heavily implied.
- A **premise** is a statement from which another statement can be inferred or a statement that leads the reader to a conclusion. A premise would always be explicitly stated within a passage of text.

Hence a conclusion is shown/implied/proven by a premise. Similarly, a premise shows/indicates/establishes a conclusion.

Consider for example: *My mom, being a woman, is clever as all women are clever.*

**Premise 1:** My mom is a woman + **Premise 2:** Women are clever = **Conclusion:** My mom is clever.

This is fairly straightforward as it's a very short passage and the conclusion is explicitly stated. Sometimes the latter may not happen.

Consider: My mom is a woman and all women are clever.

Here the conclusion is not explicitly stated, yet both premises still stand and can be used to reach the same conclusion as in the first statement.

You may sometimes be asked to identify if any of the options cannot be "reliably concluded". This is effectively asking you to identify why an option **cannot** be the conclusion.

There are many reasons why a statement cannot be reliably concluded from a passage of text but the most common ones are:

1.  Over-generalising

    *My mom is clever therefore all women are clever.*
2.  Being too specific or narrow:

    *All kids like candy thus my son also likes candy.*
3.  Confusing correlation and causation:

    *Example: Lung cancer is much more likely in patients who drink water. Hence, water causes lung cancer.*
4.  Confusing cause and effect:

    *Example: Lung cancer patients tend to smoke so it follows that having lung cancer must make people want to smoke.*

Note how conjunctives like hence, thus, therefore, and it follows give you a clue as to when a conclusion is being stated in a passage. More examples of these phrases that indicate a conclusion include: it follows that, implies that, whence, entails that.

Similarly, words and phrases like "because, as indicated by, in that, given that, due to the fact that" usually identify premises from which a conclusion or linking statement could be drawn.

**Assumptions + Flaws:**

Other types of critical thinking questions may require you to identify assumptions and flaws in the reasoning given to reach a conclusion in a passage of text. Before proceeding with examples, let's clarify the definitions:

- An assumption is a reasonable assertion that can be made based on the available evidence. It is an unstated piece of information that the rest of the argument relies upon.

- A flaw is an element of an argument that is inconsistent with the rest of the available evidence. A flaw undermines the crucial components of the overall argument being made.

Consider for example: My mom is clever because all doctors are clever.
**Premise 1:** Doctors are clever. **Assumption:** My mom is a doctor. **Conclusion:** My mom is clever.
Note that the assumption will **never** be explicitly stated within a passage of text.

In this short passage, the conclusion follows naturally even though there is only one premise because of the assumption. The argument relies on the assumption to work.
If you are unsure if a given answer option is an assumption, just ask yourself:
1) *Is it in the passage?* If the answer is **no,** then proceed to ask:
2) Does the conclusion rely on this piece of information in order to work? — If the answer is **yes** — then you've identified an assumption.

You may sometimes be asked to identify flaws in an argument — it is important to be aware of the types of flaws to look out for. In general, these are broadly similar to the flaws discussed earlier in the conclusion section (over-generalising, being too specific, confusing cause and effect, confusing correlation and causation). Remember that an assumption may also be a flaw, generating an inappropriate or inconsistent conclusion.

Note that an argument may be sound (no flawed reasoning or assumptions) and still reach a conclusion that you know is false. For instance, a sound argument may arrive at the conclusion that the earth is flat. The important thing to remember is that Section 1 of the BMAT is testing your ability to analyse the components of an argument and **not** testing your knowledge - Section 2 is a test of knowledge.

For example, consider this short extract again: *my mom is clever because all doctors are clever.*
What if the mother was not actually a doctor? The argument would then break down as the assumption would be incorrect or **flawed**.

---

*Top tip!* Don't get confused between premises and assumptions. A **premise** is a statement that is explicitly stated in the passage. An **assumption** is an inference that is made from the passage and will never be stated.

---

### Strengthening and Weakening Arguments:

You may be asked to identify an answer option that would <u>most</u> strengthen or weaken the argument being made in the passage. Normally, you'd also be told to assume that each answer option is true – even if you know them to be false (flat earth, pink elephants etc). Before we can discuss how to strengthen and weaken arguments, it is important to understand what constitutes a good argument:

1.  **Evidence:** arguments which are heavily based on value judgements and subjective statements tend to be weaker than those based on facts, statistics and the available evidence.
2.  **Logic**: a good argument should flow, and the constituent parts should fit well into an overriding view or belief. There should not be any questionable jumps to conclusions from flawed assumptions or premises.
3.  **Balance:** a good argument must concede that there are other views or beliefs (counter-argument). The key is to carefully dismantle these ideas and explain why they are wrong. Look out for words like 'the majority, often, usually' to signal an argument that is more balanced than one using 'always, every, never' etc.

Thus, when asked to strengthen an argument, look for options that would: increase the evidence basis for the argument, support or add a premise, address the counter-arguments.

Similarly, when asked to weaken an argument, look for options that would: decrease the evidence basis for the argument or create doubt over existing evidence, undermine a premise, strengthen the counter-arguments.

In order to be able to strengthen or weaken arguments, you must completely understand the conclusion of a passage. This means you can quickly test the impact of each answer option on the conclusion to see which one strengthens or weakens it the most i.e. is the conclusion stronger/weaker if I assume this information to be true and included in the passage.

Often, you'll have to decide which option strengthens/weakens the passage most. To do this, you can determine the most powerful part of a given argument and compare the impact of the additional statements. Is it the evidence provided in the original argument? Is this additional information fully addressing any counter-arguments, to make the argument watertight? Perhaps the additional statement proves that a counter argument is more powerful than the conclusion in the passage, or reveals a major flaw in the logic. The best way to learn how to tackle these questions is through practice, as eventually you will learn to recognise the patterns in the questions. Thankfully, you have plenty of time for these questions so can consider the options carefully in the exam.

# CRITICAL THINKING QUESTIONS

**Question 1-6 are based on the passage below:**

People have tried to elucidate the differences between the genders for many years. Are they societal pressures or genetic differences? In the past it has always been assumed that it was programmed into our DNA to act in a certain more masculine or feminine way but now evidence has emerged that may show it is not our genetics that determine the way we act, but that society pre-programmes us into gender identification. Although it is generally acknowledged that not all boys and girls are the same, why is it that most young boys like to play with trucks and diggers while young girls prefer dolls and pink?

The society we live in has always been an important factor in our identity, from cultural differences, the languages we speak, the food we eat, to the clothes we wear. All of these factors influence our identity. New research shows that the people around us may prove to be the biggest influence on our gendered behaviour. It shows our parents buying gendered toys may have a much bigger influence than the genes they gave us. Girls are being programmed to like the same things as their mothers and this has lasting effects on their personality. Young girls and boys are forced into their gender stereotypes through the clothes they are bought, the hairstyle they wear and the toys they are given to play with.

The power of society to influence gendered behaviour explains the cases where children have been born with different external sex organs to those with the organs matching their sex determining chromosomes. Despite the influence of their DNA they identify as the gender they have always been told they are. Once the difference has been detected, how then are they ever to feel comfortable in their own skin? The only way to prevent society having such a large influence on gender identity is to allow children to express themselves, wear what they want and play with what they want without fear of not fitting in.

**Question 1:**
What is the main conclusion from the first paragraph?
A. Society controls gendered behaviour.
B. People are different based on their gender.
C. DNA programmes how we act.
D. Boys do not like the same things as girls because of their genes.

**Question 2:**
Which of the following, if true, points out the flaw in the first paragraph's argument?
A. Not all boys like trucks.
B. Genes control the production of hormones.
C. Differences in gender may be due to an equal combination of society and genes.
D. Some girls like trucks.

**Question 3:**

According to the passage, how can culture affect identity?

A.  Culture can influence what we wear and how we speak.

B.  Our parents act the way they do because of culture.

C.  Culture affects our genetics.

D.  Culture usually relates to where we live.

**Question 4:**

Which of these is most implied by the passage?

A.  Children usually identify with the gender they appear to be.

B.  Children are programmed to like the things they do by their DNA.

C.  Girls like dollies and pink because their mothers do.

D.  It is wrong for boys to have long hair like girls.

**Question 5:**

What does the passage say is the best way to prevent gender stereotyping?

A.  Mothers spending more time with their sons.

B.  Parents buying gender-neutral clothes for their children.

C.  Allowing children to act how they want.

D.  Not telling children if they have different sex organs to their chromosomal sex.

**Question 6:**

What, according to the passage, is the biggest problem for children born with different external sex organs to those born with sex organs matching their sex chromosomes?

A.  They may have other problems with their DNA.

B.  Society may not accept them for who they are.

C.  They may wish to be another gender.

D.  They are not the gender they are treated as which can be distressing.

**Questions 7-11 are based on the passage below:**

New evidence has emerged to say that the most important factor in a child's development could be their napping routine. It has come to light that regular napping could be the key factor in determining toddlers' memory and learning abilities. This new countrywide survey of 1000 toddlers, all born in the same year, showed around 75% had regular 30-minute naps. Parents cited the benefits of their child having a regular routine (including mealtimes) such as decreased irritability, and stated the only downfall of regular naps was occasional problems with sleeping at night. Research indicating that toddlers were 10% more likely to suffer regular nighttime sleep disturbances when they regularly napped supported the parents' view.

Those who regularly took 30-minute naps were more than twice as likely to remember simple words such as those of new toys than their non-napping counterparts, who also had higher incidences of memory impairment, behavioural problems and learning difficulties. Toddlers who regularly had 30-minute naps were tested on whether they were able to recall the names of new objects the following day, and then compared to a control group who did not regularly nap. These potential links between napping and memory, behaviour and learning ability provides exciting new evidence in the field of child development.

**Question 7:**
If 5% of 100 toddlers who did not nap were able to remember a new teddy's name, how many out of 100 regularly napping toddlers would be expected to remember?

A. 8          B. 9          C. 10          D. 12

**Question 8:**
Assuming that the incidence of nighttime sleep disturbances is the same for all toddlers independent of all characteristics other than napping, what is the percentage of toddlers who suffer regular nighttime sleep disturbances as a result of napping?

A. 10%          B. 14%          C. 20%          D. 50%

**Question 9:**
Using the information from the passage above, which of the following is the most plausible alternative reason for the link between memory and napping?

A. Children who have bad memory abilities are also likely to have trouble sleeping.
B. Children who regularly nap are born with better memories.
C. Children who do not nap were unable to concentrate on the memory testing exercises for the study.
D. Parents who enforce a routine of napping are more likely to conduct memory exercises with their children.

**Question 10:**
Which of the following is most strongly indicated?

A. Families have more enjoyable mealtimes when their toddlers regularly nap.
B. Toddlers have better routines when they nap.
C. Parents enforce napping to improve their toddlers' memory ability.
D. Napping is important for parents' routines.

**Question 11:**
Which of the following, if true, would strengthen the conclusion that there is a causal link between regular napping and improved memory in toddlers?

A. Improved memory is also associated with regular mealtimes.
B. Parents who enforce regular napping are more inclined to include their children in studies.
C. Toddlers' memory development is so rapid that even a few weeks can make a difference to performance on tests.
D. There is a significant improvement and more consistency in memory test performance amongst toddler playgroups with a higher incidence of napping, compared to playgroups where napping is discouraged.

**Question 12:**

Tom's father says to him: 'You must work for your A-levels. That is the best way to do well in your A-level exams. If you work especially hard for geography, you will definitely succeed in your geography A-level exam'.

Which of the following is the best statement Tom could say to prove a flaw in his father's argument?
A. 'It takes me longer to study for my history exam, so I should prioritise that.'
B. 'I do not have to work hard to do well in my geography A-level.'
C. 'Just because I work hard, does not mean I will do well in my A-levels.'
D. 'You are putting too much importance on studying for A-levels.'
E. 'You haven't accounted for the fact that geography is harder than my other subjects.'

**Question 13:**

Today the NHS is increasingly struggling to be financially viable. In the future, the NHS may have to reduce the services it cannot afford. The NHS is supported by government funds, which come from those who pay tax in the UK. Recently the NHS has been criticised for allowing fertility treatments to be free, as many people believe these are not important and should not be paid for when there is not enough money to pay the doctors and nurses.

Which of the following is the most accurate conclusion of the statement above?
A. Only taxpayers should decide where the NHS spends its money.
B. Doctors and nurses should be better paid.
C. The NHS should stop free fertility treatments.
D. Fertility treatments may have to be cut if NHS finances do not improve.

**Question 14:**

'We should allow people to drive as fast as they want. By allowing drivers to drive at fast speeds, through natural selection the most dangerous drivers will kill only themselves in car accidents. These people will not have children, hence only safe people will reproduce and eventually the population will only consist of safe drivers.'

Which one of the following, if true, most weakens the above argument?
A. Dangerous drivers harm others more often than themselves by driving too fast.
B. Dangerous drivers may produce children who are safe drivers.
C. The process of natural selection takes a long time.
D. Some drivers break speed limits anyway.

**Question 15:**
In the winter of 2014, the UK suffered record levels of rainfall, which led to catastrophic damage across the country. Thousands of homes were damaged and even destroyed, leaving many homeless in the chaos that followed. The government faced harsh criticism that they had failed to adequately prepare the country for the extreme weather.

The government regularly assesses the likelihood of adverse events such as extreme weather happening in the future and balance the risk against the cost of advanced measures to reduce the impact should they occur. This is then compared to the cost of the event with no preparative defences in place. The risk of flooding is usually low, so it could be argued that the costs associated with anti-flooding measures would have been pre-emptively unreasonable. Should the government be expected to prepare for every conceivable threat that could come to pass? Are we to put in place expensive measures against a seismic event as well as a possible extra-terrestrial invasion?

Which of the following best expresses the main conclusion of the statement above?
A. The government has an obligation to assess risks and costs of possible future events.
B. The government should spend money to protect against potential extra-terrestrial invasions and seismic events.
C. The government should have spent money to protect against potential floods.
D. The government was justified in not spending heavily to protect against flooding.
E. The government should assist people who lost their homes in the floods.

**Question 16:**
Sadly, the way in which children interact with each other has changed over the years. While children once used to play sports and games together in the street, they now sit alone in their rooms on the computer playing games on the internet. In the past, young children learned human interaction from active games with their friends, yet this is no longer the case. How then, when these children are grown up, will they be able to socially interact with their colleagues?

Which one of the following is the conclusion of the above statement?
A. Children who play computer games now interact less outside of them.
B. The internet can be a tool for teaching social skills.
C. Computer games are for social development.
D. Children should be made to play outside with their friends to develop their social skills for later in life.
E. Adults will in the future play computer games as a means of interaction.

**Question 17:**

Between 2006 and 2013 the British government spent £473 million on Tamiflu antiviral drugs in preparation for a flu pandemic, despite there being little evidence to support the effectiveness of the drug. The antivirals were stockpiled for a flu pandemic that never fully materialised. Only 150,000 packs of Tamiflu were used during the swine flu episode in 2009, and it is unclear if this improved outcomes. Therefore, this money could have been much better spent on drugs that would actually benefit patients.

Which option best summarises the author's view in the passage?

A.  Drugs should never be stockpiled, as they may not be used.

B.  Spending millions of pounds on drugs should be justified by strong evidence showing positive effects.

C.  We should not prepare for flu pandemics in the future.

D.  The recipients of Tamiflu in the swine flu pandemic had no difference in symptoms or outcomes to patients who did not receive the antivirals.

**Question 18:**

High BMI and central obesity are risk factors associated with increased morbidity and mortality. Many believe the development of cheap, easily accessible fast-food outlets is partly responsible for the increase in rates of obesity. Unhealthy weight is commonly associated with a generally unhealthy lifestyle, such as a lack of exercise. The best way to tackle the growing problem of obesity is for the government to tax unhealthy foods so they are no longer a cheap alternative.

Why is the solution given, to tax unhealthy foods, not a logical conclusion from the passage?

A.  Unhealthy eating is not exclusively confined to low-income families.

B.  A more general approach to unhealthy lifestyles would be optimal.

C.  People do not only choose to eat unhealthy food because it is cheaper.

D.  People have personal responsibility for their own health.

E.  E. None of the above

**Question 19:**

As people are living longer, care in old age is becoming a larger burden. Many elderly people require carers to come into their home numerous times a day or need full time residential care. It is not right that the NHS should be spending vast funds on the care of people who are sufficiently wealthy to fund their own care. Some argue that they want their savings kept aside to give to their children; however this is not a right, simply a luxury. It is not right that people should be saving and depriving themselves of necessary care, or worse, making the NHS pay the bill, so they have money to pass on to their offspring. People need to realise that there is a financial cost to living longer.

Which of the following statements is the main conclusion of the above passage?

A.  We need to take personal financial responsibility for our care in old age.

B.  Caring for the elderly is a significant burden on the NHS.

C.  The reason people are reluctant to pay for their own care is that they want to pass money onto their offspring.

D.  The NHS should limit care to the elderly to reduce their costs.

E.  People shouldn't save their money for old age.

**Question 20:**

There is much interest in research surrounding production of human stem cells from non-embryo sources for potential regenerative medicine, and a huge financial and personal gain at stake for researchers. In January 2014, a team from Japan published two papers in *Nature* that claimed to have developed totipotent stem cells from adult mouse cells by exposure to an acidic environment. However, there has since been much controversy surrounding these papers. Problems included: inability by other teams to replicate the results of the experiment, an insufficient protocol described in the paper and issues with images in one of the papers. It was dishonest of the researchers to publish the papers with such problems. A requirement of a scientific paper is a sufficiently detailed protocol, so that another group could replicate the experiment.

Which statement is most implied in this passage?

A. Research is fuelled mainly by financial and personal gains.

B. The researchers should take responsibility for publishing the paper with such flaws.

C. Rivalry between different research groups makes premature publishing more likely.

D. The discrepancies were in only one of the papers published in January 2014.

**Question 21:**

The placebo effect is a well-documented medical phenomenon in which a patient's condition improves after being given an ineffectual treatment that they believe to be a genuine treatment. It is frequently used as a control during trials of new drugs/procedures, with the effect of the drug being compared to the effect of a placebo. If the drug on trial does not have a greater effect than the placebo, then it is classed as ineffective. However, this analysis discounts the fact that the drug treatment still has more of a positive effect than no action, and so we are clearly missing out on the potential to improve certain health conditions. It follows that where there is a demonstrated placebo effect, but treatments are ineffective, we should still give treatments, as there will still be some benefit to the patient.

Which of the following best expresses the main conclusion of this passage?

A. In situations where drugs are no more effective than a placebo, we should still give drugs, as they will be more effective at improving a patient's condition than not taking action.

B. Our current analysis discounts the fact that even if drug treatments have no more effect than a placebo, they may still be more effective than no action.

C. The placebo effect is a well-recognised medical phenomenon.

D. Drug treatments may have negative side effects that outweigh their benefit to patients.

E. Placebos are better than modern drugs.

**Question 22:**

The speed limit on motorways and dual carriageways has been 70mph since 1965, but this is an out-dated policy and needs to change. Since 1965, car brakes have become much more effective, and many safety features have been introduced into cars, such as seatbelts (which are now compulsory to wear), crumple zones and airbags. Therefore, it is clear that cars no longer need to be restricted to 70mph, and the speed limit can be safely increased to 80mph without causing more road fatalities.

Which of the following best illustrates an assumption in this passage?
A. The government should increase the speed limit to 80mph.
B. If the speed limit were increased to 80mph, drivers would not begin to drive at 90mph.
C. The safety systems introduced reduce the chances of fatal road accidents for cars travelling at higher speeds.
D. The roads have not become busier since the 70mph speed limit was introduced.
E. The public wants the speed limit to increase.

**Question 23:**

Despite the overwhelming scientific evidence for the theory of evolution, and even acceptance of the theory by many high-ranking religious ministers, there are still sections of many major religions that do not accept evolution as true. One of the most prominent of these in western society is the Intelligent Design movement, which promotes a religious-based idea as if it were a theory based on strong scientific evidence. Intelligent Design proponents often point to complex issues of biology as proof that God is behind the design of human beings, much like a watchmaker is inherent in the design of a watch.

One part of anatomy that has been identified as supposedly supporting Intelligent Design is fingerprints, with some proponents arguing that they are a mark of individualism created by God, with no apparent function except to identify each human being as unique. This is incorrect, as fingerprints do have a well documented function — namely channelling away water to improve grip in wet conditions. In wet conditions, hairless, smooth skinned hands would struggle to grip smooth objects. The individualism of fingerprints is accounted for by the complexity of thousands of small grooves on each digit. Development is inherently affected by stochastic or random processes, meaning that the body is unable to uniformly control its development to ensure that fingerprints are the same in each human being. Clearly, the presence of individual fingerprints does nothing to support the so-called-theory of Intelligent Design.

Which of the following best illustrates the main conclusion of this passage?
A. Fingerprints have a well-established function.
B. Evolution is supported by overwhelming scientific proof.
C. Fingerprints do not offer any support to the notion of Intelligent Design.
D. The individual nature of fingerprints is explained by stochastic processes inherent in development that the body cannot uniformly control.
E. Intelligent design is a credible and scientifically rigorous theory.

**Question 24:**

High levels of alcohol consumption are known to increase the risk of many non-infectious diseases, such as cancer, atherosclerosis and liver failure. James is a PhD student, and is analysing the data from a large-scale study of over 500,000 people to further investigate the link between heavy alcohol consumption and health problems. In the study, participants were asked about their alcohol consumption, and then their medical history was recorded. His analysis displays surprising results, concluding that those with high alcohol consumption have a *decreased* risk of cancer. James decides that those carrying out the study must have incorrectly recorded the data.

Which of the following is **NOT** a potential reason why the study has produced these surprising results?

A. Previous studies were incorrect, and high alcohol consumption does lower the risk of cancer.

B. The studies analysed didn't take account of other cancer risk factors in comparing those with high and low alcohol consumption.

C. James has made some errors in his analysis, and thus his conclusions are erroneous.

D. The participants involved in the study did not truthfully report their alcohol consumption, leading to false conclusions being drawn.

E. The study's control group data was mixed up with the test group data.

**Question 25:**

A train is scheduled to depart from Newcastle at 3:30pm. It stops at Durham, Darlington, York, Sheffield, Peterborough and Stevenage before arriving at Kings Cross station in London, where the train completes its journey. The total length of the journey between Newcastle and Kings Cross was 230 miles, and the average speed of the train during the journey (including time spent stood still at calling stations) is 115mph. Therefore, the train will complete its journey at 5:30pm.

Which of the following is an assumption made in this passage?

A. The various stopping points did not increase the time taken to complete the journey.

B. The train left Newcastle on time.

C. The train travelled by the most direct route available.

D. The train was due to end its journey at Kings Cross.

E. There were no signalling problems encountered on the journey.

**Question 26:**

There have been many arguments over the last couple of decades about government expenditure on healthcare in the devolved regions of the UK. It is often argued that, since spending on healthcare per person is higher in Scotland than in England, people in Scotland will be healthier. However, this view fails to take account of the different needs of these two populations within the UK. For example, one major factor is that Scotland gets significantly colder than England. The cold weakens the immune system, leaving people in Scotland at much higher risk of infectious disease. Thus, Scotland requires higher levels of healthcare spending per person simply to maintain the health of the population at a similar level to that of England.

Which of the following is a conclusion that can be drawn from this passage?

A.  The higher healthcare spending per person in Scotland does not necessarily mean people living in Scotland are healthier.

B.  Healthcare spending should be increased across the UK.

C.  Wales requires more healthcare spending per person simply to maintain population health at a similar level to England.

D.  It is unfair on England that there is more spending on healthcare per person in Scotland.

E.  Scotland's healthcare budget is a controversial topic.

**Question 27:**

Vaccinations have been hugely successful in reducing the incidence of several diseases throughout the 20th century. One of the most spectacular achievements was arguably the global eradication of smallpox, once a deadly worldwide killer, during the 1970s. Fortunately, there was a highly effective vaccine available for smallpox, and a major factor in its eradication was an aggressive vaccination campaign. Another disease that is potentially eradicable is polio. However, although there is a highly effective vaccine for polio available, attempts to eradicate it have so far been unsuccessful. It follows that we should plan and execute an aggressive vaccination campaign for polio, in order to ensure that this disease too is eradicated.

Which of the following is the main conclusion of this passage?

A.  Polio is a potentially eradicable disease.

B.  An aggressive vaccination campaign was a major factor in the eradication of smallpox.

C.  Both polio and smallpox have been eradicated by effective vaccination campaigns.

D.  We should execute an aggressive vaccination campaign for polio.

E.  The eradication of smallpox remains one of the most spectacular achievements of medical science.

**Question 28:**

The Y chromosome is one of two sex chromosomes found in the human genome, the other being the X chromosome. As the Y chromosome is only found in males, it can only be passed from father to son. Additionally, the Y chromosome does not exchange sections with other chromosomes during cell division (as happens with most chromosomes), meaning it is passed on virtually unchanged through the generations. All of this makes the Y chromosome a fantastic tool for genetic analysis, both to identify individual lineages and to investigate historic population movement. The identification of Genghis Khan as a descendant of up to 8% of males in 16 populations across Asia is just one famous achievement of genetic research using the Y chromosome, and provides further evidence of its utility.

Which of the following best illustrates the main conclusion of this passage?

A.  The Y chromosome is a useful tool for genetic analysis.
B.  Mutations in the Y chromosome will be passed onto sons but not daughters.
C.  X chromosome linked genetic diseases are more common than Y chromosome linked diseases.
D.  Y chromosomal analysis is a recent achievement that will help scientists investigate the movements of populations over time.
E.  Analysis of the Y chromosome will enable scientists to determine the family tree of Genghis Khan.

**Question 29:**

In order for a bacterial infection to be cleared, a patient must be treated with antibiotics. Rachel has a minor lung infection, which is thought by her doctor to be a bacterial infection. She is treated with antibiotics, but her condition does not improve. Therefore, it must not be a bacterial infection.

Which of the following best illustrates a flaw in this reasoning?

A.  It assumes that a bacterial infection would definitely improve after treatment with antibiotics.
B.  It ignores the other conditions that could potentially be treated by antibiotics.
C.  It assumes that antibiotics are necessary to treat bacterial infections.
D.  It ignores the actions of the immune system, which may be sufficient to clear the infection regardless of what has caused it.
E.  It assumes that antibiotics are the only option to treat a bacterial infection.

**Question 30:**

The link between smoking and lung cancer has been well established for many decades by overwhelming numbers of studies and conclusive research. The answer is clear and simple; the single best measure that can be taken to avoid lung cancer is to not smoke, or to stop smoking if one has already started. However, despite the evidence and clearly communicated health risks, many smokers continue to smoke, and seek to minimise their risk of lung cancer by focusing on other, less important risk factors, such as exercise and healthy eating. This approach is obviously severely flawed, and the fact that some smokers feel this is a good way to reduce their risk of lung cancer shows that they are delusional.

Which of the following best illustrates the main conclusion of this passage?
A.  Eating healthily and exercising can also help to reduce the risk of lung cancer.
B.  Some smokers consider exercise and healthy eating an easier option than cessation of smoking.
C.  The best way to minimise risk of lung cancer is avoidance of smoking.
D.  The link between lung cancer and smoking is undeniable.
E.  Banning smoking would reduce the incidence of lung cancer.

**Question 31:**

The government should invest more money into outreach schemes in order to encourage more people to go to university. These schemes allow students to meet other people who went to university, which they may not always be able to do otherwise, even on open days.

Which of the following is the best conclusion of the above argument?
A.  Outreach schemes are an effective way for encouraging people to go to university.
B.  People will not go to university without seeing it first.
C.  The government wants more people to go to university.
D.  Meeting people who went to a university is a more effective way to encourage students than university open days.
E.  It is easier to meet people at university on outreach schemes than on open days.

**Question 32:**

The illegal drug cannabis was recently upgraded from a class C drug to class B, which means it will be taken less in the UK, because people will know it is more dangerous. It also means if people are caught in possession of the drug they will face a longer prison sentence, which will also discourage its use.

Which **TWO** statements if true, most weaken the above argument?
A.  Class C drugs are cheaper than class B drugs.
B.  Upgrading drugs in other countries has not reduced their use.
C.  People who take illegal drugs do not know what class they are in.
D.  Cannabis was not the only class C drug before it was upgraded.
E.  Even if they are caught possessing class B drugs, people do not think they will go to prison.

**Question 33:**

Schools with better sports programmes such as high-performing football and netball teams tend to have better academic results, less bullying and have overall happier students. Thus, if we want schools to have the best results, reduce bullying and increase student happiness, teachers should start more sports clubs.

Which one of the following best demonstrates a flaw in the above argument?

A. Teachers may be too busy to start sports clubs.
B. Better academic results may be a precondition of better sports teams.
C. Better sports programmes may prevent students from spending time with their family.
D. Some sports teams may be seen to encourage internal bullying.
E. Sport teams that do not perform well lead to increased bullying.

**Question 34:**

The legal age for purchasing alcohol in the UK is 18. This should be lowered to 16 because the majority of 16-year-olds drink alcohol anyway without any fear of repercussions. Even if the police catch a 16-year-old buying alcohol, they are unable to enforce any consequences. If the drinking limit was lowered the police could spend less time trying to catch underage drinkers and deal with other more important crimes. There is no evidence to suggest that drinking alcohol at 16 is any more dangerous than at 18.

Which one of the following, if true, most weakens the above argument?

A. Most 16-year-olds do not drink alcohol.
B. If the legal drinking age were lowered to 16, more 15-year-olds would start purchasing alcohol.
C. Most 16-year-olds do not have enough money to buy alcohol.
D. Most 16-year-olds are able to purchase alcohol currently.

**Question 35:**

There has been a recent change in the way the government helps small businesses. Previously small businesses were given non-repayable grants to help them grow their profits. Now, small businesses only receive government loans that must be repaid with interest when the business turns a certain amount of profit. The government wants to support small businesses, but studies have shown they are less likely to prosper under the new scheme as they have been deterred from taking government money for fear of loan repayments.

Which one of the following can be concluded from the passage above?

A. Small businesses do not want government money.
B. The government cannot afford to give out grants to small businesses any longer.
C. All businesses avoid accumulating debt.
D. The government's change in policy is likely to do more harm than good to small businesses.
E. Big businesses do not need government money.

**Questions 36-41 are based on the passage below:**

Despite the innumerable safety measures in place within medical practice, there can still be disastrous results or 'never events'. Safety measures can fail when the weaknesses in the layers of defence align to create a clear path for failure. This is known as the 'Swiss cheese model of accident causation'. One such occurrence occurred where the wrong kidney was removed from a patient due to a failure in the line of defences designed to prevent such an incident occurring.

When a kidney is diseased it is removed to prevent further complications. This operation, known as a 'nephrectomy', is regularly performed by experienced surgeons. Where normally the consultant who knew the patient would have conducted the procedure, in this case he passed the responsibility to his registrar, who was also well experienced but had not met the patient previously. The person who had copied out the patient's notes had poor handwriting had accidentally written the 'R' for 'right' in such a way that it was read as an 'L' and subsequently copied, and not noticed by anyone who further reviewed the notes.

The patient had been put under anaesthetic before the registrar had arrived and so he proceeded without checking the procedure with the patient, as he normally would have done. The nurses present noticed this error but said nothing, fearing repercussions for questioning a senior medical professional. A medical student was present who had met the patient on the ward previously. The student tried to alert the registrar to the mistake he was about to make, however the registrar shouted at the student that she should not interrupt surgery; she did not know what she was talking about and asked her to leave. Consequently, the surgery proceeded with the end result being that the patient's healthy left kidney was removed, leaving them with only their diseased right kidney, which would eventually lead to the patient's premature death. Frightening as these cases appear what is perhaps scarier is the thought of how those reported may be just the 'tip of the iceberg'.

When questioned about his action to allow his registrar to perform the surgery alone, the consultant had said that it was normal to allow capable registrars to do this. 'While the public perception is that medical knowledge steadily increases over time, this is not the case with many doctors reaching their peak in the middle of their careers.' He had found that his initial increasing interest in surgery had enhanced his abilities, but with time and practice the similar surgeries had become less exciting and so his lack of interest had correlated with worsening outcomes, thus justifying his decision to devolve responsibility in this case.

**Question 36:**
Which of the following, if true, most weakens the argument above?
A. Only the most severe adverse events in clinical practice will be reported.
B. Doctors undergo extensive training to reduce risks.
C. Thousand of operations happen every year with no problems.
D. Some errors are unavoidable.
E. The patient could have passed away even if the operation had been a complete success.

**Question 37:**
Which one of the following is the overall conclusion of the passage above?
A. The error that occurred was a result of the failure of safety precautions in place.
B. Surgery should only be performed by surgeons who know their patients well.
C. The human element to medicine means errors will always occur.
D. The safety procedures surrounding surgical procedures need to be reviewed.
E. Some doctors are overconfident.

**Question 38:**

Which of the following is attributed as the original cause of the error?

A. The medical student not having asserted herself.

B. The poor handwriting in the chart.

C. The hierarchical system of medicine.

D. The registrar not having met the patient previously.

E. The lack of surgical skill possessed by the registrar.

**Question 39:**

What does the 'tip of the iceberg' refer to in the passage?

A. Problems we face every day.

B. The probable large numbers of medical errors that go unreported.

C. The difficulties of surgery.

D. Reported medical errors.

E. Problems within the NHS.

You may use the graphs below once, more than once, or not at all.

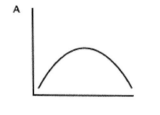
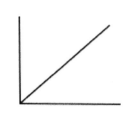
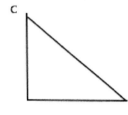
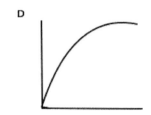
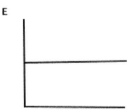
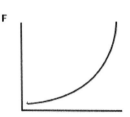

**Question 40:**

Which graph best describes the consultants' performance versus emotional investment in cases over his career?

A. A          B. B          C. C          D. D          E. E          F. F

**Question 41:**

Which graphs best describe the medical knowledge acquired over time?

| Option | Public Perception | Consultant's Perception |
|---|---|---|
| A | B | B |
| B | B | D |
| C | D | B |
| D | D | D |
| E | F | B |

**Question 42:**

Sadly, in recent times, the number of people taking less exercise and having an associated sedentary lifestyle has increased in the developed world. The lack of opportunity for exercise is endemic and these countries have also seen a rise of diseases such as diabetes even in young people. In these developed countries, conditions usually associated with old age, like high blood pressure, are rapidly increasing in younger patients. These are however still uncommon in undeveloped countries, where most people are physically active throughout the entirety of their lives.

Which one of the following can be concluded from the passage above?
A. Exercise has a greater effect on old people than young people.
B. Maintenance of good health is associated with lifelong exercise.
C. Changes in lifestyle will be necessary to cause increased life expectancies in developed countries.
D. Exercise is only beneficial when continued into old age.
E. Obesity and diabetes are the result of lack of exercise.

**Questions 43 - 45 are based on the passage below:**

'Midwives should now encourage women to give birth at home as often as possible. Not only is there evidence to suggest that normal births at home are as safe as in hospital, but it removes the medicalisation of childbirth that has emerged over the years. With the increase in availability of health resources we now use services such as a full medical team for a natural process that women have been completing single-handedly for thousands of years. Midwives are extensively trained to assist women during labour at home and are capable of assessing when there is a problem that requires a hospital environment. Expensive hospital births must and should move away from being standard practice, especially in an era where the NHS has far more demands on its services that it can currently afford.'

**Question 43:**

Which one of the following is the most appropriate conclusion from the statement?
A. People are over dependent on healthcare.
B. Some women prefer to have their babies in hospital.
C. Having a baby in hospital can actually be more risky than at home.
D. Childbirth has been over-medicalised.
E. Encouraging women to have their babies at home may relieve some of the financial pressures on the NHS.

**Question 44:**

Which one of the following, if true, most weakens the argument presented in the passage above?
A. Some women are scared of home births.
B. Home births are associated with poorer outcomes.
C. Midwives do not like performing home visits.
D. Some home births result in hospital births anyway.
E. We should have more midwives than doctors.

**Question 45:**

Which one of the following describes what the statement cites as the cause for the 'medicalisation of childbirth'?

A.  Women fear giving birth without a full medical team present.
B.  Midwives are incapable of aiding childbirth without help.
C.  Giving birth at home is not as safe as it used to be.
D.  Easy access to and availability of health services.
E.  Women only used to give birth at home because they could not do so at hospital.

**Question 46:**

We need to stop focusing so much attention on the dangers of fires. In 2011 there were only 242 deaths due to exposure to smoke, fire and flames, while there were 997 deaths from hernias. We need to think more proportionally as these statistics show that campaigns such as 'fire kills' are unnecessary. In comparison to the risk of death from hernias, clearly shows that fires are not as dangerous as they are perceived to be.

Which of the following statements identify a weakness in the above argument?

1.  More people may die in fires if there were no campaigns about their danger and how to prevent them.
2.  The smoke of a fire is more dangerous than its flames.
3.  There may be more people with hernias than those in fires.

A.  1 only
B.  2 only
C.  2 and 3 only
D.  1 and 2 only
E.  1 and 3 only

**Question 47:**

School students were surveyed to find out if there was any correlation between the sports students played and the subjects they liked. The findings were as follows: some football players liked maths and some of them liked history. All students liked English. None of the basketball players liked history, but all of them, as well as some rugby players, liked chemistry. All rugby players like geography.

Based on the findings, which one of the below must be true?

A.  Some of the footballers liked maths and history.
B.  Some of the rugby players liked three subjects.
C.  Some rugby players liked history.
D.  Some of the footballers liked English but did not like maths and history.
E.  Some basketball players like more than 3 subjects.

**Question 48:**

The control of illegal drug use is becoming increasingly difficult. New 'legal highs' are being manufactured which have a slightly different molecular structure to illegal compounds, so they are not technically illegal. These new 'legal highs' are being brought onto the street at a rate of at least one per week, and so the authorities cannot keep up. Some health professionals therefore believe that knowledge of the legal classification of street drugs is less important than knowledge of the potentially dangerous side effects. The fact that these new compounds are legal may however mean that the public are not aware of their equally high risks.

Which of the following are implied by the argument?
1. Some health professionals believe there is no value in making drugs illegal.
2. The major problem in controlling illegal drug use is the rapid manufacture of new drugs that are not classified as illegal.
3. The general public are not worried about the risks of legal or illegal highs.
4. There is no longer a good correlation between risk of drug taking and the legal status of the drug.

A. 1 only
B. 2 only
C. 1 and 4
D. 2 and 4
E. 2 and 3
F. 1, 2, 3 and 4

**Question 49:**

WilderTravel Inc. is a company which organises wilderness travel holidays, with activities such as trekking, mountain climbing, safari tours and wilderness survival courses. These activities carry inherent risks, so the directors of the company are drawing up a set of health regulations with the aim of minimising the risks by ensuring that nobody with medical conditions participates in activities that might put their health in jeopardy. They consider the following guidelines:

'Persons with pacemakers, asthma or severe allergies are at significant risk of heart attack in low oxygen environments'. People undertaking mountain climbing activities with WilderTravel frequently encounter environments with low oxygen levels. The directors therefore decide that in order to ensure the safety of customers on WilderTravel holidays, one step that must be taken is to bar those with pacemakers, asthma or allergies from partaking in mountain climbing.

Which of the following best illustrates a flaw in this reasoning?
A. Participants should be allowed to assess the safety risks themselves, and should not be barred from activities if they decide the risk is acceptable.
B. They have assumed that all allergies carry an increased risk of heart attack, when the guidelines only say this applies to those with severe allergies.
C. The directors have failed to consider the health risks of people with these conditions taking part in other activities.
D. People with these conditions could partake in mountain climbing with other holiday organisers, and thus be exposed to danger of heart attack.

**Question 50:**
St John's Hospital in Northumbria is looking to recruit a new consultant cardiologist, and interviews a series of candidates. The interview panel determines that 3 candidates are clearly more qualified for the role than the others, and they invite these 3 candidates for a second interview. During this second interview, and upon further examination of their previous employment records, it becomes apparent that candidate 3 is the most proficient at surgery of the 3, whilst candidate 1 is the best at patient interaction and explaining the risks of procedures. Candidate 2, meanwhile, ranks between the others in both these aspects of care.

The hospital director tells the interviewing team that the hospital already has a well-renowned team dedicated to patient interaction, but the surgical success record at the hospital is in need of improvement. The director issues instructions that, therefore, it is more important that the new candidate is proficient at surgery, and skills in patient interaction are less of a concern.

Which of the following is a conclusion that can be drawn from the Director's comments?
A. The interviewing team should hire candidate 2, in order to achieve a balance of good patient relations with good surgical records.
B. The interviewing team should hire candidate 1, in order to ensure good patient interactions, as these are a vital part of a doctor's work.
C. The interviewing team should ignore the hospital director and assess the candidates further to see who would be the best fit.
D. The interviewing team should hire candidate 3, in order to ensure that the new candidate has excellent surgical skills, to boost the hospital's success in this area.

**Question 51:**
Every winter in Britain, there are thousands of urgent callouts for ambulances in snowy conditions. The harsh conditions mean that ambulances cannot drive quickly, and are delayed in reaching patients. These delays cause many injuries and medical complications, which could be avoided with quicker access to treatment. Despite this, very few ambulances are equipped with winter tyres or special tyre coverings to help the ambulances deal with snow. Clearly, if more ambulances were fitted with winter tyres, then we could avoid many medical complications that occur due to delays each winter.

Which of the following is an assumption made in this passage?
A. Fitting winter tyres would allow ambulances to reach patients more quickly.
B. Ambulance trusts have sufficient funding to equip their vehicles with winter tyres.
C. Many medical complications could be avoided with quicker access to medical care.
D. There are no other alternatives to winter tyres that would allow ambulances to reach patients more quickly in snowy conditions.

**Question 52:**

Vaccinations have been one of the most outstanding and influential developments in medical history. Despite the huge successes, there is a strong anti-vaccination movement active in some countries, particularly the USA, which claims that vaccines are harmful and ineffective.

There have been several high-profile events in recent years where anti-vaccination campaigners have been refused permission to enter countries for campaigns, or have had venues refuse to host them due to the nature of their campaigns. Many anti-vaccination campaigners have claimed this is an affront to free speech, and that they should be allowed to enter countries and obtain venues without hindrance. However, although free speech is desirable, an exception must be made here because the anti-vaccination campaign spreads misinformation, causing vaccination rates to drop.

When this happens, preventable infectious diseases often begin to increase, causing avoidable deaths, particularly in children. Thus, in order to protect people, we must continue to block the anti-vaccine campaigners from spreading misinformation freely by pressuring venues not to host anti-vaccination campaign events.

Which of the following best illustrates the principle that this argument follows?

A. Free speech is always desirable and must not be compromised under any circumstances.

B. The right to protection from infectious diseases by vaccination is more important than the right to freedom of speech.

C. The right of free speech does not apply when the party speaking is lying or spreading misinformation.

D. Public health programmes that achieve significant success in reducing the incidence of disease should be promoted.


**Question 53:**

In order for a tumour to grow larger than a few centimetres, it must first establish its own blood supply by promoting angiogenesis. Roger has a tumour in his abdomen, which is investigated at the Royal General Hospital. During the tests, they detect newly formed blood vessels in the tumour, showing that it has established its own blood supply. Thus, we should expect the tumour to grow significantly, and become larger than a few centimetres. Action must be taken to deal with this.

Which of the following best illustrates a flaw in this reasoning?

A. It assumes that the tumour in Roger's abdomen has established its own blood supply.

B. It assumes that a blood supply is necessary for a tumour to grow larger than a few centimetres.

C. It assumes that nothing can be done to stop the tumour once a blood supply has been established.

D. It assumes that a blood supply is sufficient for the tumour to grow larger than a few centimetres.

**Question 54:**

In this year's Great North Run, there are several dozen people running to raise money for the Great North Air Ambulance (GNAA), as part of a large national fundraising campaign. If the runners raise £500,000 between them, then the GNAA will be able to add a new helicopter to its fleet. However, the runners only raise a total of £420,000. Thus, the GNAA will not be able to get a new helicopter.

Which of the following best illustrates a flaw in this passage?

A. It has assumed that the GNAA will not be able to acquire a new helicopter without the runners raising £500,000.

B. It has assumed that the GNAA wishes to add a new helicopter to its fleet.

C. It has assumed that the GNAA does not have better things to spend the money on.

D. It has assumed that only people running in the Great North Run are raising money for the GNAA.

**Question 55:**

Many courses, spanning universities, colleges, apprenticeship institutions and adult skills courses should be subsidised by the government. This is because they improve the skills of those attending them. It has been well demonstrated that the more skilled people are, the more productive they are economically. Thus, government subsidies of many courses would increase overall economic productivity, and lead to increased growth.

Which of the following would most weaken this argument?

A. The UK already has a high level of growth and does not need to accelerate this growth.

B. Research has demonstrated that higher numbers of people attending adult skills courses results in increased economic growth.

C. Research has demonstrated that the cost of many courses (to those taking them) has little effect on the number of people undertaking the courses.

D. Employers often seek to employ those with greater skill-sets, and appoint them to higher positions.

**Question 56:**

Pluto was once considered the 9th planet in the solar system. However, further study of the planet led to it being reclassified as a dwarf planet in 2006. One key factor in this reclassification was the discovery of many objects in the solar system with similar characteristics to Pluto, which were also placed into this new category of 'dwarf planet'. Some astronomers believe that Pluto should remain classified as a planet, along with the many entities similar to Pluto that have now been discovered. Considering all of this, it is clear that if we were to reclassify Pluto as a planet, and maintain consistency with classification of astronomical entities, then the number of planets would significantly increase.

Which of the following best illustrates the main conclusion of this passage?

A. If Pluto is classified as a planet, then many other entities should also be planets, as they share similar characteristics.

B. Some astronomers believe Pluto should be classified as a planet.

C. Pluto should not be classified as a planet, as this would also require many other entities to be classified as planets to ensure consistency.

D. If Pluto is to be classified as a planet, then the number of objects classified as planets should increase significantly.

## Question 57:

Two trains depart from Birmingham at 5:30 pm. One of the trains is heading to London, whilst the other is heading to Glasgow. The distance from Birmingham to Glasgow is three times larger than the distance from Birmingham to London, and the train to London arrives at 6:30 pm. Thus, the train to Glasgow will arrive at 8:30pm.

Which of the following is an assumption made in this passage?

A. Both trains depart at the same time.

B. Both trains depart from Birmingham.

C. Both trains travel at the same speed.

D. The train heading to Glasgow has to travel three times as far as the train heading to London.

## Question 58:

Carcinogenesis, oncogenesis and tumorigenesis are various names given to the generation of cancer, with the term literally meaning 'creation of cancer'. In order for carcinogenesis to happen, there are several steps that must occur. Firstly, a cell (or group of cells) must achieve immortality, and escape senescence (the inherent limitation of a cell's lifespan). Then they must escape regulation by the body, and begin to proliferate in an autonomous way. They must also become immune to apoptosis and other cell death mechanisms. Finally, they must avoid detection by the immune system, or survive its responses to unfamiliar genetic material. If a single one of these steps fails to occur, then carcinogenesis will not be able to occur.

Which of the following is a conclusion that can be reliably drawn from this passage?

A. Carcinogenesis is a multi-step process that occurs in discrete stages and in a specific order.

B. If all the steps mentioned occur, then carcinogenesis will occur.

C. The immune system is unable to tackle cells that have escaped regulation by the body.

D. There are various mechanisms by which carcinogenesis can occur.

E. Carcinogenesis occurs over a period of months to years, as there are multiple steps.

**Question 59:**

P53 is one of the most crucial genes in the body, responsible for detecting DNA damage and halting cell replication until repair can occur. If repair cannot take place, P53 will signal for the cell to kill itself. These actions are crucial to prevent carcinogenesis, and a loss of functional P53 is identified in over 50% of all cancers. The huge importance of P53 towards protecting the cell from damaging mutations has led to it deservedly being known as 'the guardian of the genome'. The implications of this name are clear – any cell that has a mutation in P53 is at serious risk of developing a potentially dangerous mutation.

Which of the following **CANNOT** be reliably concluded from this passage?
A.  P53 is responsible for detecting DNA damage.
B.  Most cancers have lost functional P53.
C.  P53 deserves its name 'guardian of the genome'.
D.  A cell that has a mutation in P53 will develop damaging mutations.
E.  None of the above.

**Question 60:**

Sam is buying a new car, and deciding whether to buy a petrol or a diesel model. He knows he will drive 9,000 miles each year. He calculates that if he drives a petrol car, he will spend £500 per 1,000 miles on fuel, but if he buys a diesel model, he will only spend £300 per 1,000 miles on fuel. He calculates, therefore, that if he purchases a diesel car, then this year he would make a saving of £1800, compared to if he bought the petrol car.

Which of the following is **NOT** an assumption that Sam has made?
A.  The price of diesel will not fluctuate relative to that of petrol.
B.  The cars will have the same initial purchase cost.
C.  The cars will have the same costs for maintenance and garage expenses.
D.  The cars will use the same amount of fuel.
E.  All of the above are assumptions.

**Question 61:**

In the UK, cannabis is classified as a Class B drug, with a maximum penalty of up to 5 years imprisonment for possession, or up to 14 years for possession with intent to supply. The justification for drug laws in the UK is that classified drugs are harmful, addictive, and destructive to people's lives. However, plentiful medical evidence indicates that cannabis is relatively safe, non-addictive and overall harmless. In particular, it is certainly shown to be less dangerous than alcohol, which is commonly sold and advertised across the UK. The fact that alcohol can be widely sold and advertised, but cannabis, a less harmful drug, is banned highlights the gross inconsistencies in UK drugs policy.

Which of the following best illustrates the main conclusion of this passage?

A. Cannabis is a less dangerous drug than alcohol, so it should be made more widely available.
B. In order to ensure consistency in the UK drug policy, we should either ban alcohol, or make cannabis widely available.
C. Cannabis is considered harmful and addictive, which is why it is a Class B drug.
D. The UK government's policy on drugs is grossly inconsistent.
E. Alcohol can be advertised in the UK, whereas cannabis cannot.

## Question 62:

Every year in Britain, there are thousands of accidents in the home such as burns, broken limbs and severe cuts, which cause a large number of deaths and injuries. Despite this, very few households maintain a sufficient first aid kit equipped with bandages, burn treatments, splints and saline to clean wounds. If more households stocked sufficient first aid supplies, many of these accidents could be avoided.

Which of the following best illustrates a flaw in this argument?

A. It ignores the huge cost associated with maintaining good first aid supplies, which many households cannot afford.
B. It implies that presence of first aid equipment will lead to fewer accidents.
C. It ignores the many accidents that could not be treated even if first aid supplies were readily available.
D. It neglects to consider the need for trained first aid persons in order for first aid supplies to help in reducing the severity of injuries caused by accidents.

## Question 63:

Researchers at SmithJones Inc., an international pharmaceuticals firm, are investigating a well-known historic compound, which is thought to reduce levels of DNA replication by inhibiting DNA polymerases. It is proposed that this may be able to be used to combat cancer by reducing the proliferation of cancer cells, allowing the immune system to combat them before they spread too far and cause significant damage. Old experiments have demonstrated the effectiveness of the compound via monitoring DNA levels with a dye that stains DNA red, thus monitoring the levels of DNA present in cell clusters. They report that the compound is observed to reduce the rate at which DNA replicates. However, it is known that if researchers use the wrong solutions when carrying out these experiments, then the amount of red staining will decrease, suggesting DNA replication has been inhibited, even if that is not the case. As several researchers previously used this wrong solution, we can conclude that these experiments are flawed, and do not reflect what is actually happening.

Which of the following best illustrates a flaw in this argument?

A. From the fact that the compound inhibits DNA replication, it cannot be concluded that it has potential as an anticancer drug.
B. From the fact that the wrong solutions were used, it cannot be concluded that the experiments may produce misleading results.
C. From the fact that the experiments are old, it cannot be concluded that the wrong solutions were used.
D. From the fact that the compound is old, it cannot be concluded that it is safe.

**Question 64:**

Rotherham football club are currently top of the league, with 90 points. Their closest competitors are South Shields football club, with 84 points. Next week, the teams will play each other, and after this, they each have two games left before the end of the season. Each win is worth 3 points, a draw is worth 1 point, and a loss is worth 0 points. Thus, if Rotherham beat South Shields, they will win the league (as they will then be 9 points clear, and South Shields would only be able to earn 6 more points).

In the match of Rotherham vs. South Shields, Rotherham are winning until the 85th minute, when Alberto Simeone scores an equaliser for South Shields, and South Shields then go on to win the match. Thus, Rotherham will not win the league.

Which of the following best illustrates a flaw in this passage's reasoning?
A. It has assumed that Alberto Simeone scored the winning goal for South Shields.
B. It has assumed that beating South Shields was necessary for Rotherham to win the league, when in fact it was only sufficient.
C. Rotherham may have scored an equaliser later in the game, and not lost the match.
D. It has failed to consider what other teams might win the league.

**Question 65:**

Oakville Supermarkets is looking to build a new superstore, and a meeting of its directors has been convened to decide where the best place to build the supermarket would be. The Chair of the Board suggests that the best place would be Warrington, a town that does not currently have a large supermarket, and would thus give them an excellent share of the grocery shopping market.
However, the CEO notes that the population of Warrington has been steadily declining for several years, whilst Middlesbrough has recently been experiencing high population growth. The CEO therefore argues that they should build the new supermarket in Middlesbrough, as they would then be within range of more people, and so it would have more potential customers.

Which of the following best illustrates a flaw in the CEO's reasoning?
A. Middlesbrough may already have other supermarkets, so the new superstore may get a lower share of the town's shoppers.
B. Despite the recent population changes, Warrington may still have a larger population than Middlesbrough.
C. Middlesbrough's population is projected to continue growing, whilst Warrington's is projected to keep falling.
D. Many people in Warrington travel to Liverpool or Manchester, two nearby major cities, in order to do their shopping.

**Question 66:**

Global warming is a key challenge facing the world today, and the changes in weather patterns caused by this phenomenon have led to the destruction of many natural habitats, causing many species to become extinct. Recent data shows that extinction events have been occurring at a faster rate over the last 40 years than at any other point in the earth's history, exceeding the great Permian mass extinction, which wiped out 96% of life on earth. If this rate continues, over 50% of species on earth will be extinct by 2100. It is clear that in the face of this huge challenge, conservation programmes will require significantly increased levels of funding in order to prevent most of the species on earth from becoming extinct.

Which of the following are assumptions in this argument?
1. The rate of extinction events seen in the last 40 years will continue to occur without a step-up in conservation efforts.
2. Conservation programmes cannot prevent further extinctions without increased funding.
3. Global warming has caused many extinction events, directly or indirectly.

A. 1 only
B. 2 only
C. 3 only
D. 1 and 2
E. 1 and 3

**Question 67:**

After an election in Britain, the new government is debating what policy to adopt on the railway system, and whether it should be entirely privatised, or whether public subsidies should be used to supplement costs and ensure that sufficient services are run. Studies in Austria, which has high public funding for railways, have shown that the rail service is used by many people, and is rated highly by the population. However, this is clearly down to the fact that Austria has many mountainous and high-altitude areas, which experience significant amounts of snow and ice. This makes many roads impassable by car.. Thus, rail is often the only way to travel, explaining the high passenger numbers and approval ratings. Thus, the high public subsidies clearly have no effect.

Which of the following, if true, would weaken this argument?

1. France also has high public subsidy of railways, but does not have large areas where travel by road is difficult. The French railway also has high passenger numbers and approval ratings.
2. Italy also has high public subsidy of railways, but the local population dislike using the rail service, and it has poor passenger numbers.
3. There are many reasons affecting the passenger numbers and approval ratings of a given country's rail service.

A. 1 only
B. 2 only
C. 3 only
D. 1 and 2
E. 1 and 3

**Question 68:**

In 2001-2002, 1,019 patients were admitted to hospital due to obesity. This figure was more than 11 times higher by 2011-12 when there were 11,736 patients admitted to hospital with the primary reason for admission being obesity. Data has shown higher percentages of both men and women were either obese or overweight in 2011 compared to 1993, with the percentage of overweight men climbing from 58% to 65%, and female rates of obesity increasing from 49% to 58%. Rates of adult obesity have increased even more steeply within the period from 2001-2012 – 13% to 24% for men and 16% to 26% for women.

Studies in 2011 found that nearly a third of children between 2 – 15 years were either overweight or obese, although this was not significantly higher than in 2008. Lifestyles are also becoming less healthy, with a decline in both children and adults eating the recommended portions of fruit and vegetables each day or taking the recommended amount of exercise each week. The ease and availability of cheap fast-food outlets may be partly to blame for the rising number of obese people. Education is required to teach people the importance of a healthy lifestyle, however people must take some personal responsibility for their health.

Using only information from the passage, which of the following statements is correct?
A. In 2011, there was a higher proportion of obese men than women.
B. Obesity rates are rising steeply for both males and females of all age groups.
C. A combination of education and personal responsibility is needed to improve the population's health
D. The main reason people eat fast food is because it's cheaper than healthy alternatives.

**Question 69:**

Tobacco companies sell cigarettes despite being fully aware that cigarettes cause significant harm to the health and wellbeing of those that smoke them. Diseases caused or aggravated by smoking cost billions of pounds for the NHS to treat each year and have an enormous impact on the individuals affected by smoking related diseases. This is extremely irresponsible behaviour from the tobacco companies. Tobacco companies should be taxed, and the money raised put towards funding the NHS.

Which of the following conclusions **CANNOT** be drawn from the above?
A. There is a connection between lung cancer and smoking.
B. People who smoke are more likely to also drink.
C. There is a connection between oral cancer and smoking.
D. All smokers drink excessively.
E. All of the above.

## Question 70:

Investigations in the origins of species suggest that humans and the great apes have the same ancestors. This is suggested by the high degree of genetic similarity between humans and chimpanzees (estimated at 99%). At the same time there is an 84% homology between the human genome and that of pigs. This raises the interesting question of whether it would be possible to use pig or chimpanzee organs for the treatment of human disease.

Which conclusion can be reasonably drawn from the above article?

A. Pigs and chimpanzees have a common ancestor.

B. Pigs and humans have a common ancestor.

C. It can be assumed that chimpanzees will develop into humans if given enough time to evolve.

D. There seems to be great genetic homology across a variety of species.

E. Organs from pigs or chimpanzees present a good alternative for human organ donation.

## Question 71:

Poor blood supply to a part of the body can cause damage to the affected tissue. There are a variety of known risk factors for vascular disease. Diabetes is a major risk factor. Other risk factors are more dependent on the individual as they represent individual choices such as smoking, poor dietary habits as well as little to no exercise. In some cases infarction of the limbs and in particular the feet can become very bad and extensive with patches of tissue dying. This is known as necrosis and is marked by the skin of the affected area of the body (often fingers or toes) turning black. Necrotic tissue is usually removed in surgery.

Which of the following statements **CANNOT** be concluded from the information in the above passage?

A. Smoking causes vascular disease.

B. Diabetes causes vascular disease.

C. Vascular disease always leads to infarctions.

D. Necrotic tissue must be removed surgically.

E. Necrotic tissue only occurs following severe infarction.

F. All of the above.

**Question 72:**

People who can afford to pay for private education should not have access to the state school system. This would allow more funding to be reserved for educating students from lower income backgrounds. More funding would provide better resources for students from lower income backgrounds, and will help to bridge the gap in educational attainment between students from higher income and lower income backgrounds.

Which of the following statements, if true, would most strengthen the above argument?

A.  Educational attainment is a significant factor in determining future prospects.
B.  Providing better resources for students has been demonstrated to lead to an increase in educational attainment.
C.  Most people who can afford to do so choose to purchase private education for their children.
D.  A significant gap exists in educational attainment between students from high and low income backgrounds.
E.  Most schools currently receive funding according to the number of students in the school.

**Question 73:**

Increasing numbers of people are choosing to watch films on DVD in recent years. In the past few years, cinemas have lost customers, causing them to close down. Many cinemas have recently closed, removing an important focal point for many local communities and causing damage to the local economy. Therefore, we should ban DVDs in order to help local communities.

Which of the following best states an assumption made in this argument?

A.  Cinemas have closed because of reduced profits due to people choosing to watch DVDs instead.
B.  Cinemas being forced to close causes damage to local communities.
C.  DVDs are improving local communities by allowing people to meet up and watch films together.
D.  Sales of DVDs have increased due to economic growth.
E.  Local communities have called for DVDs to be banned.

**Question 74:**

Aeroplanes are the fastest form of transport available. An aeroplane can travel a given distance in less time than a train or a car. John needs to travel from Glasgow to Birmingham. If he wants to arrive as soon as possible, he should travel by aeroplane.

Which of the following best illustrates a flaw in this argument?

A.  One day, cars that travel as fast as aeroplanes could be developed
B.  Travelling by air is often more expensive.
C.  It ignores the time taken to travel to an airport and check in to a flight, which may mean he will arrive later if travelling by aeroplane.
D.  John may not own a car, and thus may not have any option.
E.  John may not be legally allowed to make the journey.

**Question 75:**

During autumn, spiders frequently enter homes to escape the cold weather. Many people dislike spiders and seek ways to prevent them from entering properties, leading to spider populations falling as they struggle to cope with the cold weather. Studies have demonstrated that when spider populations fall, the population of flies rises. Higher numbers of flies are associated with an increase in food poisoning cases. Therefore, people must not seek to prevent spiders from entering their homes.

Which of the following best illustrates the main conclusion of this argument?

A. People should not dislike spiders being present in their homes.

B. People should seek alternative methods to prevent flies from entering their homes.

C. People should actively encourage spiders to occupy their homes to increase biodiversity.

D. People should accept the presence of spiders in their homes to reduce the incidence of food poisoning.

E. Spiders should be cultivated and used as a biological pest control to combat flies.

**Question 76:**

Each year, thousands of people acquire infections during prolonged stays in hospital. Concurrently, bacteria are becoming resistant to antibiotics at an ever-increasing rate. In spite of this, progressively fewer pharmaceutical companies are investing in research into new antibiotics, and the number of antibiotics coming onto the market is decreasing. As a result, the number of antibiotics that can be used to treat infections is falling. If pharmaceutical companies were pressured into investing in new antibiotic research, many lives could be saved.

Which of the following best illustrates a flaw in this argument?

A. It assumes the infections acquired during stays at hospital are resulting in deaths.

B. It ignores the fact that many people never have to stay in hospital.

C. It does not take into account the fact that antibiotics do not produce much profit for pharmaceutical companies.

D. It ignores the fact that some hospital-acquired infections are caused by organisms that cannot be treated by antibiotics, such as viruses.

E. It assumes that bacterial resistance to antibiotics has not been happening for some time.

**Question 77:**

Katherine has shaved her armpits most of her adult life, but has now decided to stop. She explains her reasons for this to John, saying she does not like the pressures society puts on women to be shaven in this area. John listens to her reasons, but ultimately responds 'just because you explain why I should find your hairiness attractive, it does not mean I will. I find you unattractive, as I do not like girls with hair on their armpits.'

What assumption has John made?

A. That just because he finds Katherine unattractive, he would find other girls with unshaven armpits unattractive.

B. That Katherine is trying to make John find her armpit hair attractive.

C. That Katherine will never conceal her armpit hair.

D.  Katherine must be wrong, because she is a woman.

E. That Katherine thinks women should stop shaving.

**Question 78:**

Medicine and the availability of powerful drugs have improved significantly over the last century. Better medical practice results in a reduction in the death rate from all causes. However, as people age, they are more likely to suffer from infectious diseases.

Many developing countries have a high rate of deaths from infectious diseases. Sunita argues that this is a result of better medical practices in developing countries. Better medicine has given rise to an ageing population, which explains why there is a higher rate of death from infectious diseases.

However, this cannot be the case. In developing countries, most people do not live to old age. In fact, it is common for people in developing countries to die from infectious diseases at a young age. Therefore, an ageing population cannot be the reason behind the high rate of death from infectious disease in developing countries. Since better medicine reduces the death rate from all causes, it is clear that better medicine would lead to a reduction in the death rate from infectious disease in developing countries.

Which of the following best states the main conclusion of this argument?

A. We can expect that improvements in medicine seen over the last century will improve.

B. Better medicine is not responsible for the increased prevalence of infectious disease in third world countries.

C. Better medicine has caused the overall death rate of third world countries to increase.

D. Better medicine will cause a decrease in the rate of death from infectious disease in third world countries.

E. As people get older, they suffer from infectious disease more commonly.

**Question 79:**

Bristol and Cardiff are two cities with similar demographics, and are located in a similar area of the country. Bristol has higher demand for housing than Cardiff. Therefore, a house in Bristol will cost more than a similar house in Cardiff.

Which of the following best illustrates an assumption in the statement above?

A. House prices will be higher if demand for housing is higher.

B. People can commute from Cardiff to Bristol.

C. Supply of housing in Cardiff will not be lower than in Bristol.

D. Bristol is a better place to live.

E. Cardiff has sufficient housing to provide for the needs of its communities.

**Question 80:**

Jellicoe Motors is a small motor company in Sheffield, employing three people. The company is hiring a new mechanic and interviews several candidates. New research into production lines has indicated that having employees with a good ability to work as part of a team boosts the productivity and profits of a company. Therefore, Jellicoe motors should hire a candidate with good team-working skills.

Which of the following best illustrates the main conclusion of this argument?

A. Jellicoe Motors should not hire a new mechanic.

B. Jellicoe motors should hire a candidate with good team-working skills in order to boost their productivity and profits.

C. Jellicoe motors should hire several new candidates in order to form a good team, and boost their productivity.

D. If Jellicoe motors does not hire a candidate with good team-working skills, they may struggle to be profitable.

E. Jellicoe motors should not listen to the new research.

**Question 81:**

Research into new antibiotics is seldom profitable for pharmaceutical firms. As a consequence, many firms are not investing in antibiotic research, and very few new antibiotics are being produced. However, with bacteria becoming increasingly resistant to current antibiotics, new drugs are desperately needed to avoid running the risk of thousands of deaths from bacterial infections. Therefore, the UK government must provide financial incentives for pharmaceutical companies to invest in research into new antibiotics.

Which of the following best expresses the main conclusion of this argument?

A. If bacteria continue to become resistant to antibiotics, there could be thousands of deaths from bacterial infections.

B. Pharmaceutical firms are not investing in new antibiotic research due to a lack of potential profit.

C. If the UK government invests in research into new antibiotics, thousands of lives will be saved.

D. The pharmaceutical firms should invest in areas of research that are profitable and ignore antibiotic research.

E. The UK government must provide financial incentives for pharmaceutical firms to invest into antibiotic research if it wishes to avoid risking thousands of deaths from bacterial infections.

**Question 82:**

People in developing countries use far less water per person than those in developed countries. It is estimated that at present, people in the developing world use an average of 30 litres of water per person per day, whilst those in developed countries use on average 70 litres of water per person per day. It is estimated that for the current world population, an average water usage of 60 litres per person per day would be sustainable, but any higher than this would be unsustainable.

The UN has set development targets such that in 20 years, people living in developing countries will be using the same amount of water per person per day as those living in developed countries. Assuming the world population stays constant for the next 20 years, if these targets are met the world's population will be using water at an unsustainable rate.

Which of the following, if true, would most weaken the argument above?

A. The prices of water bills are dropping in developed countries like the UK.

B. The level of water usage in developed countries is falling and may be below 60 litres per person per day in 20 years.

C. The total population of all developing countries is less than the total population of all developed countries.

D. Climate change is likely to decrease the amount of water available for human use over the next 20 years.

E. The UN's development targets are unlikely to be met.

**Question 83:**

An advert for a senior management post states "we need someone who can keep a cool head in a crisis and react quickly to events". The applicant says he suffers from a phobia of flying, and panics especially when an aircraft is landing and that therefore he would prefer not to travel abroad on business if it could be avoided. The interview panel conclude he is obviously a very nervous type of person who would clearly go to pieces and panic in an emergency and fail to provide the leadership qualities necessary for the job. Therefore, they decide this person is not a suitable candidate for the post.

Which of the following highlights the biggest flaw in the argument above?
A. It falsely assumes that phobias are untreatable or capable of being eliminated.
B. It falsely assumes that the person appointed to the job will need to travel abroad.
C. It falsely assumes that a specific phobia indicates a general tendency to panic.
D. It falsely assumes that people who stay cool in a crisis will be good leaders.
E. It fails to take into account other qualities the person might have for the post.

**Question 84:**

There are significant numbers of people attending university every year: as many as 45% of 18-year-olds. As a result, there are many more graduates entering the workforce with better skills and better earning potential. Going to university makes economic sense and we should encourage as many young people to attend as possible.

Which of the following highlights the biggest flaw in the argument above?
A. There are no more university places left.
B. Students can succeed without going to university.
C. Not all degrees equip students with the skills needed to earn higher salaries.
D. Some universities are better than others.

**Question 85:**

Young people spend too much time watching television, which is bad for them. Watching excessive amounts of TV is linked to obesity, social exclusion and can cause eye damage. If young people were to spend just one evening a week playing sport or going for a walk, the benefits would be signficant. They would lose weight, feel better about themselves and it would be a sociable activity. Exercise is also linked to strong performance at school and so young people would be more likely to perform well in their exams.

Which of the following highlights the biggest flaw in the argument above?
A. Young people can watch sport on television.
B. There are many factors that affect exam performance.
C. Television does not necessarily have any damaging effect.
D. Television and sport are not linked.

**Question 86:**

Campaigners pushing for the legalisation of cannabis present many arguments to support their cause. Most claim there is little evidence of any adverse affects to health caused by cannabis use, that many otherwise law-abiding people are users of cannabis and that in any case, prohibition of drugs does not reduce their usage. Legalising cannabis would also reduce crime associated with drug trafficking and would provide an additional revenue stream for the government.

Which of the following best represents the conclusion of the passage?
A. Regular cannabis users are unlikely to have health problems.
B. Legalising cannabis would be good for cannabis users.
C. There are multiple reasons to legalise cannabis.
D. Prohibition is an effective measure to reduce drugs usage.
E. Drug associated crime would reduce if cannabis was legal.

**Question 87:**

Mohan has been offered a new job in Birmingham, starting in several months with a fixed salary. In order to ensure he can afford to live in Birmingham on his new salary, Mohan compares the prices of some houses in Birmingham. He finds that a 2-bedroom house will cost £200,000. A 3-bedroom house will cost £250,000. A 4-bedroom house with a garden will cost £300,000.

Mohan's bank tells him that if he is earning the salary of the job he has been offered, they will grant him a mortgage for a house costing up to £275,000. After a month of deliberation, Mohan accepts the job and decides to move to Wolverhampton. He begins searching for a house to buy. He reasons that he will not be able to purchase a 4-bedroomed house.

Which of the following is NOT an assumption that Mohan has made?
A. A house in Wolverhampton will cost the same as a similar house in Birmingham.
B. A different bank will not offer him a mortgage for a more expensive house on the same salary.
C. The salary for the job could increase, allowing him to purchase a more expensive house.
D. A 4-bedroom house without a garden will not cost less than a 4-bedroom house with a garden.
E. House prices in Birmingham will not have fallen in the time between now and Mohan purchasing a house.

**Question 88:**

We should teach the Holocaust in schools. It is important that young people see what it was like for Jewish people under Nazi rule. If we expose the harsh realities to impressionable people, then this will help improve tolerance of other races. It will also prevent other such terrible events happening again.

Which is the best conclusion?
A. We should teach about the Holocaust in schools.
B. The Holocaust was a tragedy.
C. The Nazis were evil.
D. We should not let terrible events happen again.
E. Educating people is the best solution to the world's problems.

**Question 89:**

The popular series 'Game of Thrones' should not be allowed on television because it shows scenes of a disturbing nature, in particular scenes of rape. Children may find themselves watching the programme on TV, and then going on to commit the terrible crime of rape, mimicking what they have watched.

Which of the following best illustrates a flaw in this argument?

A. Children may also watch the show on DVD.

B. Adults may watch the show on television.

C. Watching an action does not necessarily lead to recreating the action yourself.

D. There are lots of non-violent scenes in the show.

**Question 90:**

The TV series 'House of Cards' teaches us all a valuable lesson: the world is not a place that rewards kind behaviour. The protagonist of the series, Frank Underwood, uses intrigue and guile to achieve his goals, and through clever political tactics he is able to climb in rank. If he were to be kinder to people, he would not be able to be so successful. Success is dependent on his refusal to conform to conventional morality. The TV series should be shown to small children in schools, as it could teach them how to achieve their dreams.

Which of the following is an assumption made in the argument?

A. Children pay attention to school lessons.

B. The TV series is sufficiently entertaining.

C. One cannot both obey a moral code and succeed.

D. Frank Underwood is a likable character.

**Question 91:**

Freddy makes lewd comments about a female passer-by's body to his friend, Neil, loud enough for the woman in question to hear. Neil is uncomfortable with this, and states that it is inappropriate for Freddy to make these comments, and that Freddy is being sexist. Freddy refutes this, and Neil retorts that Freddy would not make these comments about a man's body. Freddy replies by saying 'it is not sexist, I am a feminist, I believe in equality for men and women.'

Which of the following describes a flaw made in Freddy's logic?

A. A self-proclaimed feminist could still say a sexist thing.

B. The female passer-by in question felt uncomfortable.

C. Neil, too, considers himself a feminist.

D. It would still not be OK to make lewd comments at male passers-by.

E. Lewd comments are always inappropriate.

**Question 92:**

The release of $CO_2$ from consumption of fossil fuels is the main reason behind global warming, which is causing significant damage to many natural environments across the globe. One significant source of $CO_2$ emissions is cars, which release $CO_2$ as they use up petrol. In order to tackle this problem, many car companies have begun to design cars with engines that do not use as much petrol. However, engines which use less petrol are not as powerful, and less powerful cars are not attractive to the public. If a car company produces cars which are not attractive to the public, they will not be profitable.

Which of the following best illustrates the main conclusion of this argument?
A. Car companies which produce cars that use less petrol will not be profitable.
B. The public prefer more powerful cars.
C. Car companies should prioritise profits over helping the environment.
D. Car companies should seek to produce engines that use less petrol but are still just as powerful.
E. The public are not interested in helping the environment.

**Question 93:**

Automobiles have grown to become an environmental hazard. Previously a prized possession, there are now over 1.4 billion vehicles worldwide, with the number unlikely to decrease anytime soon. In town centres especially, cars have caused many problems for local councils, the public and the air we breathe. With increasing awareness of the damage to the environment we are causing through fossil fuel use, the currently unrestricted use of cars must now be restrained. How many more lung problems and worrying environmental studies will emerge before significant changes are brought in?

Which of the following best illustrates the main conclusion of this argument?
A. The general health of the world population is at risk because so many people use cars.
B. We need to place more restrictions on parking in town centres.
C. The price of automobiles needs to be increased.
D. It is in everyone's best interests to reduce car usage worldwide.
E. We need to be more aware of the environmental issues caused by cars.

**Question 94:**

If Schweikart do not raise lawyers' salaries, then the morale of their lawyers will fall, leading to a decline in productivity. This means less work is done, so less money is made, and eventually the whole firm could go bankrupt. Higher salaries could help make the firm bigger and more successful, as some case studies from other companies have shown.

Which of the following best illustrates the main conclusion of this argument?
A. The employers will have to accept some decrease in productivity.
B. Fall in productivity could mean the end of Schweikart.
C. The morale of the lawyers is dangerously low right now.
D. If salaries are not raised, the firm could go bankrupt.
E. If salaries are raised, the firm will be bigger and more successful.

**Question 95:**

Bushfires in Australia this year emitted 900 million tonnes of $CO_2$ into the atmosphere. Some scientific studies have suggested that the whole planet must release under 100 million tonnes of $CO_2$ every year from now on if we are to avoid further global warming. When forest vegetation burns, the amount of $CO_2$ released into the atmosphere can be taken back up again by the plants as they regrow over many years. Bushfires in Australia burn most fiercely in seasons when the air is drier, as it was this year. Rain arrived in Australia recently, and the number of new fires has dropped significantly.

Which of the following is a conclusion that can be drawn from this passage?
A. The Australian bushfires will probably not release as much carbon dioxide next time they occur, as they were so big and devastating this year.
B. Further global warming and climate change would not occur if bushfires could be prevented or controlled in a better way.
C. As a result of these bushfires, it is likely that some carbon dioxide released into the atmosphere will remain there for some time.
D. The bushfires in Australia will prevent the world targets for carbon emissions being reached.
E. Australia is the world's biggest contributor of carbon emissions.

**Question 96:**

If we are not the only life in the universe, other life must exist on planets of a similar size and with similar terrain to Earth. The hypothetical planet would need to orbit at the right distance from a star to make the climate tolerable for living organisms. Until now, technology has not been able to discover planets like these. China built a new bubble-scope so technologically advanced that for the first time in history astronomers will be able to see if there are any Earth-sized planets in the habitable zones around stars - the region where the temperature is right for liquid water to exist on the surface. If the bubble-scope finds that these planets exist, we can say that there is life on planets other than Earth.

Which of the following is the best statement of the flaw in the above argument?
A. It assumes that it is necessary to have technologically advanced telescopes to see other planets.
B. It assumes that the presence of liquid water is sufficient for life to exist.
C. It assumes that planets of a similar size to Earth will have life similar to that on Earth.
D. It assumes that the Bubble-scope is good enough to see Earth-sized planets in the habitable zones.
E. It assumes life must exist elsewhere in the universe.

**Question 97:**

The government was criticised for failing to prepare for heavy snowfall last winter. The economy faced a downturn because workers were simply unable to get to work. Others felt that these occasional economic costs should be accepted. Since the probability of heavy snow in the UK is very low, it could be argued that the massive cost of investing in preventative measures would not be a wise use of a finite government budget. Governments must make a judgement on the probability of potential events occurring, assessing risk, the cost of preventative measures and the cost of the event happening. Sometimes, the cost of preventative measures is too high when the risk is low, so it is not worth the investment. The recent extreme weather is an example of this.

Which of the following best illustrates the main conclusion of this argument?
A. The Government should compensate businesses for the money lost and help to bring the economy back to its previous level.
B. The Government should have spent more on preventative measures for the extreme snowfall.
C. Heavy snowfall in the UK is unusual.
D. The Government was right not to take the preventative measures necessary to get us through extreme snowfall.
E. The Government deserves its criticism for the handling of recent extreme weather.


**Question 98:**

Countries with a thriving arts sector (including architecture, film, literature and music) tend to be less authoritarian, fairer and more economically powerful. They also tend to have happier and more psychologically balanced citizens. If we want to live in a less authoritarian, fairer and more economically powerful society, we should request that the Government financially support the arts.

Which of the following illustrates a flaw in the above argument?
A. A thriving arts sector may positively influence the mental health of citizens.
B. There may be other more important uses of Government spending.
C. Some of the traditional arts are outdated and have no place in modern society.
D. Some of the arts may be seen as totalitarian.
E. A robust economy may be a prerequisite of a thriving traditional arts sector.


**Question 99:**

When GCSE results come out again next summer, there will inevitably be controversy and criticism about the standard of education in this country. If the results are slightly above average, people will say that the GCSEs are too easy nowadays – not that people are smarter. Alternatively, if the results are slightly below average, then people will raise the issue of state funding for education – rather than arguing it shows a natural fluctuation in ability. In conclusion, there will be negative stories in the media either way, so we should not pay attention to these news stories.

Which of the following is the best statement of the flaw in the above argument?
A. It does not establish that GCSEs are a varying level of difficulty year upon year.
B. The options are either slightly above average or below – the results could also stay roughly the same.
C. It makes an undeserved attack on journalism.
D. The fact that a negative story is inevitable does not mean that it should be ignored.
E. It makes a future prediction without any hard evidence.

**Question 100:**

Infant road deaths and serious injuries have decreased by 29.8% in the past decade. Nonetheless, we should not assume that guidance for road safety is no longer essential for students. One study shared its results from 2009: almost 1900 young boys and 900 girls were killed or seriously injured in road traffic accidents as pedestrians. On top of this, 750 young cyclists were killed or seriously injured, more than 450 of whom were boys.

Assuming that 2009 is a representative year for road accidents involving infant pedestrians and cyclists, which one of the following is a conclusion that can be drawn from the passage?

A. Boys are more than twice as likely as girls to be killed or seriously injured as cyclists.
B. Boys are more than twice as likely as girls to be killed or seriously injured as pedestrians.
C. Girls are usually supervised as adults, whereas boys are more reckless and thus are subject to more accidents on the road.
D. There are more boys than girls who ride bicycles and walk on the streets.
E. Lessons in road safety specifically designed for boys would be beneficial in reducing these worrying numbers.

**Question 101:**

The conduct of the public has been a major contributing factor to the disinclination of doctors to work outside of regular office hours. When doctors only dealt with actual medical emergencies on call, the workload was under control. The state has contributed to making the public think they should now be entitled to medical care 24 hours a day, no matter how insignificant or non-urgent the problem is. Only some of these minor problems should be dealt with at GP surgeries or by NHS 111.

Which of the following best illustrates the main conclusion of this argument?

A. The State should encourage doctors to offer separate urgent and non-urgent surgeries outside of office hours.
B. The public are having difficulty drawing a line between which medical problems require hospital assistance and medical care, and which do not.
C. Doctors should turn away patients who come with non-urgent problems to their surgeries outside of office hours.
D. The problems with providing medical care outside of office hours are partly due to the general public.
E. There needs to be a change in the rules for what defines an urgent medical problem.

**Question 102:**

Vast increases in the cost of bringing a case to court introduced last week are an outrage on the general public's access to legal representation. It means that justice is treated as a commodity. Fees are set to increase by more than 700% for claims of a quarter of a million pounds or more. This deters small businesses and ordinary people from taking cases to court, for fear of the financial loss if they lose, bankrupting anyone who tries to get justice. All civil settlements are affected. If justice is not accessible for most ordinary people, the government must change things. The civil courts are the cornerstone of a just and fair society.

Which of the following best illustrates the main conclusion of this argument?

A. The civil courts are crucial to fairness and justice in society.
B. The government needs to rethink its policies, or justice will simply be inaccessible to most due to cost.
C. Capitalism is corrupting the justice system.
D. The planned increase in court fees aids people's ability to seek justice.
E. Small businesses and individuals will not use civil courts anymore to resolve matters.

**Question 103:**

Studies reveal that families from more affluent socio-economic backgrounds tend to have children who score highly in IQ tests. It seems unlikely that there is a direct relationship between money and IQ. These studies did not record whether the link between family income and children's IQ scores was affected by the parents' profession. A much more likely explanation is that intelligence tends to result in higher income, since a certain level of intelligence is needed for higher paid and skilled careers such as medicine, law, banking or engineering. If these studies found that the children of high earners in sport, music and entertainment did not generally have high IQ scores, we could conclude that the intelligence level of children is largely genetically inherited from their parents.

Which of the following is the main assumption underlying this argument?
A. High IQ scores are not found in children of parents in the sports, entertainment and music industries.
B. Children of affluent families are likely to have a much better education than others.
C. To get into professions that are higher paid and more skilled, all that is needed is a high level of intelligence.
D. IQ is a representative test for intelligence.
E. Careers in entertainment, music and sport do not require high levels of intelligence.

**Question 104:**

One cohort of medical researchers have a unique chance to analyse human brains due to the recent contributions of brain post-mortems. Dissection of these brains and the analysis of synapses may add evidence to the hypothesis of cognitive reserve. This states that when a person gets older, they gradually lose some brain synapses, leading to declining cognitive function. Those who have led an active lifestyle with respect to their brain are thought to have created more synapses, creating a resistance to the natural degradation of synapses as they age. Having a healthy lifestyle when younger should make it feasible to maintain a higher standard of cognitive ability into old age. This sort of lifestyle includes eating a healthy diet, reading and exercising regularly.

Which of the following can be reliably be concluded from this passage??
A. Reading, eating well and keeping active will ensure quality of life in old age.
B. Declining brain performance in old age is not understood very well because of the limited resources scientists have.
C. Scientists should encourage the public to donate their brains for medical research after death.
D. The decline in brain synapses in old age is due to poor lifestyle choices made in youth.
E. On average, those older people who have lived an active lifestyle are expected to have a higher number of synapses in their brain.

**Question 105:**

Everyone who lives in the UK is entitled to free healthcare. It is paid for by everyone who pays tax. Some people who use a lot of drugs and drink a lot of alcohol use this free healthcare service a lot more than others who lead healthy lives. This is unfair, as healthy people should not have to pay for the healthcare of people who use drugs and drink lots of alcohol. These people who use the healthcare system a lot more than others should therefore pay for their treatments.

Which of the following best illustrates the principle underlying this argument?
A. People who earn more should get their treatment faster than others.
B. People who drive more should pay more road tax.
C. All channels on television should be provided in one bundle, not on separate subscriptions.
D. If people have leftover mobile data on their monthly plan, it should rollover onto the next month.
E. People should have to empty their own bins in designated disposal sites, so those with less waste have less to do.

**Question 106:**

A journalist says; "we should impose a tariff on imported vegetables so that they cost consumers more than domestic vegetables. Otherwise, growers from other countries who can grow vegetables more cheaply will put domestic vegetable growers out of business. This will result in farmland being converted for more lucrative industrial uses and the consequent vanishing of a unique way of life."

Which of the following principles does the journalist's recommendation most closely conform to?
A. Government intervention sometimes creates more economic efficiency than free markets.
B. A country should put the interests of its own citizens ahead of those of citizens of other countries.
C. Social concerns should sometimes take precedence over economic efficiency.
D. The interests of producers should always take precedence over those of consumers.
E. A country should put its own economic interest over that of other countries.

**Question 107:**

A columnist said that; "there should be complete freedom of thought and expression. That means there is nothing wrong with exploiting unsavoury popular tastes for the sake of financial gain."

Which of the following judgments conforms most closely to the principle the columnist is expressing?
A. There should be no laws restricting which books are published, but publishing books that pander to people with depraved tastes is not necessarily morally acceptable.
B. The public have the freedom to purchase whatever recordings are produced, but that does not mean that the government may not limit the production of recordings.
C. People who produce depraved movies have the freedom to do so, but they should be discouraged.
D. The government should grant artists the right to create whatever works of art they want to create so long as no one considers those works to be depraved.
E. If we are all free to say what we like, we are free to say things which are offensive to others if it benefits us.

**Question 108:**

Lions do not tolerate an attack by one lion on another if the latter demonstrates submission by baring its throat. The same is true of tigers and domesticated cats. So, it would be erroneous to deny that animals have rights on the grounds that only human beings are capable of obeying moral rules.

What is the underlying structure of this argument?

A. It provides counterexamples to refute the premise on which this particular conclusion is based.

B. It establishes inductively that all animals possess some form of morality.

C. It casts doubt on the principle that being capable of obeying moral rules is a necessary condition for having rights.

D. It establishes a claim by showing that the denial of that claim entails a logical contradiction.

E. It provides evidence suggesting that the concept of morality is often applied too broadly.

**Question 109:**

When a nation is on the brink of financial crisis, its government must violate free market principles in order to prevent economic collapse by limiting the extent to which foreign investors and lenders can withdraw their money. After all, the right to free speech does not include the right to shout "Fire!" in a crowded theatre, and the harm done when investors and lenders rush madly to get their money out before anyone else does can be just as real as the harm resulting from a stampede in a theatre.

What is the underlying structure of this argument?

A. It uses an analogy to show that a set of principles should not be adhered to in every circumstance.

B. It makes a claim by arguing that the truth of that claim best explains the observed facts.

C. It presents numerous experimental results as evidence for a general principle.

D. It attempts to demonstrate that the explanation of a phenomenon is flawed by showing that it fails to explain a particular instance of that phenomenon.

E. It applies an empirical generalisation to reach a conclusion about a particular case.

**Question 110:**

The most advanced kind of moral motivation is based solely on abstract principles. This form of motivation is in contrast to calculated self-interest or the desire to adhere to societal norms and conventions.

The actions of which of the following individuals exhibit the most advanced kind of moral motivation, as described above?

A. Jay gave money to a local charity after walking past a charity collection box at work because he worried that not doing so would make him look stingy.

B. Will gave money to a local charity after walking past a charity collection box at work as he believed that doing so would improve his employer's opinion of him.

C. Harvey's employers engaged in an illegal but profitable practice that caused serious environmental damage. He did not report this to the authorities out of fear his employers would retaliate against him.

D. Rachel's employers engaged in an illegal but profitable practice that caused serious environmental damage. She reported it to the authorities out of a belief that protecting the environment is always more important than money.

E. Lee's employers engaged in an illegal but profitable practice that caused serious environmental damage. He reported it to the authorities because several colleagues pressured him to do so.

**Question 111:**

José claims that the Northeast Faithville Neighbourhood Federation opposes the new electricity system and uses this as evidence of citywide opposition. The Federation passed a resolution opposing it, but less than 10% of members voted, and 40% of those who voted, voted in favour of the system. The opposing votes represent less than 1% of the population of Faithville. One should not assume that so few votes represent the majority view.

Which of the following most accurately describes the author's form of argument?
A. Attempting to cast doubt on a conclusion by claiming the statistical sample on which the conclusion is based is too small to be dependable.
B. Criticizing a view on grounds that the view is based on evidence that is impossible to dispute.
C. Questioning a conclusion based on vote results, on the grounds that people with certain views are more likely to vote.
D. It is in everyone's best interests to reduce car usage worldwide.
E. Attempting to refute an argument by showing that, contrary to what has been claimed, the truth of the premise does not guarantee the truth of the conclusion.

**Question 112:**

All sharks in the Atlantic Ocean have flat parts on their bodies, called fins. All dolphins in the Pacific Ocean also have fins. Therefore, they are similar.

Which of the following most closely parallels the reasoning of this argument?
A. Sharks and dolphins are similar; however, they have many differences.
B. All sharks have teeth, dolphins are similar to sharks, therefore they must have teeth.
C. Bats and eagles must be similar because every bat has wings, and so does every eagle.
D. All dogs have eyes, and all cats have eyes.
E. Some rats have fur, and all mammals have fur; therefore, rats are mammals.

**Question 113:**

If I have promised to keep a secret and someone asks me a question, I cannot answer truthfully without breaking this promise. I cannot keep and break the same promise. So, one cannot be obliged to answer all questions truthfully and to keep all promises.

Which of the following arguments is the most similar in its reasoning to the argument above?
A. If business hours are extended, we will have to hire new employees or have current staff work overtime. Both options would increase labour costs. We cannot afford to do this, so we will have to keep business hours as they are.
B. Some politicians gain votes by making extravagant promises, but this deceives people. Since the only way for some politicians to be popular is by deception, and all politicians need to be popular, it follows that some must deceive.
C. If we put an effort into making a report look good, the client might think we did so because we thought the proposal would not stand on its own merits. But if we do not try to make it look good, they might think we are not serious about our business. So, whatever we do, we risk criticism from the client.
D. It is claimed that we have the right to say whatever we want. We also have an obligation to be civil to others. But civility requires that we are not always able to say what we want. Therefore, it cannot be true that we have the right to say whatever we want while still being civil.
E. If creditors have legitimate claims against a business, and they have resources to pay those debts, then they are obliged to pay them. Also, if this is the case, then a court will enforce it. But the courts did not force this business to pay its debts, so either the creditors did not have sufficient legitimate claims, or the business did not have sufficient resources.

**Question 114:**

Phone companies frequently request consumer information about human factors, such as whether the phone is comfortable to hold or whether a set of features are easy to use. However, designer interaction with consumers is superior to survey data; the data may tell the designer why a feature on last year's model had a lower rating, but it will not explain how that feature needs to be changed to increase the rating.

Which of the following arguments is the most similar in its reasoning to the argument above?
A. Designers aim to create features that will appeal to specific market niches.
B. A phone will have unappealing features if consumers are not consulted during the design stage.
C. Consumer input affects external rather than internal design components of phones.
D. Getting consumer input for design changes can help contribute to successful product design.
E. Phone companies always conduct extensive post-market surveys.

**Question 115:**

Someone living in a cold climate buys a winter coat that is stylish but not warm in order to appear sophisticated. People are sometimes willing to sacrifice practicality and comfort for the sake of appearances.

Which of the following situations and explanations are most similar to the above passage?

A. A performer convinces his entertainment company to purchase an expensive outfit so he can impress the audience more.

B. A woman sets her thermostat at a low temperature in the winter because she is concerned about environmental damage caused by using fossil fuels to heat her home.

C. Someone buys a particular wine even though their favourite wine tastes better and is easier to find because they think the other wine will impress their dinner guests more.

D. A parent buys a car seat for their child because it is more colourful and comfortable for the child than other seats on the market, though no safer.

E. A man buys a car to commute to work even though public transport is already quick and reliable.

**Question 116:**

Chris owns a car dealership which has donated cars to driver education programmes for over 5 years. He finds the statistics on car accidents disturbing and wants to do something to encourage better driving in young drivers. Some people show support by buying cars from Chris' dealership.

Which of the following is best illustrated by the passage?

A. The only way to reduce traffic accidents is through driver education programmes.

B. Altruistic actions sometimes have additional positive consequences for those who perform them.

C. Young drivers are the group most likely to benefit from driver education programs.

D. It is usually in one's best interest to perform actions that benefit others.

E. An action must have broad community support if it is to be successful.

**Question 117:**

In academia, sources are always cited when used in articles or presentations. In open-source software, the code in which the program is written can be viewed and modified by individual users for their purposes without getting permission. In contrast, the use of proprietary software is kept secret, and modifications can only be made by the producer, for a fee. This shows that open-source software better matches the values embodied in academic scholarship and since scholarship is central to the mission of universities, universities should use only open-source software.

Which of the following most closely conforms to the reasoning above?

A. Whatever software tools are the most advanced and can achieve the goals of academic scholarship are the ones that should be used in universities.

B. Universities should use the type of software technology that is cheapest, as long as it is adequate for their purposes.

C. Universities should choose the type of software technology that best matches the values embodied in the activities central to the mission of universities.

D. The form of software technology that best matches the values embodied in the activities central to the mission of universities is the form of software technology most efficient for universities to use.

E. A university should not pursue any activity that would block the achievement of academic goals at that university.

**Question 118:**

Every business strives to increase its productivity, as this increases profits for the owners and the probability that the business will survive. Not all efforts to increase productivity are beneficial to the business as a whole. A lot of the time, attempts to increase productivity decrease the number of employees, which clearly harms the dismissed employees as well as the sense of security of the employees kept at the company.

Which of the following best illustrates the main conclusion of this argument?

A. Reducing the number of employees in a business undermines the sense of security of the retained employees.
B. Every business makes efforts to increase productivity.
C. Interests align only if the employees of a business are also its owners, which enables measures that are beneficial to the overall business.
D. Some measures taken by a business to increase productivity fail to be beneficial to the overall business.
E. If an action taken to secure the survival of a business fails to enhance employee welfare, that action cannot be good for the overall business.

**Question 119:**

A recent report suggests that Saino's pre-packaged meals are lacking nutritional value. But this report was commissioned by Tesoc, Saino's largest corporate rival. Some primary drafts of the report were submitted for approval to Tesoc's public relations department. Due to the obvious bias of this report, it is clear that Saino's pre-packaged meals really are nutritious.

Which of the following best outlines the flaw in this argument?

A. It treats evidence of an apparent bias as actual evidence that the report's claims are false.
B. It draws a conclusion based solely on an unrepresentative sample of Saino's products.
C. It fails to take into account the possibility that Saino's has just as much motivation to create negative publicity for Tesoc as Tesoc has to create negative publicity for Saino's.
D. It fails to provide evidence that Tesoc's pre-packaged meals are not more nutritious than Saino's meals are.
E. It assumes that Tesoc's public relations department would not approve a draft of a report that was hostile to Tesoc's products.

**Question 120:**

No one with a criminal conviction can be appointed to the board. An undergraduate degree is necessary for appointment to the executive board. Therefore, Jim – who has a master's degree as well as a bachelor's degree – cannot be accepted as the new executive administrator, as he has a criminal conviction.

Which of the following is an assumption of the above argument?

A. Anyone with a bachelor's degree without a criminal conviction is eligible for appointment to the executive board.
B. Only candidates eligible for appointment to the executive board can be accepted for the position of executive administrator.
C. A bachelor's degree is not necessary for acceptance for the role of executive administrator.
D. If Jim did not have a criminal conviction, he would be accepted for the position of executive administrator.
E. The criminal charge on which Jim was convicted is relevant to the duties of the role of executive administrator.

**Question 121:**

Whenever possible, all scientific experiments should be performed using a double-blind protocol. This helps prevent common misinterpretations of trial results due to expectations and opinions that scientists already hold. Clearly scientists should be extremely diligent in trying to avoid such misinterpretations.

Which of the following best expresses the main conclusion of this argument?
A. Double blind experiments are an effective way of ensuring scientific objectivity.
B. Whenever they can, scientists should refrain from interpreting evidence based on previously formed expectations.
C. The objectivity of scientists may be impeded when interpreting experimental evidence on the basis of expectations and opinions they already have.
D. It is advisable for scientists to use double blind techniques in as many experiments as they can.
E. Scientists sometimes fail to adequately consider the risk of misinterpreting evidence on the basis of prior expectations and opinions.

**Question 122:**

Aluminium soft drink cans all contain the same amount of aluminium. At dispoal and manufacture, the cans are divided into several groups. Fifty percent of the aluminium in Group B was recycled from cans in Group A, a group of used aluminium soft drink cans. Since all the cans from Group A were recycled into cans in Group B, and since the amount of material other than aluminium in the cans is negligible, it follows that Group B has twice as many cans as Group A.

Which of the following best illustrates the main assumption of this argument?
A. The aluminium of cans in Group B cannot be recycled further.
B. Recycled aluminium is of poorer quality than unrecycled aluminium.
C. All of the aluminium of an aluminium can is recovered when the can is recycled.
D. Aluminium soft drink cans are more easily recycled than other cans made of different materials.
E. None of the soft drinks from Group A had been made from recycled aluminium.

**Question 123:**

A policy has been developed to avoid many serious cases of influenza. This goal will be met by the annual vaccination of high-risk individuals. This means everyone over 65 years old and/or with a chronic disease will be offered a vaccine. The vaccination produced each year only prevents the strain deemed most prevalent that year. Every year a vaccine will be necessary for all high-risk individuals to prevent serious influenza.

Which of the following best expresses the main assumption of this argument?
A. The number of individuals in the high-risk group will not significantly change every year.
B. The likelihood that a serious influenza epidemic will occur varies every year.
C. No vaccine against the influenza virus protects against more than one strain of the virus.
D. Every year, the strain deemed most prevalent will be one that had not previously been deemed most prevalent.
E. Every year, the vaccine will have fewer side effects than the previous year's vaccine, since technology will improve year by year.

**Question 124:**
At a recent conference on non-profit management, several computer experts maintained that the most significant threat faced by large institutions such as universities and hospitals is unauthorised access to confidential data. In light of this testimony, we should make the protection of our clients' confidentiality our highest priority.

Which of the following best is a flaw in this argument?
A. It confuses the causes of a problem with the appropriate solutions to it.
B. It relies on the testimony of experts whose expertise is not shown to be sufficient to support their general claim.
C. It assumes a correlation between two phenomena is evidence that one is the cause of the other.
D. It draws a general conclusion about a group, based on data about an unrepresentative sample.
E. It infers that a property belonging to large institutions belongs to all institutions.

**Question 125:**
My friends say I will have a road accident one day because I drive my sports car recklessly. But I have done some research, and it says minivans and larger sedans have very low accident rates compared to sports cars. So, trading my sports car in for a minivan would reduce my risk of having an accident.

Which of the following best expresses the main flaw of the passage?
A. It infers a cause from a correlation.
B. It relies on a sample that is too narrow.
C. It misinterprets evidence that a result is likely as evidence that the result is certain.
D. It mistakes a condition sufficient for bringing about a result for a condition necessary for doing so.
E. It relies on an unreliable source.

**Question 126:**
An action is morally right if it would be reasonably expected to increase the overall wellbeing of the people affected by it. An action is morally wrong if and only if it can be reasonably expected to reduce the wellbeing of the people affected by it. Therefore, actions that would be reasonably expected to leave the overall wellbeing of the people affected by them unchanged are also morally right.

Which of the following best the ain assumption of the passage above?
A. Only morally wrong actions can be reasonably expected to reduce the overall wellbeing of the people affected by them.
B. No action is both right and wrong.
C. Any action that is not morally wrong is morally right.
D. There are actions reasonably expected to leave the overall wellbeing of the people affected by them unchanged.
E. Only morally right actions have good consequences.

**Question 127:**

Many companies have started to decorate their halls with motivational posters in the hope of boosting the motivation and producitivity of their employees. However, almost all of these employees are already motivated to work productively. Therefore, although these companies use motivational posters it is unlikely to achieve their intended purpose.

Which of the following best expresses the main flaw of the passage?

A.  It fails to consider whether companies that do not currently use motivational posters would increase their employees' motivation to work productively if they began to use the posters.
B.  It takes for granted that companies that decorate their halls with motivational posters are representative of companies in general.
C.  It fails to consider whether even if motivational posters do not have one particular benefit for companies, they may have similar effects that are equally beneficial.
D.  It does not adequately address the possibility that employee productivity is strongly affected by factors other than their motivation.
E.  It fails to consider that even if employees are already motivated to work productively, motivational posters may increase that motivation.

**Question 128:**

An entomologist observed ants carrying particles to neighbouring ant colonies and inferred that the ants were bringing food to their neighbours. However, further research revealed that the ants were emptying their own colony's dump site. Therefore, the entomologist was wrong.

A.  Which of the following best illustrates the main assumption of this argument?
B.  Ant colonies do not interact in the same way human societies do.
C.  There is only weak evidence for the view that ants have the capacity to make use of objects as gifts.
D.  Ant dumping sites do not contain particles that could be used as food.
E.  The ants to whom the particles were brought never carried the particles into their own colonies.

**Question 129:**

Febrooze leaves clothes fluffy and soft to touch – combine this with its fresh odour and it is a delight. We conducted a test with over a hundred consumers to prove it is indeed the best clothes product out there. Each person was given one towel washed with Febrooze and one towel washed without it. 99% of these consumers preferred the Febroozed towel. Therefore, Febrooze is the most effective fabric softener available.

The reasoning in the passage is most vulnerable to criticism because it fails to consider which of the following points?

A.  If any of the consumers tested are allergic to fabric softeners.
B.  If Febrooze is more or less harmful to the environment than other fabric softeners.
C.  If Febrooze is cheaper or more expensive than other fabric softeners.
D.  If the consumers tested find the benefits of using fabric softeners worth the expense.
E.  If the consumers tested had the chance to evaluate fabric softeners other than Febrooze.

**Question 130:**

The government pays for individual medical needs through a healthcare system, requiring all citizens to pay for this service through taxes. Since it is individuals who need medical attention that primarily benefit from this, the government should ensure individuals who have the medical attention bear the cost and should impose an end-user fee on medical care.

Which one of the following principles would do most to justify the conclusion of the argument?
A. The government should avoid any actions that might alter the behaviour of taxpayers.
B. Any rational healthcare system must base the amount of the cost on the usage involved.
C. The people who stand to benefit from a service should always be made to bear the cost of a service.
D. Government based medical care for individuals should be provided only when it does not reduce incentives for individuals to seek medical care.
E. The choice of not accepting an offered service should be available, even if there is no charge.

**Question 131:**

Most people can tell whether a sequence of words in their own dialect is grammatically correct or not, yet few people who can do so are able to specify the relevant grammatical rules.

Which of the following best illustrates the principle underlying the argument above?
A. Some people are able to write coherent and accurate narrative descriptions of events, but these people are not necessarily capable of composing emotionally moving and satisfying poems.
B. Engineers who apply the principles of physics to design buildings and bridges must know a great deal more than the physicists who discovered these principles.
C. Some people are able to tell whether any given piece of music is a waltz, but the majority of these people cannot state the defining characteristics of a waltz.
D. Those travellers who most enjoy their journeys are not always those most capable of vividly describing details of those journeys to others.
E. Quite a few people know the rules of chess, but only a small number of them can play chess well.

**Question 132:**

A robber comes to your house and steals your computer. You lose all your pictures and music. Later, the robber turns himself in to police. He apologises, says the robbery was a moment of weakness, and repents. The robber is prepared to accept whatever punishment the law thinks appropriate. This is the robber's third crime, and he will go to jail for life if found guilty. Unfortunately, the computer was broken in the robbery, and you can't get any data back. The police come to you and ask if you want to press charges. You say no.

Which of the following sufficiently illustrates the principle underlying the argument above?
A. Anyone who repents of a crime deserves mercy and should not be punished.
B. All convicted criminals must be sent to jail.
C. You should not have mercy for a criminal who does not repent.
D. You should only punish a criminal if they cause irreparable damage.
E. You should only have mercy for a criminal if they repent.

**Question 133:**

Hospitals, universities, labour unions, and other institutions may well have public purposes and be quite successful at achieving them even though each of their individual staff members does what he or she does only for selfish reasons.

Which of the following best illustrates the principle underlying the argument above?
A.  What is true of some social organisations is not necessarily true of all such organisations.
B.  An organisation can have a property that not all of its members possess.
C.  People often claim altruistic motives for actions that are in fact selfish.
D.  Many social institutions have social consequences unintended by those who founded them.
E.  Often an instrument created for one purpose will be found to serve another purpose just as effectively.

**Question 134:**

When drivers are sleep deprived, there are definite behavioural changes, such as slower response times to stimuli and a reduced ability to concentrate, but self-awareness of these changes is poor. Most drivers think they can tell when they are about to fall asleep, but they cannot.

Select the answer option that does not illustrate the same principle as the passage above:
A.  People who have been drinking alcohol are not good judges of whether they are too drunk to drive.
B.  Primary school students who dislike arithmetic are not good judges of whether multiplication tables should be included in the school's curriculum.
C.  Industrial workers who have just been exposed to noxious fumes are not good judges of whether they should keep working.
D.  People who have just donated blood and have become faint are not good judges of whether they are ready to walk out of the facility.
E.  People who are being treated for schizophrenia are not good judges of whether they should continue their medical treatment.

**Question 135:**

One of our local television stations has been criticised for its recent coverage of the personal problems of a local politician's nephew, but the coverage was in fact good journalism. The information was accurate. Furthermore, the newscast had significantly more viewers than it normally does, because many people are curious about the politician's nephew's problems.

Which of the following principles, if valid, would most help to justify the reasoning above?
A.  Journalism deserves to be criticised if it does not provide information that people want.
B.  Any journalism that intentionally misrepresents the facts of a case deserves to be criticised.
C.  Any journalism that provides accurate information on a subject about which there is considerable interest is good journalism.
D.  Good journalism will always provide people with information that they desire or need.
E.  Journalism that neither satisfies the public's curiosity nor provides accurate information can never be considered good journalism.

**Question 136:**

Because people are generally better at detecting mistakes in others' work than in their own, a prudent principle is that one should always have one's own work checked by someone else.

Which of the following provides the best illustration of the principle above?

A.  The best primary school maths teachers are not those for whom maths was always easy. Teachers who had to struggle through maths themselves are better able to explain maths to students.

B.  One must make a special effort to clearly explain one's views to someone else; people normally find it easier to understand their own views than to understand others' views.

C.  Juries composed of legal novices, rather than panels of lawyers, should be the final arbiters in legal proceedings. People who are not legal experts are in a better position to detect good legal arguments by lawyers than are other lawyers.

D.  People should always have their writing proofread by someone else. Someone who does not know in advance what is going to be said is in a better position to spot typographical errors.

E.  Two people going out for dinner will have a more enjoyable meal if they order for each other. By allowing someone else to choose, one opens oneself up to new and exciting dining experiences.

**Question 137:**

All beagles bark a lot when they are not supposed to. All pugs do not bark often. Each of Amy's dogs is a cross between a beagle and a pug, so these dogs are moderate barkers that bark some of the time.

Which of the following parallels the reasoning in the argument above?

A.  All of Faith's dresses are very well made. All of Hannah's dresses are very badly made. Half of the dresses in this closet are very well made and half are very badly made. So, half of these dresses must be Faith's and half are Hannah's.

B.  All students at Wonn School live in Blue County. All students at Perrie School live in Bong County. Members of the Edwards family attend both Wonn and Perrie School. Therefore, some members of the Edwards family live in Blue County and some live in Bong County.

C.  All stenographers know shorthand. All engineers know calculus. Tom has worked as both a stenographer and an engineer, so he knows both shorthand and calculus.

D.  All mercury is extremely toxic to humans. All glycols are nontoxic to humans. This household cleaner is a mixture of mercury and glycols, so is moderately toxic.

E.  All students who study a lot get good grades. But some students who do not study a lot also get good grades. Michael studies some of the time, so has pretty good grades.

**Question 138:**

We should accept the proposal to demolish the old railway station because the local historical society, who intensely oppose this, is dominated by people who have no commitment to long-term economic wellbeing. Preserving old buildings blocks the progress of new development, which is crucial for economic health and wellbeing.

Which of the following is the flawed reasoning in the passage above most similar to?
A. We should try to protect works of art that are of national cultural significance. They might not be recognised as such by all taxpayers or critics, nevertheless, we should expend whatever money is needed to procure all such works as they become available.
B. Documents of importance to local heritage should be preserved for future generations. If even one of these documents is lost or damaged, the integrity of the overall historical record will be damaged.
C. You should have your hair cut only once a month. Beauticians often suggest that their customers have haircuts twice a month in order to generate more business for themselves.
D. The committee should endorse the plan to postpone construction of the new motorway. Many local residents who would be affected are opposed to it, and the committee has an obligation to avoid alienating those residents.
E. One should not borrow even small sums of money unless strictly necessary. Once one borrows small sums, the interest starts to accumulate. The longer one takes to repay, the more one owes, and eventually a small debt has become a large one.

**Question 139:**

It has been scientifically established that all dogs do indeed bark. As a result, any animal that barks is a dog. So, if a person hears an animal bark, that person can safely conclude that the animal is a dog.

Which of the following arguments most closely parallels the flawed reasoning above?
A. Only high interest debt is debt that should be avoided. Debt that is not high interest should not be avoided.
B. All high interest debt should be avoided. Debt that isn't high interest need not be avoided. So, people should prefer low interest debt.
C. All debt that should be avoided is high interest debt because all high interest debt should be avoided. Debt that should be avoided must be high interest debt.
D. High interest debt should sometimes be avoided. As a result, some debt that should be avoided is high interest debt. So, a person can safely conclude that high interest debt should be avoided.
E. If all high interest debt should be avoided, and if some debt is high interest, then some debt should be avoided.

**Question 140:**

Everyone who thinks the Raiders should win the title thought that Jackie would win the award for Most Valuable Payer, but Jackie did not get this award. Therefore, anyone who believes the Raiders will win the title is wrong.

Which of the following arguments contains similarly flawed reasoning?

A.  Anyone who thinks exercising after eating is a good idea has never taken a health class. But Paulo has never taken a health class and knows he should not eat before exercising. Therefore, taking a health class is not necessary for you to know eating before exercise is a bad idea.

B.  Anyone who believes seagull migration is based on advanced spatial recognition patterns believes that most bird species have highly developed frontal cortices. But it has been proven that most bird species do not have highly developed frontal cortices. Therefore, the belief that seagulls migrate based on advanced spatial recognition patterns is false.

C.  Anyone who thinks animals deserve better treatment believes animals are capable of moral judgment. You do not believe that animals deserve better treatment, so you do not think they are capable of moral judgment.

D.  Anyone who thinks chickens are ugly thinks ducks are also ugly. Since there is no reason to think ducks are ugly, there is no reason to think chickens are ugly.

E.  If you believe in the tooth fairy, then you do not believe in blood sucking vampires. Since Calum believes in blood sucking vampires, he cannot believe in the tooth fairy.

**Question 141:**

Winning requires the willingness to cooperate, which in turn requires motivation. So, you will not win if you are not motivated.

Which of the following is most similar to the argument above?

A.  Being healthy requires exercise, but exercise involves risk of injury. So, paradoxically, anyone who wants to be healthy will not exercise.

B.  Learning requires making some mistakes, and you must learn if you are to improve. So, you will not make mistakes without there being a noticeable improvement in your skills.

C.  Our political party will retain its status only if it raises more money, but raising more money requires increased campaigning. So, our party will not retain its status unless it increases campaigning.

D.  Getting a ticket requires waiting in line. Waiting in line requires patience. So, if you do not wait in line, you lack patience.

E.  You can repair your own bicycle only if you are enthusiastic. And if you are enthusiastic, you will also have mechanical aptitude. So, if you are not able to repair your own bicycle you lack mechanical aptitude.

**Question 142:**

The national Sooper Plate was held last weekend. In order to win the tournament, a contestant must answer three questions correctly and consecutively. Angela answered three questions correctly and consecutively, so she must have won the Sooper Plate.

Which of the following arguments contains similar reasoning to the passage above?
A. To win the county swim meet, a swimmer needs to win three heats. Dave won the swim meet, so he must have won three heats.
B. Good doctors spend time getting to know their patients as people, not just their medical history. Doctor Smith is a bad doctor, so he must not know his patients on a personal level.
C. Daniel likes to win tournaments. He enters a new tournament every week, even if he is completely unskilled in the tasks involved. He has even won a few trophies.
D. People who win tournaments are confident. People with confidence are usually successful at work. It must follow then, that people who win tournaments are successful at work.
E. When a television station is owned by a large conglomerate, it often has to edit its news to be favourable to its parent company and all of its related products. The local independent station, channel 7, never runs a bad story about SOD Industries. It must be owned by SOD Industries, and so is incapable of fair reporting.

**Question 143:**

If Max Landsy is healthy, it is highly unlikely the Tokes will win their match-up with the Patties. But in fact, the Tokes did win the match-up, so it's highly unlikely that Max Landsy was healthy.

The pattern of reasoning in the passage is most similar to that in which of the following arguments?
A. If the football cup was not fixed, the winning team would have been highly unlikely to win the whole thing. Thus, since this team was highly unlikely to win, the tournament was probably fixed.
B. If the Prime Minister was a speaker at the event, it's highly unlikely that the Sun would cover the event. It's very unlikely that the Prime Minister did speak, since as it turns out, the Sun did cover the event.
C. If the dice were not loaded, Oliver, who planned to win the roulette 5 times in a row, would have been highly unlikely to win the roulette 5 times in a row. Since he was unlikely to win, the dice were probably loaded.
D. If the star player is raring to go, it is highly likely her team will win their crucial match to win the league title. They did win. It was reported that it was an outstanding team effort to win.
E. If the first-choice keeper has an illness, it is highly unlikely that The United would win their match against The City. The City did in fact win this match, so it follows that the first choice keeper was not playing.

**Question 144:**

Although birds have long been considered much less intelligent than humans and apes, new research has shown that some species of birds have similar thinking skills to apes. Crows can create and use tools and are socially sophisticated when finding and protecting food. How is a bird with a walnut-sized brain capable of this higher level of cognition? The answer is that both crows and apes have much bigger brains than you would expect from the size of their bodies. The same pattern is found in other intelligent animals, including humans, parrots and chimps.

Which of the following can be drawn as a conclusion from this passage?
A.  Apes are not as similar to humans as had been thought.
B.  Crows are more intelligent than other species of birds.
C.  Animals that cannot create tools are not intelligent.
D.  Relative brain size is a better indicator of intelligence than absolute brain size.
E.  It could be argued that birds are as intelligent as apes.

**Question 145:**

There is a higher than average risk of death or injury to young drivers and their passengers. In 2007, 32 per cent of car driver deaths and 40 per cent of car passenger deaths occurred in people aged between 17 and 24. Young male drivers were much more likely to be killed or seriously injured than young female drivers. In order to reduce the number of road accidents and the numbers of people killed or injured, young people should not be allowed to drive until they reach the age of 24

Which of the following is an assumption upon which this argument depends?
A.  Young people would not accept the raising of the legal driving age.
B.  Most of the accidents involving young people were the fault of the young drivers.
C.  The driving test does not effectively test the skill of drivers.
D.  The majority of drivers aged between 17 and 24 drive dangerously.
E.  Amongst drivers aged between 17 and 24, there are more male drivers than female drivers.

**Question 146:**

Some disabled people find it difficult to gain access to some of our older public buildings because the entrances have steps. The problem is most often solved by installing ramps. All public buildings should be accessible to everyone therefore they must all install ramps.

Which of the following identifies the flaw in this argument?
A.  Disabled people must have access to all buildings not just public ones so all buildings should have ramps.
B.  Installing ramps in all public buildings would be extremely expensive.
C.  It is unreasonable to suggest that disabled people should be able to access all public buildings.
D.  Some older public buildings without ramps may already be accessible to disabled people.
E.  Inaccessible public buildings should be replaced by buildings accessible to all.

**Question 147:**

If more workers worked for only four days each week there would be fewer commuters, and therefore less traffic congestion and less pollution. Fewer people would be unemployed because there would be more work to go around. There is evidence that part-time workers are absent from work less often than full-time workers, so a person working a four-day week is likely to be more productive. Less work means less pressure, which means less stress and happier people.

Which of the following can be drawn as a conclusion from this passage?
A.  People choosing to work a four-day week would have to take a 20% pay cut.
B.  There would be less pressure on the health services if most workers were on a four-day week.
C.  The economy would be more competitive if people worked more productively.
D.  The government should enforce a four-day working week.
E.  There would be many benefits to working a four-day week.

## Question 148:

Some types of migratory birds that are unable to fly long distances without resting have to use the shortest distance over water in their flights to and from Africa, and so they cross at the Strait of Gibraltar. It is essential for these birds, some of which are very rare, that the route remains open. For that reason, it is important that plans to build electricity-generating wind farms on the hills surrounding the Strait of Gibraltar do not go ahead.

Which of the following is an assumption upon which this argument depends?
A.  The birds that migrate across the Strait of Gibraltar are close to extinction.
B.  Electricity-generating wind farms have to be built on hills.
C.  The planned wind farms will make it dangerous for migratory birds to use their usual route.
D.  Other species of bird can fly further and can thus use other routes in their migration.
E.  There are no plans to build wind farms at other places along the coast.

## Question 149:

When mobile phones were first introduced there were concerns about the microwave radiation they produced, and the effects that these could have on the brain, given that phones are held close to the ear while being used. These concerns have ultimately been shown to be unfounded, as mobile phones are more frequently used for sending text messages than for making phone calls. Sending a text message does not require the phone to be anywhere near to the brain so it cannot cause any problems.

Which of the following identifies the flaw in this argument?
A.  It ignores research showing that microwaves from the phones cannot penetrate far enough to reach the brain.
B.  It ignores evidence suggesting that text messaging is only popular in certain age groups.
C.  It does not consider uses of mobile phones other than making phone calls and sending text messages.
D.  It does not consider other technology such as wireless internet which could cause similar problems.
E.  It ignores the possible effects of the phone calls that are still made.

## Question 150:

A comparison is sometimes made between fast-food restaurants and factories. This is because fast-food is a mass-produced, heavily processed product, and restaurant workers' jobs are as routine and boring as those in manufacturing. Not only does fast-food taste the same everywhere, but all workers involved are on low wages and have little power to improve their conditions.

Which of the following best expresses the main conclusion of this argument?
A.  Workers who do routine and boring jobs are often poorly paid.
B.  Mass production in factories leads to poor working conditions.
C.  It is not unrealistic to compare fast-food restaurants with factories.
D.  All fast-food tastes the same because it is heavily processed.
E.  Working in a fast-food restaurant is no different from working in a factory..

# SECTION 1: PROBLEM SOLVING

Section 1 problem solving questions are arguably the hardest to prepare for. However, there are some useful techniques you can employ to solve some types of questions much more quickly:

### Construct Equations

Some of the problems in Section 1 are quite complex and you'll need to be comfortable with turning prose into equations and then manipulating them. For example, when you read "Mark is twice as old as Jon" – this should immediately register as M = 2J. Once you get comfortable forming equations from the text, you can start to approach some of the harder questions in this book (and past papers) which may require you to form and solve simultaneous equations. Consider the following example:

Nick has a sleigh that contains toy horses and clowns. He counts 44 heads and 132 legs in his sleigh. Given that horses have one head and four legs, and clowns have one head and two legs, calculate the difference between the number of horses and clowns.

| | | |
|---|---|---|
| A. 0 | C. 22 | E. 132 |
| B. 5 | D. 28 | F. More information is needed. |

To start with, let C= Clowns and H= Horses.
For Heads: $C + H = 44$; For Legs: $2C + 4H = 132$
This now sets up your two equations that you can solve simultaneously.
$C = 44 - H$ so $2(44 - H) + 4H = 132$
Thus, $88 - 2H + 4H = 132$;
Therefore, $2H = 44$; $H = 22$
Substitute back in to give $C = 44 - H = 44 - 22 = 22$
Thus, the difference between horses and clowns $= C - H = 22 - 22 = 0$

It's important you are able to do these types of questions quickly (and **without resorting to trial & error**) as they are commonplace in Section 1 of the BMAT.

### Diagrams

When a question asks about timetables, orders or sequences, draw out diagrams. By doing this, you can organise your thoughts and help make sense of the question.

"Mordor is West of Gondor but East of Rivendale. Lorien is midway between Gondor and Mordor. Erebus is West of Mordor. Eden is not East of Gondor."

*Which of the following **cannot** be concluded?*
A. Lorien is East of Erebus and Mordor.
B. Mordor is West of Gondor and East of Erebus.
C. Rivendale is west of Lorien and Gondor.
D. Gondor is East of Mordor and East of Lorien
E. Erebus is West of Mordor and West of Rivendale.

Whilst it is possible to solve this in your head, it becomes much more manageable if you draw a quick diagram and plot the positions of each town:

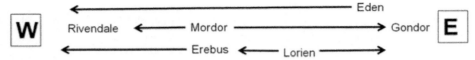

Now, it's a simple case of going through each option and seeing if it is correct according to the diagram. You can now easily see that Option E- Erebus cannot be west of Rivendale.

Don't feel that you have to restrict yourself to linear diagrams like this either – for some questions you may need to draw tables or even Venn diagrams. Consider this example:

Slifers and Osiris are not legendary. Krakens and Minotaurs are legendary. Minotaurs and Lords are both divine. Humans are neither legendary nor divine.

A. Krakens may be only legendary or legendary and divine.
B. Humans are not divine.
C. Slifers are only divine.
D. Osiris may be divine.
E. Humans and Slifers are the same in terms of both qualities.

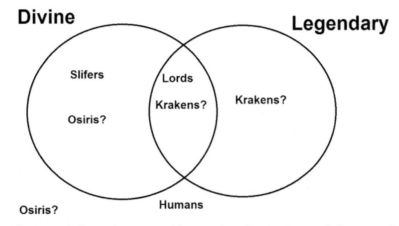

**Constructing a Venn diagram** allows us to quickly see that the position of Osiris and Krakens aren't certain. Thus, A and D must be true. Humans are neither so B is true. Krakens may be divine so A is true. E cannot be concluded as Slifers are divine but are humans are not. Thus, E is False.

### Spatial Reasoning

There are usually 1-2 spatial reasoning questions every year. They usually give nets for a shape or a patterned cuboid and ask which of the answer options are possible from rotations of the original shape. Unfortunately, they are extremely difficult to prepare for because the skills necessary to solve these types of questions can take a very long time to improve. The best thing you can do to prepare is to familiarise yourself with the basics of how cube nets work and what the effect of transformations are e.g. what happens if a shape is reflected in a mirror etc.

It is also a good idea to try to learn to draw basic shapes like cubes from multiple angles if you can't do so already. Finally, remember that if the shape is straightforward like a cube, it might be easier for you to draw a net, cut it out and fold it yourself to see which of the options are possible. Another option is to practice rotating small cube or cuboidal objects such as dice or erasers, to understand the 3D relationships between the 6 faces better.

# PROBLEM SOLVING QUESTIONS

**Question 151:**

Pilbury is south of Westside, which is south of Harrington. Twotown is north of Pilbury and Crewville but not further north than Westside. Crewville is:
A.   South of Westside, Pilbury and Harrington but not necessarily Twotown.
B.   North of Pilbury, and Westside.
C.   South of Westside and Twotown, but north of Pilbury.
D.   South of Westside, Harrington and Twotown but not necessarily Pilbury.
E.   South of Harrington, Westside, Twotown and Pilbury.

**Question 152:**

The hospital coordinator is making the rota for the ward for next week; two of Drs Evans, James and Luca must be working on weekdays, none of them on Sundays and all of them on Saturdays. Dr Evans works 4 days a week including Mondays and Fridays. Dr Luca cannot work Monday or Thursday. Only Dr James can work 4 days consecutively, but he cannot do 5.

What days does Dr James work?
A.   Saturday, Sunday and Monday.
B.   Monday, Tuesday, Wednesday, Thursday and Saturday.
C.   Monday, Thursday Friday and Saturday.
D.   Tuesday, Wednesday, Friday and Saturday.
E.   Monday, Tuesday, Wednesday, Thursday and Friday.

**Question 153:**

Michael, a taxi driver, charges a call out rate and a rate per mile for taxi rides. For a 4-mile ride he charges £11, and for a 5 mile ride, £13.

How much does he charge for a 9-mile ride?
A.  £15            B.  £17            C.  £19            D.  £20            E.  £21

**Question 154:**

Goblins and trolls are not magical. Fairies and goblins are both mythical. Elves and fairies are magical. Gnomes are neither mythical nor magical.

Which of the following is **FALSE**?
A.   Elves may be only magical or magical and mythical.
B.   Gnomes are not mythical.
C.   Goblins are only mythical.
D.   Trolls may be mythical.
E.   Gnomes and goblins are the same in terms of both qualities.

**Question 155:**

Jessica runs a small business making bespoke wall tiles. She has just had a rush order for 100 tiles placed that must be ready for today at 7pm. The client wants the tiles packed all together, a process which will take 15 minutes. Only 50 tiles can go in the kiln at any point, and they must be put in the kiln to heat for 45 minutes. The tiles then sit in the kiln to cool before they can be packed, a process which takes 20 minutes. While tiles are in the kiln Jessica is able to decorate more tiles at a rate of 1 tile per minute.

What is the latest time Jessica can start making the tiles?
A.  2:55pm
B.  3:15pm
C.  3:30pm
D.  3:45pm

**Question 156:**

Pain nerve impulses are twice as fast as normal touch impulses. If Yun touches a boiling hot pan this message reaches her brain, 1 metre away, in 1 millisecond.

What is the speed of a normal touch impulse?
A.  5 m/s
B.  20 m/s
C.  50 m/s
D.  200m/s
E.  500 m/s

**Question 157:**

A woman has two children, Melissa and Jack. Their birthdays are 3 months apart, both being on the 22nd of the month. The woman wishes to continue the trend of her children's names beginning with the same letter as the month they were born. If her next child, Alina is born on the 22nd 2 months after Jack's birthday, how many months after Alina is born will Melissa have her next birthday?

A.  2 months
B.  4 months
C.  5 months
D.  6 months
E.  7 months

**Question 158:**

Policemen work in pairs. PC Carter, PC Dirk, PC Adams and PC Bryan must work together but not for more than seven days in a row, which PC Adams and PC Bryan now have.  PC Dirk has worked with PC Carter for 3 days in a row. PC Carter does not want to work with PC Adams if it can be avoided.

Who should work with PC Bryan?
A.  PC Carter
B.  PC Dirk
C.  PC Adams
D.  Nobody is available under the guidelines above.

**Question 159:**

My hairdressers charges £30 for a haircut, £50 for a cut and blow-dry, and £60 for a full hair dye. They also do manicures, of which the first costs £15, and includes a bottle of nail polish, but are subsequently reduced by £5 if I bring my bottle of polish. The price is reduced by 10% if I book and pay for the next 5 appointments in advance and by 15% if I book at least the next 10.

I want to pay for my next 5 cut and blow-dry appointments, as well as for my next 3 manicures. How much will it cost?

A.  £170
B.  £255
C.  £260
D.  £285
E.  £305

**Question 160:**

Alex, Bertha, David, Gemma, Charlie, Elena and Frankie are all members of the same family consisting of three children, two of whom, Frankie and Gemma are girls. No other assumption of gender based on name can be established. There are also four adults. Alex is a doctor and is David's brother. One of them is married to Elena, and they have two children. Bertha is married to David; Gemma is their child.

Who is Charlie?

A. Alex's daughter          C. Gemma's brother          E. Gemma's sister
B. Frankie's father          D. Elena's son

**Question 161:**

At 14:30 three medical students were asked to examine a patient's heart. Having already watched their colleague, the second two students were twice as fast as the first to examine. During the 8 minutes break after the final student had finished, they were told by their consultant that they had taken too long and so should go back and do the examinations again. The second time, all the students took half as long as they had taken the first time with the exception of the first student who, instead took the same time as his two colleagues' second attempt. Assuming there was a one-minute change over time between each student and they were finished by 15:15, how long did the second student take to examine the first time?

A. 3 minutes          B. 4 minutes          C. 6 minutes          D. 7 minutes          E. 8 minutes

**Question 162:**

I pay for 2 chocolate bars that cost £1.65 each with a £5 note. I receive 8 coins change, only 3 of which are the same.

Which **TWO** coins do I not receive in my change?
A. 1p          C. 20p          E. £2
B. 2p          D. 10p

**Question 163:**

Two 140m long trains are running at the same speed in opposite directions. If they cross each other in 14 seconds, then what is the speed of each train?
A. 10 km/hr          B. 18 km/hr          C. 32 km/hr          D. 36 km/hr          E. 42 km/hr

**Question 164:**

Anil has to refill his home's swimming pool. He has four hoses which all run at different speeds. Alone, the first would completely fill the pool with water in 6 hours, the second in two days, the third in three days and the fourth in four days.

Using all the hoses together, how long will it take to fill the pool to the nearest quarter of an hour?
A. 4 hours 15 minutes          C. 4 hours 45 minutes          E. 5 hours 15 minutes
B. 4 hours 30 minutes          D. 5 hours

**Question 165:**

An ant is stuck in a 30 cm deep ditch. When the ant reaches the top of the ditch, he will be able to climb out straight away. The ant is able to climb 3 cm upwards during the day, but falls back 2 cm at night.

How many days does it take for the ant to climb out of the ditch?

A.  27          B.  28          C.  29          D.  30          E.  31

**Question 166:**

When buying his ingredients, a chef gets a discount of 10% when he buys 10 or more of each item, and a 20% discount when he buys 20 or more. On one order he bought 5 sausages and 10 oranges, and paid £8.50. On another, he bought 10 sausages and 10 apples and paid £9, on a third he bought 30 oranges and paid £12.

How much would an order of 2 oranges, 13 sausages and 12 apples cost?

A.  £12.52          B.  £12.76          C.  £13.52          D.  £13.76          E.  £13.80

**Question 167:**

My hairdressers encourage all of their clients to become members. By paying an annual membership fee, the cost of haircuts decreases. VIP membership costs £125 annually with a £10 reduction on each haircut. Executive VIP membership costs £200 for the year with a £15 reduction per haircut. At the moment I am not a member and pay £60 per haircut. I know how many haircuts I have a year, and I work out that by becoming a member on either programme it would work out cheaper, and I would save the same amount of money per year on either programme.

How much will I save this year by buying membership?

A.  £10          B.  £15          C.  £25          D.  £30          E.  £50

## Question 168:

If criminals, thieves and judges are represented below:

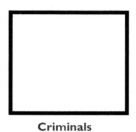 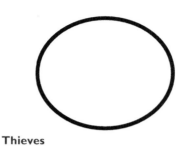 

| Criminals | Thieves | Judges |

Assuming that judges must have a clean record, all thieves are criminals and all those who are guilty are convicted of their crimes, which of one of the following best represents their interaction?

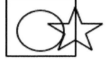

A.

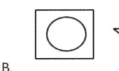

B.

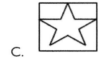

C.

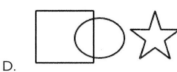

D.

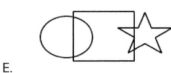

E.

## Question 169:

The months of the year have been made into number codes. The code is comprised of three factors, including two of these being related to the letters that make up the name of the month. No two months would have the same first number. But some such as March, which has the code 3513, have the same last number as others, such as May, which has the code 5313. October would be coded as 10715 while February is 286.

What would be the code for April?
A. 154          B. 441          C. 451          D. 514          E. 541

## Question 170:

A mother gives yearly birthday presents of money to her children, based on their age and their exam results. She gives them £5 each, plus £3 for every year they are older than 5, and a further £10 for every A they achieved in their results. Josie is 16 and gained 9 As in her results. Although Josie's brother Carson is 2 years older, he receives £44 less a year for his birthday.

How many more As did Josie get than Carson?
A. 2          B. 3          C. 4          D. 5          E. 10

**Question 171:**

Apples are more expensive than pears, which are more expensive than oranges. Peaches are more expensive than oranges. Apples are less expensive than grapes.

Which **two** of the following must be true?
A. Grapes are less expensive than oranges.
B. Peaches may be less expensive than pears.
C. Grapes are more expensive than pears.
D. Pears and peaches are the same price.
E. Apples and peaches are the same price.

**Question 172:**

What is the minimum number of straight cutting motions needed to slice a cylindrical cake into 8 equally sized pieces?
A. 2       B. 3       C. 4       D. 5       E. 6       F. 8

**Question 173**

Three friends, Mark, Russell and Tom had agreed to meet for lunch at 12 PM on Sunday. Daylight saving time (GMT+1) had started at 2 AM the same day, where clocks should be put forward by one hour. Mark's phone automatically changes the time, but he does not realise this so when he wakes up he puts his phone forward an hour and uses his phone to time his arrival to lunch. Tom puts all of his clocks forward one hour at 7 AM. Russell forgets that the clocks should go forward, wakes at 10 AM, and doesn't change his clocks. All of the friends arrive on time as far as they are concerned.

Assuming that none of the friends realise any errors before arriving, which **TWO** of the following statements are **FALSE**?
A. Tom arrives at 12 PM (GMT +1).
B. All three friends arrive at the same time.
C. There is a 2-hour difference between when the first and last friend arrive.
D. Mark arrives late.
E. Mark arrives at 1 PM (GMT+3).

**Question 174:**

A class of young students has a pet spider. Deciding to play a practical joke on their teacher, one day during morning break one of the students put the spider in their teacher's desk. When first questioned by the headteacher, Mr Jones, the five students who were in the classroom during morning break all lied about what they saw. Realising that the students were all lying, Mr Jones called all 5 students back individually and, threatened with suspension, all the students told the truth. Unfortunately, Mr Jones only wrote down the student's statements not whether they had been told in the truthful or lying questioning.

The students' two statements appear below:

**Archie**: "It wasn't Edward. "
     "It was Bella."

**Darcy**: "It was Charlotte"
     "It was Bella"

**Edward**: "It was Darcy"
     "It wasn't Archie"

**Charlotte**: "It was Edward."
     "It wasn't Archie"

**Bella**: "It wasn't Charlotte."
     "It wasn't Edward."

Who put the spider in the teacher's desk?

A. Edward      C. Darcy      E. More information needed.
B. Bella      D. Charlotte

**Question 175:**

Dr Massey wants to measure out 0.1 litres of solution. Unfortunately, the lab assistant dropped the 200 ml measuring cylinder, and so the scientist only has a 300 ml and a half litre-measuring beaker. Assuming he cannot accurately use the beakers to measure anything less than their full capacity, what is the minimum volume he will have to use to be able to ensure he measures the right amount?

A. 100 ml      C. 300 ml      E. 600 ml
B. 200 ml      D. 400 ml

**Question 176:**

Francis lives on a street with houses all consecutively numbered evenly. When one adds up the value of all the house numbers it totals 870.

In order to determine Francis' house number:
1. The relative position of Francis' house must be known.
2. The number of houses in the street must be known.
3. At least three of the house numbers must be known.

A. 1 only       B. 2 only       C. 3 only       D. 1 and 2       E. 2 and 3

**Question 177:**

There were 20 people exercising in the cardio room of a gym. Four people were about to leave when suddenly a man collapsed on one of the machines. Fortunately, a doctor was on the machine beside him. Emerging from his office, one of the personal trainers called an ambulance. In the 5 minutes that followed before the two paramedics arrived, half of the people who were leaving, left upon hearing the commotion, and eight people came in from the changing rooms to hear the paramedics pronouncing the man dead.

How many living people were left in the room?
A. 25       B. 26       C. 27       D. 28       E. 29

**Question 178:**

A man and woman are in an accident. They both suffer the same trauma, which causes both of them to lose blood at a rate of 0.2 litres/minute. At normal blood volume the man has 8 litres and the woman 7 litres, and people collapse when they lose 40% of their normal blood volume.

Which **TWO** of the following are true?
A. The man will collapse 2 minutes before the woman.
B. The woman collapses 2 minutes before the man.
C. The total blood loss is 5 litres.
D. The woman has 4.2 litres of blood in her body when she collapses.
E. The man's blood loss is 4.8 litres when he collapses.

**Question 179:**

Jenny, Helen and Rachel have to run a distance of 13 km. Jenny runs at a pace of 8 kmph, Helen at a pace of 10 kmph, and Rachel 11 kmph.

If Jenny sets off 15 minutes before Helen, and 25 minutes before Rachel, what order will they arrive at the destination?
A. Jenny, Helen, Rachel.       C. Helen, Jenny, Rachel.       E. Jenny, Rachel, Helen.
B. Helen, Rachel, Jenny.       D. Rachel, Helen, Jenny.

**Question 180:**

On a specific day at a GP surgery 150 people visited the surgery, and common complaints were recorded as a percentage of total patients. Each patient could use their appointment to discuss up to 2 complaints. The split of complaints was as follows: 56% flu-like symptoms, 48% pain, 20% diabetes, 40% asthma/COPD and 30% high blood pressure.

Which statement **must** be true?

A. A minimum of 8 patients complained of pain and flu-like symptoms.

B. No more than 45 patients complained of high blood pressure and diabetes.

C. There were a minimum of 21 patients who did not complain about flu-like symptoms or high blood pressure.

D. There were actually 291 patients who visited the surgery.

E. None of the above.

**Question 181:**

The prices of all products in a store were marked up by 15%. The products were subsequently reduced in a sale, with quoted savings of 25% from the higher price. What is the true reduction from the original price?

A. 5%         C. 13.75%         E. 20%

B. 10%        D. 18.25%

**Question 182:**

A recipe states it makes 12 pancakes and requires the following ingredients: 2 eggs, 100g plain flour, and 300ml milk. Steve is cooking pancakes for 15 people and wants to have sufficient mixture for 3 pancakes each.

What quantities should Steve use to ensure this whilst using whole eggs?

A. 2½ eggs, 125g plain flour, 375ml milk

B. 3 eggs, 150g plain flour, 450 ml milk

C. 7½ eggs, 375g plain flour, 1125 ml milk

D. 8 eggs, 400g plain flour, 1200 ml milk

E. 12 eggs, 600g plain flour, 1800 ml milk

**Question 183:**

Spring Cleaning cleaners buy industrial bleach from a warehouse and dilute it twice before using it domestically. The first dilution is by 9:1 and then the second, 4:1.

If the cleaners require 6 litres of diluted bleach, how much warehouse bleach do they require?

A. 30 ml        C. 166 ml        E. 1,200 ml

B. 120 ml       D. 666 ml

**Question 184:**

During a GP consultation in 2015, Ms Smith tells the GP about her grandchildren. Ms Smith states that Charles is the middle grandchild and was born in 2002. In 2010, Bertie was twice the age of Adam, and in 2015 there are 5 years between Bertie and Adam. Charles and Adam are separated by 3 years.

How old are the 3 grandchildren in 2015?
A. Adam = 16, Bertie = 11, Charles = 13
B. Adam = 5, Bertie = 10, Charles = 8
C. Adam = 10, Bertie = 15, Charles = 13
D. Adam = 10, Bertie = 20, Charles = 13
E. Adam = 11, Bertie = 10, Charles = 8

**Question 185:**

Kayak Hire charges a fixed flat rate and then an additional half-hourly rate. Peter hires a kayak for 3 hours and pays £14.50, and his friend Kevin hires 2 kayaks for 4 hrs 30 mins each and pays £41.

How much would Tom pay to hire one kayak for 2 hours?
A. £8          C. £15          E. £35.70
B. £10.50     D. £33.20

**Question 186:**

A ticketing system uses a common digital display of numbers 0 – 9. The number 7 is showing. However, a number of the light elements are not currently working.

Which set of digits is possible given the configuration of a common digital display?
A. 3, 4, 7          B. 0, 1, 9          C. 2, 7, 8          D. 0, 5, 9          E. 3, 8, 9

**Question 187:**

A team of 4 builders take 12 days of 7 hours' work to complete a house. The company decides to recruit 3 extra builders.

How many 8 hour days will it take the new workforce to build a house?
A. 2 days          C. 7 days          E. 12 days
B. 6 days          D. 10 days

**Question 188:**

All astragalus are fabacaea as are all gummifer. Acacia are not astragalus. Which of the following statements is true?

A. Acacia are not fabacaea.                    D. Some acacia may be fabacaea.
B. No astragalus are also gummifer.           E. Gummifer are all acacia.
C. All fabacae are astragalus or gummifer.

**Question 189:**

The Smiths want to reupholster both sides of their seating cushions (dimensions shown on diagram). The fabric they are using costs £10/m, can only be bought in whole metre lengths and has a standard width of 1m. Each side of a cushion must be made from a single piece of fabric. The seamstress changes a flat rate of £25 per cushion. How much will it cost them to reupholster 4 cushions?

A. £20
B. £80
C. £110
D. £130
E. £150

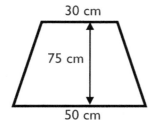

30 cm

75 cm

50 cm

Negligible Thickness

**Question 190:**

Lisa buys a cappuccino from either Milk or Beans Coffee shops each day. The quality of the coffee is the same but she wishes to work out the relative costs once the loyalty scheme has been taken into account. At Milk, a regular cappuccino is £2.40, and at Beans, £2.15. However, the loyalty scheme in Milk gives Lisa a free cappuccino for every 9 drinks she buys, whereas Beans use a points system of 10 points per full pound spent (each point is worth 1p) which can be used to cover the cost of a full cappuccino.

If Lisa buys a cappuccino each day of September, which coffee shop would work out cheaper, and by how much?

A. Milk, by £4.60
B. Beans by £6.30
C. Beans, by £4.60
D. Beans, by £2.45
E. Milk, by £2.45

**Question 191:**

Paula needs to be at a meeting in Notting Hill at 11 am. The route requires her to walk 5 minutes to the 283 bus, which takes 25 minutes, and then change to the 220 bus which takes 14 minutes. Finally, she walks for 3 minutes to her meeting. If the 283 bus comes every 10 minutes, and the 220 bus at 0 minutes, 20 minutes and 40 minutes past the hour, what is the latest time she can leave and still be at her meeting on time?

A. 09.45    B. 09.58    C. 10.01    D. 10.05    E. 10.10

**Question 192:**

Two trains, a high-speed train A and a slower local train B, travel from Manchester to London. Train A travels the first 20 km at 100 km/hr and then at an average speed of 150km/hr. Train B travels at a constant average speed of 90 km/hr. If train B leaves 20 minutes before train A, at what distance will train A pass train B?

A. 75 km    B. 90 km    C. 100 km    D. 120 km    E. 150 km

**Question 193:**

The university gym has an upfront cost of £35 with no contracted monthly fee, but classes are charged at £3 each. The local gym has no joining fee and is £15 per month including all classes. What is the minimum number of classes I need to attend in a 12 month period to make the local gym cheaper than the university gym?

A. 40    B. 48    C. 49    D. 50    E. 55    F. 60

**Question 194:**

"All medicines are drugs, but not all drugs are medicines", goes a well-known saying. If we accept this statement as true, and consider that all antibiotics are medicines, but no herbal drugs are medicines, then which of the following is definitely **FALSE**?

A. Some herbal drugs are not medicines.

B. All antibiotics are drugs.

C. Some herbal drugs are antibiotics.

D. Some medicines are antibiotics.

E. None of the above.

**Question 195:**

Sonia has been studying the routes taken by various trains travelling between London and Edinburgh on the East coast. Trains can stop at the following stations: Newark, Peterborough, Doncaster, York, Northallerton, Darlington, Durham and Newcastle. She notes the following:

- All trains stop at Peterborough, York, Darlington and Newcastle.
- All trains that stop at Northallerton also stop at Durham.
- Each day, 50% of the trains stop at both Newark *and* Northallerton.
- All designated "fast" trains make less than 5 stops. All other trains make 5 stops or more.
- On average, 16 trains run each day.

Which of the following can be reliably concluded from these observations?

A. All trains, which are not designated "fast" trains, must stop at Durham.

B. No more than 8 trains on any given day will stop at Northallerton.

C. No designated "fast" trains will stop at Durham.

D. It is possible for a train to make 5 stops, including Northallerton.

E. A train which stops at Newark will also stop at Durham.

**Question 196:**

Rakton is 5 miles directly north of Blueville. Gallford is 8 miles directly south of Haston. Lepstone is situated 5 miles directly east of Blueville, and 5 miles directly west of Gallford.

Which of the following **CANNOT** be reliably concluded from this information?

A. Lepstone is South of Rakton

B. Haston is North of Rakton

C. Gallford is East of Rakton

D. Blueville is East of Haston

E. Haston is North of Lepstone

**Question 197:**

The Eastminster Parliament is undergoing an election. There are 600 seats up for election, each of which will be elected separately by the people living in that constituency. Six parties win at least one seat in the election, the Blue Party, the Red Party, the Orange Party, the Yellow Party, the Green Party and the Purple Party. In order to form a government, a party (or coalition) must hold *over* 50% of the seats. After the election, a political analysis committee produces the following report:

- No party has gained more than 45% of the seats, so no party is able to form a government alone.
- The Red and the Blue party each gained over 40% of the seats.
- No other party gained more than 4% of the seats.
- The Yellow party did not win the fewest seats

The Red party work out that if they collaborate with the Green party and the Orange party, between the 3 of them, they will have enough seats to form a coalition government.

What is the minimum number of seats that the Green party could have?

A. 5          B. 6          C. 13          D. 14          E. 23          F. 24

**Questions 198-202 are based on the following information:**

A grandmother wants to give her five grandchildren £100 between them for Christmas this year. She wants to grade the money she gives to each grandchild exactly so that the older children receive more than the younger ones. She wants to share the money such that she will give the $2^{nd}$ youngest child as much more than the youngest, as the $3^{rd}$ youngest gets than the $2^{nd}$ youngest, as the $4^{th}$ youngest gets from the $3^{rd}$ youngest and so on. The result will be that the two youngest children together will get seven times less money than the three oldest.

$M$ is the amount of money the youngest child receives, and $D$ the difference between the amount the youngest and $2^{nd}$ youngest children receive.

**Question 198:**

What is the expression for the amount the oldest child receives?

A. M

B. M + D

C. 2M

D. $4M^2$

E. M + 4D

F. None of the above.

**Question 199:**

What is the correct expression for the total money received?

A. 5M = £100

B. 5D + 10M = £100

C. $D = \frac{M}{100}$

D. 5M + 10D = £100

E. $M = \frac{2D}{11}$

**Question 200:**

"The two youngest children together will get seven times less money than the three oldest."

Which one of the following best expresses the above statement?

A. 7(3M + 9D) = 2M + D

B. 7D = M

C. 7(2M + D) = 3M + 9D

D. 2(7M + D) = 3M + 9D

E. None of the above

**Question 201:**

Using the statement in the previous question, what is the correct expression for *M?*

A. $\frac{2D}{11}$       C. $\frac{10D}{11}$       E. None of the above

B. $\frac{2}{11}$       D. $\frac{120}{11}$

**Question 202:**

Express £100 in terms of D.

A. $£100 = \frac{120D}{11}$       C. $£100 = \frac{120}{11D}$       E. $£100 = 5M + 10D$

B. $£100 = \frac{120D}{10}$       D. $£100 = 21D$

**Question 203:**

Four young girls entered a local baking competition. Though a bit burnt, Ellen's carrot cake did not come last. The girl who baked a Madeira sponge had practised a lot, and so came first, while Jaya came third with her entry. Aleena did better than the girl who made the tiramisu, and the girl who made the Victoria sponge did better than Veronica.

Which **TWO** of the following were **NOT** results of the competition?

A. Veronica made a tiramisu       D. The Victoria sponge came in 3rd place

B. Ellen came second       E. The carrot cake came 3rd

C. Aleena made a Victoria sponge

**Question 204:**

In a young children's football league, the 5 teams were Celtic Changers, Eire Lions, Nordic Nesters, Sorten Swipers and the Whistling Winners. One of the boys playing in the league, after being asked by his parents, said that while he could remember the other teams' total points, he could not remember the score for his own team, the Eire Lions. He said that all the teams played each other and when teams lost, they were given 0 points, when they drew, 1 point, and 3 points for a win. He remembered that the Celtic Changers had a total of 2 points; the Sorten Swipers had 5; the Nordic Nesters had 8, and the Whistling Winners 1.

How many points did the boy's team score?

A. 1       C. 8       E. 11

B. 4       D. 10

**Question 205:**

T is the son of Z, Z and J are sisters, R is the mother of J and S is the son of R.

Which one of the following statements is correct?

A. T and J are cousins       D. S is the maternal uncle of T

B. S and J are sisters       E. R is the grandmother of Z.

C. J is the maternal uncle of T

**Question 206:**

John likes to shoot bottles off a wall. In the first round, he places 16 bottles on the wall and knocks off 8 bottles. 3 of the knocked off bottles are damaged and can no longer be used, whilst 1 bottle is lost. He puts the undamaged bottles back on the wall before continuing. In the second round he shoots six times and misses 50% of these shots. He damages two bottles with every shot that does not miss. 2 bottles also fall off the wall at the end. He puts up 2 new bottles before continuing. In the final round, John misses all his shots and in frustration, knocks over 50% of the remaining bottles.

How many bottles were left on the wall after the final round?

A. 2              C. 4              E. 6

B. 3              D. 5

**Questions 207 - 213 are based on the information below:**

All train lines are named after a station they serve, apart from the Oval and Rectangle lines, which are named for their recognisable shapes. Trains run in both directions.

- There are express trains that run from end to end of the St Mark's and Straightly lines taking 5 and 6 minutes respectively.
- It takes 2 minutes to change between St Mark's and both Oval and Rectangle lines, 1 minute between Rectangle and Oval.
- It takes 3 minutes to change between the Straightly and all other lines, except for the St Mark's line which only takes 30 seconds to change between.
- The Straightly line is a fast line and takes only 2 minutes between stops apart from to and from Keyton, which only takes 1 minute, and to and from Lime St which takes 3 minutes.
- The Oval line is much slower and takes 4 minutes between stops, apart from between Baxton and Marven, and also Archite and West Quays, where travelling between stops takes 5 minutes.
- The Rectangle line is a reliable line; it never runs late but as a consequence is much slower taking 6 minutes between stops.
- The St Mark's line is fast and takes 2 and half minutes between stations.
- If a passenger reaches the end of the line, it takes three minutes to change onto a train travelling back in the opposite direction.

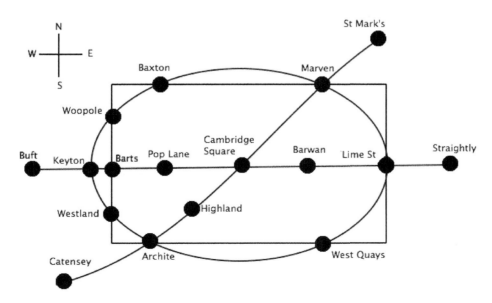

**Question 207:**
Assuming all lines are running on time, how long does it take to go from St Mark's to Archite on the St Mark's line?

A.  5 minutes
B.  6 minutes

C.  7.5 minutes
D.  10 minutes

E.  12.5 minutes

**Question 208:**
Assuming all lines are running on time, what's the shortest time it will take to go from Buft to Straightly?

A.  6 minutes
B.  10 minutes

C.  12 minutes
D.  14 minutes

E.  16 minutes

**Question 209:**
What is the shortest time it will take to go from Baxton to Pop Lane?

A.  11 minutes
B.  12 minutes

C.  13 minutes
D.  14 minutes

E.  15 minutes

**Question 210:**
Which station, even allowing for the quickest journey time, takes the longest to reach from Cambridge Square?

A.  Catensey

B.  Buft

C.  Woopole

D.  Westland

**Questions 211-213 use this additional information:**
On a difficult day there are signal problems whereby all lines except the reliable line are delayed, such that train travel times between stations are doubled. These delays have caused overcrowding at the platforms which means that while changeover times between lines are still the same, passengers always have to wait an extra 5 minutes on all of the platforms before catching the next train.

**Question 211:**
At best, how long will it now take to go from Westland to Marven?

A.  25 minutes
B.  29 minutes

C.  30 minutes
D.  33 minutes

E.  35 minutes

**Question 212:**

There is a bus that goes from Baxton to Archite and takes 27-31 minutes. Susan lives in Baxton and needs to get to her office in Archite as quickly as possible. With all the delays and lines out of service,

How should you advise Susan to enable her to get to work most quickly?
A.  Baxton to Archite via Barts using the Rectangle line.
B.  Baxton to Woopole on the Rectangle line, then Oval to Archite via Keyton.
C.  It is not possible to tell between the fastest two options.
D.  Baxton to Woopole on the Rectangle line, then Oval to Archite via Keyton.
E.  Baxton to Archite on the Oval line.
F.  Baxton to Archite using the bus.

**Question 213:**

In addition to the delays, the Oval line signals fail completely, so the line falls out of service. How long will the fastest journey now take to go from St Mark's to West Quays?

A.  35 minutes
B.  30 minutes
C.  33 minutes
D.  29 minutes
E.  30.5 minutes
F.  None of the above.

**Question 214:**

In an unusual horserace, only 4 horses competed. Each had different racing colours and numbers. Simon's horse wore number 1. Lila's horse was painted neither yellow nor blue, and the horse that wore number 3, which was wearing red, beat the horse that came in third place. Only one horse wore the same number as the position it finished in. Arthur's horse beat Simon's horse, whereas Celia's horse beat the horse that wore number 1. The horse wearing green, Celia's, came second, and the horse wearing blue wore number 4. Which one of the following must be true?

A.  Simon's horse was yellow and placed 3rd.
B.  Celia's horse was red.
C.  Celia's horse was in third place.
D.  Arthur's horse was blue.
A.  Lila's horse wore number 4.

**Question 215:**

Jessie plants a tree with a height of 40 cm.  The information leaflet states that the plant should grow by 20% each year for the first 2 years, and then 10% each year thereafter.

What is the expected height at 4 years?
A.  58.08 cm
B.  64.89 cm
C.  69.696 cm
D.  89.696 cm
E.  82.944 cm

**Question 216:**

A company is required to pay each employee 10% of their wages into a pension fund if their annual total wage bill is above £200,000. However, there is a legal loophole stating that if the company splits over two sites, the £200,000 limit applies to the total wages for each individual site. The company therefore decides to have an east site and a west site.

| Name | Annual Salary (£) |
|---|---|
| Luke | 47,000 |
| John | 78,400 |
| Emma | 68,250 |
| Nicola | 88,500 |
| Victoria | 52,500 |
| Daniel | 63,000 |

Which employees should be grouped at the same site to minimise the cost to the company?

A. John, Nicola, Luke          C. Nicola, Daniel, Luke          E. Luke, Victoria, Emma
B. Nicola, Victoria, Daniel    D. John, Daniel, Emma

**Question 217:**

A bus takes 24 minutes to travel from White City to Hammersmith with no stops. Each time the bus stops to pick up and/or drop off passengers, it takes approximately 90 seconds. This morning, the bus picked up passengers from 5 stops, and dropped off passengers at 7 stops.

What is the minimum journey time from White City to Hammersmith this morning?
A. 28 minutes          C. 34.5 minutes          E. 37.5 minutes
B. 34 minutes          D. 36 minutes            F. 42 minutes

**Question 218:**

Sally is making a Sunday roast for her family and is planning her schedule regarding cooking times. The chicken takes 15 minutes to prepare, 75 minutes to cook, and needs to stand for exactly 5 minutes after cooking. The potatoes take 18 minutes to prepare, 5 minutes to boil, then 50 minutes to roast. The potatoes must be roasted immediately after boiling, and then served immediately after roasting. The vegetables require only 5 minutes preparation time and 8 minutes boiling time before serving, and can be kept warm to be served at any time after cooking. Given that the cooker can only be cooking two items at any given time and Sally can prepare only one item at a time, what should Sally's schedule be if she wishes to serve dinner at 4pm and wants to start cooking each item as late as possible?

A. Chicken 2.25, potatoes 2.47, vegetables 2.42
B. Chicken 2.25, potatoes 2.47, vegetables 3.47
C. Chicken 2.35, potatoes 3.47, vegetables 2.47
D. Chicken 2.35, potatoes 2.47, vegetables 3.47
E. Chicken 2.45, potatoes 3.47, vegetables 2.47
F. Chicken 2.45, potatoes 2.47, vegetables 3.47

**Question 219:**

The Smiths have 4 children with a total age of 80. Paul is double the age of Jeremy. Annie is exactly halfway between the ages of Jeremy and Paul, and Rebecca is 2 years older than Paul. How old are each of the children?

A. Paul 23, Jeremy 12, Rebecca 26, Annie 19.

B. Paul 22, Jeremy, 11, Rebecca 24, Annie 16.

C. Paul 24, Jeremy 12, Rebecca 26, Annie 18.

D. Paul 28, Jeremy 14, Rebecca 30, Annie 21.

E. More information needed.

**Question 220:**

Sarah has a jar of spare buttons that are a mix of colours and sizes. The jar contains the following assortment of buttons:

|  | 10mm | 25mm | 40mm |
|---|---|---|---|
| **Cream** | 15 | 22 | 13 |
| **Red** | 6 | 15 | 7 |
| **Green** | 9 | 19 | 8 |
| **Blue** | 20 | 6 | 15 |
| **Yellow** | 4 | 8 | 26 |
| **Black** | 17 | 16 | 14 |
| **Total** | 71 | 86 | 83 |

Sarah wants to use a 25mm diameter button but doesn't mind if it is cream or yellow. What is the maximum number of buttons she will have to remove in order to guarantee picking a suitable button on the next attempt?

A. 210          C. 219          E. None of the above

B. 218          D. 239

**Question 221:**

Ben wants to optimise his score with one throw of a dart. 50% of the time he hits a segment to either side of the one he is aiming at. With this in mind, which of the following segments should he aim for?
[Ignore all double/triple modifiers]

A. 15

B. 16

C. 17

D. 18

E. 19

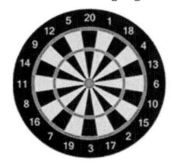

**Question 222:**

Victoria is completing her weekly shop and the total cost of the items is £8.65. She looks in her purse and sees that she has a £5 note and a large amount of change, including all types of coins. She uses the £5 note and pays the remainder using the maximum number of coins possible in order to remove some weight from the purse. However, the store has certain rules she must follow when paying:

- No more than 20p can be paid in "bronze" change (the name given to any combination of 1p pieces and 2p pieces)
- No more than 50p can be paid using any combination of 5p pieces and 10p pieces.
- No more than £1.50 can be paid using any combination of 20p pieces and 50p pieces.

Victoria pays the exact amount and does not receive any change. Under these rules, what is the *maximum* number of coins that Victoria can have paid with?

A. 30          B. 31          C. 36          D. 41          E. 46

**Question 223:**

I look at the clock on my bedside table, and I see the following digits:

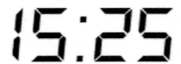

However, I also see that there is a glass of water between me and the clock, which is in front of 2 adjacent figures. I know that this means these 2 figures will appear reversed. For example, 10 would appear as 01, and 20 would appear as 05 (as 5 on a digital clock is a reversed image of a 2). Some numbers, such as 3, cannot appear reversed because there are no numbers which look like the reverse of 3.

Which of the following could be the actual time shown on the clock?

A. 15:52          B. 21:25          C. 12:55          D. 12:22          E. 21:52

**Question 224:**

Slavica has invaded Worsid, whilst Nordic has invaded Lorkdon. Worsid, spotting an opportunity to bolster its amount of land and natural resources, invades Nordic. Each of these countries is either a dictatorship or a democracy. Slavica is a dictatorship, but Lorkdon is a democracy. 10 years ago, a treaty was signed which guaranteed that no democracy would invade another democracy. No dictatorship has both invaded another dictatorship *and* been invaded by another dictatorship.

Assuming the aforementioned treaty has been upheld, what style of government is practised in Worsid?

A. Worsid is a dictatorship.
B. Worsid is a democracy.
C. Worsid does not practice either of these forms of government.
D. It is impossible to tell.

**Question 225:**

Sheila is on a shift at the local supermarket. Unfortunately, the till has developed a fault, meaning it cannot tell her how much change to give each customer. A customer is purchasing the following items, at the following costs:

* A packet of grated cheese priced at £3.25
* A whole cucumber, priced at 75p
* 750g of carrots, priced at 60p/kg
* 3 DVDs, each priced at £3.00

Sheila knows there is an offer on DVDs in the store at present, in which 3 DVDs bought together will be a third off. The customer pays with a £50 note.

How much change will Sheila need to give the customer?

A.  £36.00  B.  £36.40  C.  £36.55  D.  £39.40  E.  £39.55

**Question 226:**

Ryan is cooking breakfast for several guests at his hotel. He is frying most of the items using the same large frying pan, to get as much food prepared in as little time as possible. Ryan is cooking bacon, sausages, and eggs in this pan. He calculates how much room is taken up in the pan by each item. He calculates the following:

* Each rasher of bacon takes up 7% of the available space in the pan
* Each sausage takes up 3% of the available space in the pan.
* Each egg takes up 12% of the available space in the pan.

Ryan is cooking 2 rashers of bacon, 4 sausages and 1 egg for each guest. He decides to cook all the food for each guest at the same time, rather than cooking all of each item at once.

How many guests can he cook for at once?

A.  1  B.  2  C.  3  D.  4  E.  5

**Question 227:**

SafeEat Inc. is a national food development testing agency. The Manchester-based laboratory has a system for recording all of the laboratory employees' birthdays, and presenting them with cake on their birthday, in order to keep staff morale high. Certain amounts of petty cash are set aside each month in order to fund this. 40% of the staff have their birthday in March, and the secretary works out that £60 is required to fund the birthday cake scheme during this month.

If all birthdays cost £2 to provide a cake for, how many people work at the laboratory?

A.  45  B.  60  C.  75  D.  100  E.  150

**Question 228:**

Many diseases, such as cancer, require specialist treatment, and thus cannot be treated by a general practitioner. Instead, these diseases must be referred to a specialist after an initial, more generalised, medical assessment. Bob has had a biopsy on the 1st of August on a lump in his abdomen. The results show that it is a cancerous tumour, with a slight chance of spreading to other parts of the body, so he is referred to a waiting list for specialist radiotherapy and chemotherapy. The average waiting time in the UK for such treatment is 3 weeks, but in Bob's local district, high demand means that it takes 50% longer for each patient to receive treatment. As he is a lower risk case (due to a low risk of the disease spreading), his waiting time is extended by another 20%.

How many weeks will it be before Bob receives specialist treatment?

A. 4.5          B. 4.6          C. 5.0          D. 5.1          E. 5.4          F. 5.6

**Question 229:**

In a class of 30 seventeen-year-old students, 40% drink alcohol at least once a month. Of those who drink alcohol at least once a month, 75% drink alcohol at least once a week. 1 in 3 of the students who drink alcohol at least once a week also smoke marijuana. 1 in 3 of the students who drink alcohol less than once a month also smoke marijuana.

How many of the students in total smoke marijuana?

A. 3          B. 4          C. 6          D. 9          E. 10          F. 15

**Question 230:**

Complete the following sequence of numbers: 1, 4, 10, 22, 46, ...

A. 84          B. 92          C. 94          D. 96          E. 100

**Question 231:**

If the mean of 5 numbers is 7, the median is 8 and the mode is 3, what must the two largest numbers in the set of numbers add up to?

A. 14          C. 24          E. 35
B. 21          D. 26          F.   More information needed.

**Question 232:**

Ahmed buys 1kg bags of potatoes from the supermarket. By law, 1kg bags have to weigh between 900 and 1100 grams. In the first week, there are 10 potatoes in the bag. The next week, there are only 5. Assuming that the potatoes in the bag in week 1 are all the same weight as each other, and the potatoes in the bag in week 2 are all the same weight as each other, what is the maximum possible difference between the heaviest and lightest potato in the two bags?

A. 50g          B. 70g          C. 90g          D. 110g          E. 130g

**Question 233:**

A football tournament involves a group stage, then a knockout stage. In the group stage, groups of four teams play in a round robin format (i.e. each team plays every other team once) and the team that wins the most matches in each group proceeds through to a knockout stage. In addition, the single best performing second place team across all the groups gains a place in the knockout stage. In the knockout stage, sets of two teams play each other and the one that wins proceeds to the next round until there are two teams left, who play the final.

If we start with 60 teams, how many matches are played altogether?

A. 75       B. 90       C. 100       D. 105       E. 165

**Question 234:**

The last 4 digits of my card number are 2 times my Personal Identification Number (PIN), plus 200. The last 4 digits of my husband's card number are the last four digits of my card number doubled, plus 200. My husband's PIN is 2 times the last 4 digits of his card number, plus 200. Given that all these numbers are 4 digits long, whole numbers, and cannot begin with 0, what is the largest number my PIN can be?

A. 1,074       C. 2,348       E. 9,999

B. 1,174       D. 4,096

**Question 235:**

All women between the age 50 to 70 in the UK are invited for breast cancer screening every 3 years. Patients at Doddinghurst Surgery are invited for screening for the first time at any point between their 50th and 53rd birthday. If they ignore an invitation, they are sent reminders every 5 months. We can assume that a woman is screened exactly 1 month after she is sent the invitation or reminder that she accepts. The next invitation for screening is sent exactly 3 years after the previous screening.

If a woman accepts the screening on the second reminder each time, what is the youngest she can be when she has her 4th screening?

A. 60       B. 61       C. 62       D. 63       E. 64

**Question 236:**

Ellie gets a pay rise of $k$ thousand pounds on every anniversary of joining the company, where $k$ is the number of years she has been at the company. She currently earns £40,000, and she has been at the company for 5.5 years. What was her salary when she started at the company?

A. £25,000       C. £28,000       E. £31,000

B. £27,000       D. £30,000

**Question 237:**

Northern Line trains arrive at Kings Cross station every 8 minutes, Piccadilly Line trains every 5 minutes and Victoria Line trains every 2 minutes. If trains from all 3 lines arrived at the station exactly 15 minutes ago, how long will it be before they do so again?

A. 24 minutes       C. 40 minutes       E. 65 minutes

B. 25 minutes       D. 60 minutes

## Question 238:

If you do not smoke or drink alcohol, your risk of getting Disease X is 1 in 12. If you smoke, you are half as likely to get Disease X as someone who does not smoke. If you drink alcohol, you are twice as likely to get Disease X. A new drug is released that halves anyone's total risk of getting Disease X for each tablet taken. How many tablets of the drug would someone who drinks alcohol have to take to reduce their risk to the same level as someone who smoked but did not take the drug?

A. 0          B. 1          C. 2          D. 3          E. 4

## Questions 239 – 241 refer to the following information:

There are 20 balls in a bag. 1/2 are red. 1/10 of those balls that are not red are yellow. The rest are green except 1, which is blue.

## Question 239:

If I draw 2 balls from the bag (without replacement), what is the most likely combination to draw?
A.  Red and green                        C.  Red and red
B.  Red and yellow                       D.  Blue and yellow

## Question 240:

If I draw 2 balls from the bag (without replacement), what is the least likely (without being impossible) combination to draw?
A.  Blue and green                       C.  Yellow and yellow
B.  Blue and yellow                      D.  Yellow and green

## Question 241:

How many balls do you have to draw (without replacement) to guarantee getting at least one of at least three different colours?

A. 5          B. 12          C. 13          D. 17          E. 19

**Question 242:**

A general election in the UK resulted in a hung parliament, with no single party gaining more than 50% of the seats. Thus, the main political parties are engaged in discussion over the formation of a coalition government. The results of this election are shown below:

| Political Party | Seats won |
|---|---|
| Conservatives | 260 |
| Labour | 270 |
| Liberal Democrats | 50 |
| UKIP | 35 |
| Green Party | 20 |
| Scottish National Party | 17 |
| Plaid Cymru | 13 |
| Sinn Fein | 9 |
| Democratic Unionist Party (DUP) | 11 |
| Other | 14 (14 other parties won 1 seat each) |

There are a total of 699 seats, meaning that in order to form a government, any coalition must have at least 350 seats between them. Several of the party leaders have released statements about who they are and are not willing to form a coalition with, which are summarised as follows:

- The Conservative party and Labour party are not willing to take part in a coalition together.
- The Liberal Democrats refuse to take part in any coalition which also involves UKIP.
- The Labour party will only form a coalition with UKIP if the Green party are also part of this coalition.
- The Conservative party are not willing to take part in any coalition with UKIP unless the Liberal Democrats are also involved.

Considering this information, what is the minimum number of parties required to form a coalition government?

A. 2           B. 3           C. 4           D. 5           E. 6

**Question 243:**

On Tuesday, 360 patients attend appointments at Doddinghurst Surgery. Of the appointments that are booked in, only 90% are attended. Of the appointments that are booked in, 1 in 2 are for male patients, the remaining appointments are for female patients. Male patients are three times as likely to miss their booked appointment as female patients.

How many male patients attend appointments at Doddinghurst Surgery on Tuesday?

A. 30           B. 60           C. 130           D. 150           E. 170

**Question 244:**

Every A Level student at Greentown Sixth Form studies maths. Additionally, 60% study biology, 50% study economics and 50% study chemistry. The other subject on offer at Greentown Sixth Form is physics. Assuming every student studies 3 subjects and that there are 60 students altogether, how many students study physics?

A. 15          C. 30          E. 60
B. 24          D. 40

**Question 245:**

100,000 people are diagnosed with chlamydia each year in the UK. An average of 0.6 sexual partners are informed per diagnosis. Of these, 80% have tests for chlamydia themselves. Half of these tests come back positive.

Assuming that each of the people diagnosed has had an average of 3 sexual partners (none of them share sexual partners or have sex with each other) and that the likelihood of having chlamydia is the same for those partners who are tested and those who are not, how many of the sexual partners who were not tested (whether they were informed or not) have chlamydia?

A. 120,000          C. 136,000          E. 240,000
B. 126,000          D. 150,000

**Question 246:**

In how many different positions can you place an additional tile to make a straight line of 3 tiles?

A. 6
B. 7
C. 8
D. 9
E. 10
F. 11
G. 12

**Question 247:**

Harry is making orange squash for his daughter's birthday party. He wants to have a 200ml glass of squash for each of the 20 children attending and a 300ml glass of squash for him and each of 3 parents who are helping him out. He has 1,040ml of the concentrated squash.

What ratio of water: concentrated squash should he use in the dilution to ensure he has the right amount to go around?
A.  2:1          B.  3:1          C.  4:1          D.  5:1          E.  6:1

**Question 248:**

4 children, Alex, Beth, Cathy and Daniel are each sitting on one of the 4 swings in the park. The swings are in a straight line. One possible arrangement of the children is, left to right, Alex, Beth, Cathy, Daniel.

How many other possible arrangements are there?
A.  5          B.  12          C.  23          D.  24          E.  64

**Question 249:**

A delivery driver is looking to make deliveries in several towns. He is given the following map of the various towns in the area. The lines indicate roads between the towns, along with the lengths of these roads, where m is miles.

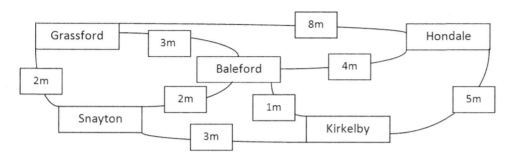

The delivery driver's vehicle has a black box which records the distance travelled and locations visited. At the end of the day, the black box recording shows that he has travelled a total of 14 miles. It also shows that he has visited one town twice, but has not visited any other town more than once. Which of the following is a possible route the driver could have taken?

A. Snayton → Baleford → Grassford → Snayton → Kirkelby
B. Baleford → Kirkelby → Hondale → Grassford → Baleford → Snayton
C. Kirkelby → Hondale → Baleford → Grassford → Snayton
D. Baleford → Hondale → Grassford → Baleford → Hondale → Kirkelby
E. None of the above.

**Question 250:**

Ellie, her brother Tom, her sister Georgia, her mum and her dad line up in height order from shortest to tallest for a family photograph. Ellie is shorter than her dad but taller than her mum. Georgia is shorter than both her parents. Tom is taller than both his parents.

If 1 is shortest and 5 is tallest, what position is Ellie in the line?
A. 1          B. 2          C. 3          D. 4          E. 5

**Question 251:**

Miss Briggs is trying to arrange the 5 students in her class into a seating plan. Ashley must sit on the front row because she has poor eyesight. Danielle disrupts anyone she sits next to apart from Caitlin, so she must sit next to Caitlin and no-one else. Bella needs to have a teaching assistant sat next to her. The teaching assistant must be sat on the left-hand side of the row. Emily does not get on with Bella, so they need to be sat apart from one another. The teacher has 2 tables which each sit 3 people, which are arranged 1 behind the other.

Who is sitting in the front right seat?
A. Ashley          C. Caitlin          E. Emily
B. Bella          D. Danielle

**Question 252:**

My aunt runs the dishwasher twice a week as standard. She also runs the dishwasher an additional time for each person who is living in the house that week. When her son is away at university, she buys a new pack of dishwasher tablets every 6 weeks, but when her son is home, she must buy a new one every 5 weeks. How many people are living in the house when her son is home?

A. 2          B. 3          C. 4          D. 5          E. 6

**Question 253:**

Dates can be written in an 8-digit form, for example 26-12-2014. How many days after 26-12-2014 would be the next time that the 8 digits were made up of exactly 4 different integers?

A. 6          B. 8          C. 10          D. 16          E. 24

**Question 254:**

Redtown is 4 miles east of Greentown. Bluetown is 5 miles north of Greentown. If every town is due North, South, East or West of at least two other towns, and the only other town is Yellowtown, how many miles away from Yellowtown is Redtown, and in what direction?

A.  4 miles east of Yellowtown.          D.  4 miles west of Yellowtown.
B.  5 miles south of Yellowtown.          E.  5 miles west of Yellowtown.
C.  5 miles north of Yellowtown.

**Question 255:**

Jenna pours wine from two 750ml bottles into glasses. The glasses hold 250ml, but she only fills them to 4/5 of capacity, except the last glass, into which she pours whatever liquid she has left. How full is the last glass compared to its capacity?

A. 1/5          B. 2/5          C. 3/5          D. 4/5          E. 5/5

**Question 256:**

There are 30 children in Miss Smith's class. Two thirds of the girls in Miss Smith's class have brown eyes, and two thirds of the class as a whole have brown hair. Given that the class is half boys and half girls, what is the difference between the minimum and maximum number of girls that could have brown eyes and brown hair?

A. 0          C. 5          E. 10
B. 2          D. 7

**Question 257:**

A biased die with the numbers 1 to 6 on it is rolled twice. The resulting numbers are multiplied together, and then their sum subtracted from this result to get the 'score' of the dice roll. If the probability of getting a negative (non-zero) score is 0.75, what is the probability of rolling a 1 on a third throw of the die?

A. 0.1          C. 0.3          E. 0.5
B. 0.2          D. 0.4

**Questions 258 - 260 are based on the following information:**

Fares on the number 11 bus are charged at a number of pence per stop that you travel, plus a flat rate. Emma, who is 21, travels 15 stops and pays £1.70. Charlie, who is 43, travels 8 stops and pays £1.14. Children (under 16) pay half the adult flat rate plus a quarter of the adult charge "per stop".

**Question 258:**

How much does 17-year-old Megan pay to travel 30 stops to college?

A. £0.85        C. £2.90        E. More information needed.
B. £2.40        D. £3.40

**Question 259:**

How much does 14-year-old Alice pay to travel 25 stops to school?

A. £0.50        C. £1.25        E. More information needed.
B. £0.75        D. £2.50

**Question 260:**

James, who is 24, wants to get the bus into town. The town stop is the 25th stop along a straight road from his house, but he only has £2.

Assuming he has to walk past the stop nearest his house, how many stops will he need to walk past before he gets to the stop he can afford to catch the bus from?

A. 4        B. 6        C. 7        D. 8        E. 9

**Questions 261 -263 are based on the following information:**

Emma mounts and frames paintings. Each painting needs a mount which is 2 inches bigger in each dimension than the painting, and a wooden frame which is 1 inch bigger in each dimension than the mount. Mounts are priced by multiplying 50p by the largest dimension of the mount, so a mount which is 8 inches in one direction and 6 in the other would be £4. Frames are priced by multiplying £2 by the smallest dimension of the frame, so a frame which is 8 inches in one direction and 6 in the other would be £12.

**Question 261:**

How much would mounting and framing a painting that is 10 x 14 inches cost?

A. £8        B. £26        C. £27        D. £34        E. £42

**Question 262:**

How much more would mounting and framing a 10 x 10 inch painting cost than mounting and framing an 8 x 8 inch painting?

A. £ 3.00        B. £ 4.00        C. £ 5.00        D. £ 6.00        E. £ 7.00

**Question 263:**

What is the largest square painting that can be framed for £40?

A.  12 inches
B.  13 inches

C.  14 inches
D.  15 inches

E.  16 inches

**Question 264:**

The word 'CREATURES' is coded as 'FTEAWUTEV', which would be coded for a second time as 'HWEAYUWEX'. What would be the second coding of the word 'MAGICAL'?

A.  QCKIGAN
B.  OCIIEAN

C.  PAJIFAN
D.  RALIHAQ

E.  RCIMGEP

**Question 265:**

Jane's mum has asked Jane to go to the shops to get some items that they need. She tells Jane that she will pay her per kilometre that she cycles on her bike to get to the shop, plus a flat rate payment for each shop she goes to. Jane receives £6 to go to the grocers, a distance of 5 km, and £4.20 to go the supermarket, a distance of 3km.

How much would she earn if she then cycles to the library to change some books, a distance of 7 km?

A.  £7.50
B.  £7.70
C.  £7.80
D.  £8.00
E.  £8.10

**Question 266:**

In 2001-2002, 1,019 patients were admitted to hospital due to obesity. This figure was more than 11 times higher by 2011-12 when there were 11,736 patients admitted to hospital with the primary reason for admission being obesity.

If the rate of admissions due to obesity continues to increase at the same linear rate as it has from 2001/2 to 2011/12, how many admissions would you expect in 2031/32?

A.  22,453
B.  23,437

C.  33,170
D.  134,964

E.  269,928

**Question 267:**

A shop puts its dresses on sale at 20% off the normal selling price. During the sale, the shop makes a 25% profit over the price at which they bought the dresses. What is the percentage profit when the dresses are sold at full price?

A.  36%
B.  42.5%

C.  56.25%
D.  64%

E.  77%

**Question 268:**

The 'Keys MedSoc committee' is made up of 20 students from each of the 6 year groups of medical students at the university. However, the president and vice-president are sabbatical roles which require students to take a year out from studying. There must be at least two general committee students from each year group as well as the specialist roles. Also, the social and welfare officers must be pre-clinical students (years 1-3) but not first years, and the treasurer must be a clinical student (years 4-6).

Which **TWO** of the following statements must be true?

1. There can be a maximum of 13 preclinical (years 1-3) students on the committee.
2. There must be a minimum of 6 $2^{nd}$ and $3^{rd}$ years.
3. There is an unequal distribution of committee members over the different year groups.
4. There can be a maximum of 10 clinical (years 4-6) students on the committee.
5. There can be a maximum of 2 first year students on the committee.
6. General committee members are equally spread across the 6 years.

A. 1 and 4          C. 2 and 4          E. 4 and 5
B. 2 and 3          D. 3 and 6

**Question 269:**

Friday the 13th is superstitiously considered an 'unlucky' day. If 13th January 2012 was a Friday, when would the next Friday the 13th be?

A. March 2012          C. July 2012          E. January has the only Friday
B. April 2012          D. August 2012                13th in 2012.

**Question 270:**

A farmer has 18 sheep, 8 of which are male. Unfortunately, 9 sheep die, of which 5 were female. The farmer decides to breed his remaining sheep in order to increase the size of his herd. Assuming every female gives birth to two lambs, how many sheep does the farmer have after all the females have given birth once?

A. 10          B. 14          C. 15          D. 16          E. 19

**Question 271:**

Piyanga writes a coded message for Nishita. Each letter of the original message is coded as a letter a specific number of characters further on in the alphabet (the specific number is the same for all letters). Piyanga's coded message includes the word "PJVN". What could the original word say?

A. CAME          B. DAME          C. FAME          D. GAME          E. LAME

**Question 272:**

A number of people get on the bus at the station, which is considered the first stop. At each subsequent stop, 1/2 of the people on the bus get off and then 2 people get on. Between the 4th and 5th stop after the station, there are 5 people on the bus.

How many people got on at the station?

A.  4                    B.  6                    C.  20                    D.  24                    E.  30

**Question 273:**

I recently moved into a new house, and I am looking to paint my new living room. The price of several different colours of paint is displayed in the table below. A small can contains enough to paint 10 m² of wall. A large can contains enough to paint 25 m² of wall.

| Colour | Cost for a Small Can | Cost for a Large Can |
|--------|----------------------|----------------------|
| Red | £4 | £12 |
| Blue | £8 | £15 |
| Black | £3 | £9 |
| White | £2 | £13 |
| Green | £7 | £15 |
| Orange | £5 | £20 |
| Yellow | £10 | £12 |

I decide to paint my room a mixture of blue and white, and I purchase some small cans of blue paint and white paint. The cost of blue paint accounts for 50% of the total cost. I paint a total of 100 m² of wall space.
I use up all the paint. How many m² of wall space have I painted blue?

A.  10 m²                B.  20 m²                C.  40 m²                D.  50 m²                E.  80 m²

**Question 274:**

Cakes usually cost 42p at the bakers. The bakers want to introduce a new offer where the amount in pence you pay for each cake is discounted by the square of the number of cakes you buy. For example, buying 3 cakes would mean each cake costs 33p. Isobel says that this is not a good offer from the baker's perspective as it would be cheaper to buy several cakes than just 1. How many cakes would you have to buy for the total cost to fall below 40p?

A.  2                    B.  3                    C.  4                    D.  5                    E.  6

**Question 275:**

The table below shows the percentages of students in two different universities who take various courses. There are 800 students in University A and 1200 students in University B. Biology, chemistry and physics are counted as "sciences".

|  | University A | University B |
|---|---|---|
| **Biology** | 23.50 | 13.25 |
| **Economics** | 10.25 | 14.5 |
| **Physics** | 6.25 | 14.75 |
| **Mathematics** | 11.50 | 17.25 |
| **Chemistry** | 30.25 | 7.00 |
| **Psychology** | 18.25 | 33.25 |

Assuming each student only takes one course, how many more students in University A than University B study a "science"?

A. 10          B. 25          C. 60          D. 250          E. 600

**Question 276:**

Traveleasy Coaches charge passengers at a rate of 50p per mile travelled, plus an additional charge of £5.00 for each international border crossed during the journey. Europremier Coaches charge £15 for every journey, plus 10p per mile travelled, with no charge for crossing international borders. Sonia is travelling from France to Germany, crossing 1 international border. She finds that both companies will charge the same price for this journey.

How many miles is Sonia travelling?
A. 10          B. 20          C. 25          D. 35          E. 40

**Question 277:**

Lauren, Amy and Chloe live in different cities across England. They decide to meet up together in London and have a meal together. Lauren departs from Southampton at 2:30pm and arrives in London at 4pm. Amy's journey lasts twice as long as Lauren's journey and she arrives in London at 4:15pm. Chloe departs from Sheffield at 1:30pm, and her journey lasts an hour longer than Lauren's journey.

Which of the following statements is definitely true?
A. Chloe's journey took the longest time.
B. Amy departed after Lauren.
C. Chloe arrived last.
D. Everybody travelled by train.
E. Amy departed before Chloe.

**Question 278:**

Emma is packing to go on holiday by aeroplane. On the aeroplane, she can take a case with dimensions of 50cm by 50cm by 20cm, which, when fully packed, can weigh up to 20kg. The empty suitcase weighs 2kg. In her suitcase, she needs to take 3 books, each of which is 0.2m by 0.1m by 0.05m in size, and weighs 1000g. She would also like to take as many items of clothing as possible. Each item of clothing has volume 1500cm³ and weighs 400 g.

Assuming each item of clothing can be squashed so as to fill any shape gap, how many items of clothing can she take in her case?

A.  28            B.  31            C.  34            D.  37            E.  40

**Question 279:**

Alex is buying a new bed and mattress. There are 5 bed shops Alex can buy the bed and mattress he wants from, each of which sells the bed and mattress for a different price as follows:

- **Bed Shop A:** Bed £120, mattress £70
- **Bed Shop B:** All beds and mattresses £90 each
- **Bed Shop C:** Bed £140, mattress £60. Mattress half price when you buy a bed and mattress together.
- **Bed Shop D:** Bed £140, mattress £100. Get 33% off when you buy a bed and mattress together.
- **Bed Shop E:** Bed £175. All beds come with a free mattress.

Which is the cheapest place for Alex to buy the bed and mattress from?

A.  Bed Shop A            C.  Bed Shop C            E.  Bed Shop E
B.  Bed Shop B            D.  Bed Shop D

**Question 280:**

In Joseph's sock drawer, there are 21 socks. 4 are blue, 5 are red, 6 are green and the rest are black. How many socks does he need to take from the drawer in order to guarantee he has a matching pair?

A.  3            B.  4            C.  5            D.  6            E.  7

**Question 281:**

Printing a magazine uses 1 sheet of card and 25 sheets of paper. It also uses ink. Paper comes in packs of 500 sheets and card comes in packs of 60 sheets. A pack of card is twice the price of a pack of paper. Each ink cartridge prints 130 sheets of either paper or card. A pack of paper costs £3. Ink cartridges cost £5 each.

How many complete magazines can be printed with a budget of £300?

A.  210            B.  220            C.  230            D.  240            E.  250

**Question 282:**

Rebecca went swimming yesterday. After a while she had covered one fifth of her intended distance. After swimming six more lengths of the pool, she had covered one quarter of her intended distance. How many lengths of the pool did she intend to complete?

A.  40            B.  72            C.  80            D.  100            E.  120

**Question 283:**

As a special treat, Sammy is allowed to eat five sweets from his very large jar. The jar contains 3 flavours of sweets – lemon, orange and strawberry. He wants to eat his five sweets in such a way that no two consecutive sweets have the same flavour.

In how many ways can he do this?
A. 32          B. 48          C. 72          D. 108          E. 162

**Question 284:**

Granny and her granddaughter Gill both had their birthday yesterday. Today, Granny's age in years is an even number and 15 times that of Gill. In 4 years' time Granny's age in years will be the square of Gill's age in years.

How many years older than Gill is Granny today?
A. 42          B. 49          C. 56          D. 60          E. 64

**Question 285:**

Pierre said, "Just one of us is telling the truth". Qadr said, "What Pierre says is not true". Ratna said, "What Qadr says is not true". Sven said, "What Ratna says is not true". Tanya said, "What Sven says is not true".

How many of them were telling the truth?
A. 0          B. 1          C. 2          D. 3          E. 4

**Question 286:**

Two entrants in a school's sponsored run adopt different tactics. Angus walks for half the time and runs for the other half, whilst Bruce walks for half the distance and runs for the other half. Both competitors walk at 3 mph and run at 6 mph. Angus takes 40 minutes to complete the course.

How many minutes does Bruce take?
A. 30          B. 35          C. 40          D. 45          E. 50

**Question 287:**

Dr Song discovers two new alien life forms on Mars. Species 8472 have one head and two legs. Species 24601 have four legs and one head. Dr Song counts a total of 73 heads and 290 legs in the area. How many members of Species 8472 are present?

A. 0          C. 72          E. 145
B. 1          D. 73

**Question 288:**

A restaurant menu states that:

*"All chicken dishes are creamy, and all vegetable dishes are spicy.  No creamy dishes contain vegetables."*

Which of the following **must** be true?

A.  Some chicken dishes are spicy.
B.  All spicy dishes contain vegetables.
C.  Some creamy dishes are spicy.
D.  Some vegetable dishes contain tomatoes.
E.  None of the above

**Question 289:**

Simon and his sister Lucy both cycle home from school.  One day, Simon is kept back in detention, so Lucy sets off for home first.  Lucy cycles the 8 miles home at 10 mph.  Simon leaves school 20 minutes later than Lucy. How fast must he cycle in order to arrive home at the same time as Lucy?

A.  10 mph          B.  14 mph          C.  17 mph          D.  21 mph          E.  24 mph

**Question 290:**

Dr. Whu buys 2000 shares in a company at a rate of 50p per share.  He then sells the shares for 58p per share. Subsequently he buys 1000 shares at 55p per share then sells them for 61p per share.  There is a charge of £20 for each transaction of either buying or selling shares.  What is Dr. Whu's total profit?

A.  £140          B.  £160          C.  £180          D.  £200          E.  £220

**Question 291:**

Jina is playing darts.  A dartboard is composed of equal segments, numbered from 1 to 20.  She takes three throws, and each of the darts lands in a numbered segment.  None land in the centre or in double or triple sections.  What is the probability that her total score with the three darts is odd?

A.  $1/4$          B.  $1/3$          C.  $1/2$          D.  $3/5$          E.  $2/3$

**Question 292:**

John Morgan invests £5,000 in a savings bond paying 5% interest per annum.  What is the value of the investment in 3 years' time?

A.  £5,250          C.  £5,750          E.  £5,788
B.  £6,125          D.  £6,442

**Question 293:**

Joe is 12 years younger than Michael.  In 5 years, the sum of their ages will be 62.  How old was Michael two years ago?

A.  20          B.  24          C.  26          D.  30          E.  32

**Question 294:**

A book has 500 pages. Vicky tears every page out that is a multiple of 4. She then tears out a fifth of the remaining pages. If the book measures 15 cm x 30cm and is made from paper of weight 110 gm$^{-2}$, how much lighter is the book now than at the start?

A. 990 g          B. 1,010 g          C. 1,250 g          D. 1,485 g          E. 1,590 g

**Question 295:**

A farmer is fertilising his crops. The more fertiliser is used, the more the crops grow. Fertiliser costs 80p per kilo. Fertilising at a rate of 0.2 kgm$^{-2}$ increases the crop yield by £1.30 m$^{-2}$. For each additional 100g of fertiliser above 200g, the extra yield is 30% lower than the linear projection of the stated rate. At what rate of fertiliser application is it no longer cost effective to increase the dose?

A. 0.5 kgm$^{-2}$          B. 0.6 kgm$^{-2}$          C. 0.7 kgm$^{-2}$          D. 0.8 kgm$^{-2}$          E. 0.9 kgm$^{-2}$

**Question 296:**

Pet-Star, Furry Friends and Creature Cuddles are three pet shops, which each sell food for various types of pets.

| Type of pet food | Amount of food required per week | Price per Kg in: | | |
|---|---|---|---|---|
| | | Pet-star | Furry Friends | Creature Cuddles |
| Guinea Pig | 3 Kg | £2 | £1 | £1.50 |
| Cat | 6 Kg | £4 | £6 | £5 |
| Rabbit | 4 Kg | £3 | £1 | £2.50 |
| Dog | 8 Kg | £5 | £8 | £6 |
| Chinchilla | 2 Kg | £1.50 | £0.50 | £1 |

Given the information above, which of the following statements can we state is definitely *not* true?
A. Regardless of which of these shops you use, the most expensive animal to provide food for will be a dog.
B. If I own a mixture of cats and rabbits, it will be cheaper for me to shop at Pet-star.
C. If I own 3 cats and a dog, the cheapest place for me to shop is at Pet-star
D. Furry Friends sells the cheapest food for the type of pet requiring the most food
E. If I only have one pet, Creature Cuddles will not be the cheapest place to shop regardless of which type of pet I have.

**Question 297:**

I record my bank balance at the start of each month for six months to help me see how much I am spending each month. My salary is paid on the 10$^{th}$ of each month. At the start of the year, I earn £1000 a month but from March inclusive I receive a pay rise of 10%.

| Date | Bank balance |
|---|---|
| January 1st | 1,200 |
| February 1st | 1,029 |
| March 1st | 1,189 |
| April 1st | 1,050 |
| May 1st | 925 |
| June 1st | 1,025 |

In which month did I spend the most money?

A. January        B. February        C. March        D. April        E. May

**Question 298:**

Amy needs to travel from Southtown station to Northtown station, which are 100 miles apart. She can travel by 3 different methods: train, aeroplane or taxi. The tables below show the different times for these 3 methods. The taxi takes 1 minute to cover a distance of 1 mile. Aeroplane passengers must be at the airport 30 minutes before their flight. Southtown airport is 10 minutes travelling time from Southtown station and Northtown airport is 30 minutes travelling time from Northtown station.

If Amy wants to arrive by 1700 and wants to set off as late as possible, what method of travel should she choose and what time will she leave Southtown station?

| | | 1400 | 1500 | 1600 |
|---|---|---|---|---|
| **Train** | Departs Southtown station | 1400 | 1500 | 1600 |
| | Arrives Northtown station | 1615 | 1650 | 1715 |
| **Flights** | Departs Southtown airport | 1610 | | |
| | Arrives Northtown airport | 1645 | | |

A. Flight, 1530          C. Taxi, 1520          E. Flight, 1610
B. Train, 1600           D. Train, 1500

**Question 299:**

In the multiplication grid below, a, b, c and d are all integers. What does d equal?

A. 18        B. 24        C. 30        D. 40        E. 45

| | c | d |
|---|---|---|
| a | 168 | 720 |
| b | 119 | 510 |

**Question 300:**

A sixth form college has 1,500 students. 48% are girls. 80 of the girls are mixed race.

If an equal proportion of boys and girls are mixed race, how many mixed-race boys are there in the college to the nearest 10?

A. 50                B. 60                C. 70                D. 80                E. 90

# SECTION 2

Section 2 is undoubtedly the most time-pressured section of the BMAT. This section tests concepts from GCSE level biology, chemistry, physics and maths. You have 27 questions to answer in 30 minutes. The questions can be quite difficult and it's easy to trip up when scientific concepts are presented in unfamiliar ways. However, Section 2 is also the section in which you can improve the most quickly in so it's well worth spending time practicing for it.

Although the vast majority of questions in section 2 aren't particularly difficult, the intense time pressure of having to do one question every minute makes this section the hardest for many students sitting the BMAT. As with section 1, the trick is to identify and complete the easier questions first whilst leaving the harder ones for the end.

In general, the biology and chemistry questions in the BMAT require the least amount of time per question whilst the maths and physics are more time consuming as they usually consist of multi-step calculations.

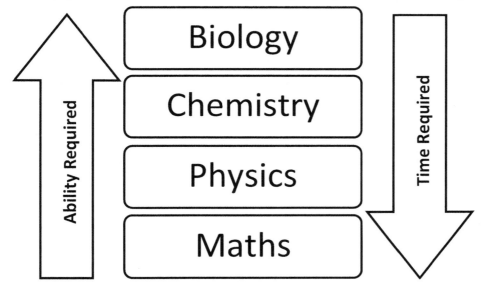

### Gaps in Knowledge

The BMAT only tests GCSE level content. However, there is a large variation in content between the GCSE exam boards meaning that you may not have covered some topics that are examinable. This is more likely if you didn't carry on with biology or physics to AS level (e.g. Newtonian mechanics and parallel circuits in physics; hormones and stem cells in biology). If you fall into this category, you are highly advised to go through the BMAT specification and ensure that you have covered all examinable topics. An electronic copy of this can be obtained from the official BMAT website at www.admissionstestingservice.org/bmat.

It is worth noting that although the content (i.e. concepts and scientific facts) tested in the BMAT is set at GCSE level, very often the questions will required *application* of this content to an unfamiliar scenario. This is designed to test your understanding as well as recall of the material, so it's paramount that you brush up on any weak areas.

The questions in this book will help highlight any particular areas of weakness or gaps in your knowledge that you may have. Upon discovering these, make sure you take some time to revise these topics before carrying on – there is little to be gained by attempting section 2 questions with huge gaps in your knowledge.

### Maths

Being confident with maths is extremely important for section 2. You won't have access to a calculator, so need to be confident manipulating numbers in your head or using pen and paper. Many students find that improving their numerical and algebraic skills usually results in big improvements in their section 1 and 2 scores. Remember that maths concepts tested in section 2 will also span physics (manipulating equations and standard form) and chemistry (mass calculations). So, if you find yourself consistently running out of time in section 2, spending a few hours on brushing up your basic maths skills (such as long division, converting between percentages and decimals…) may do wonders for you.

# SECTION 2: BIOLOGY

Thankfully, the biology questions tend to be fairly straightforward and require the least amount of time compared to other questions in Section 2. You should be able to do the majority of these well within 60 seconds. This means that you should be aiming to make up time by quickly completing biology questions, leaving more time for calculations etc. Unlike the other topics in section 2, the majority of biology questions will simply test your recall, so the trick really is to ensure that there are no obvious gaps in your knowledge.

Before going onto to do the practice questions in this book, ensure you are comfortable with the following commonly tested topics:

- Structure of animal, plant and bacterial cells
- Osmosis, diffusion and active transport
- Cell Division (mitosis + meiosis)
- Family pedigrees and Inheritance
- DNA structure and replication
- Gene technology & stem Cells
- Enzymes – function, mechanism and examples of digestive enzymes
- Aerobic and anaerobic respiration
- The central vs. peripheral nervous system
- The respiratory cycle including movement of ribs and diaphragm
- The cardiac cycle
- Hormones
- Basic immunology
- Food chains and food webs
- The carbon and nitrogen cycles

> ***Top tip!*** If you find yourself getting less than 50% of biology questions correct in this book, make sure you revisit the syllabus before attempting more questions as this is the best way to maximise your efficiency. In general, there is no reason why you shouldn't be able to get the vast majority of biology questions correct (and in well under 60 seconds) with sufficient practice.

# BIOLOGY QUESTIONS

**Question 301:**
In relation to the human genome, which of the following statements are correct?

1.  The genome is encoded by 4 different bases in DNA.
2.  The sugar backbone of the DNA strand is formed of glucose.
3.  DNA is found in the nucleus of bacteria.

A.  1 only
B.  2 only
C.  3 only
D.  1 and 2
E.  1 and 3

**Question 302:**
Animal cells contain organelles that take part in vital metabolic processes. Which of the following is true?

1.  The majority of energy production by animal cells occurs in the mitochondria.
2.  The cell wall protects the animal cell membrane from outside pressure differences.
3.  Chloroplasts are not present in animal cells.

A.  1 only
B.  2 only
C.  3 only
D.  1 and 3
E.  2 and 3

**Question 303:**
With regards to animal mitochondria, which of the following is correct?

A.  Mitochondria are not necessary for aerobic respiration.
B.  Mitochondria are enveloped by a double membrane.
C.  Mitochondria are more abundant in skeletal muscle than fat cells.
D.  The majority of DNA replication happens inside mitochondria.
E.  The majority of protein synthesis occurs in mitochondria.

**Question 304:**
In relation to bacteria, which of the following is **FALSE**?

A.  Bacteria always lead to disease.
B.  Bacteria contain plasmid DNA.
C.  Bacteria do not contain mitochondria.
D.  Bacteria have a cell wall and a plasma membrane.
E.  Some bacteria are susceptible to antibiotics.

**Question 305:**

In relation to bacterial replication, which of the following is correct?

A. Bacteria undergo sexual reproduction.
B. Bacteria have a nucleus.
C. Bacteria carry genetic information on circular plasmids.
D. Bacterial genomes are formed of RNA instead of DNA.
E. Bacteria require gametes to replicate.

**Question 306**

Which of the following statements are correct regarding active transport?

A. ATP is necessary and sufficient for active transport.
B. ATP is not necessary but is sufficient for active transport.
C. The relative concentrations of the material being transported have little impact on the rate of active transport.
D. Transport proteins are necessary and sufficient for active transport.
E. Active transport relies on transport proteins that are powered by an electrochemical gradient.

**Question 307:**

Concerning mammalian reproduction, which of the following is **FALSE**?

A. Fertilisation involves the fusion of two gametes.
B. Reproduction is sexual and the offspring display genetic variation.
C. Reproduction relies upon the exchange of genetic material.
D. Mammalian gametes are diploid cells produced via meiosis.
E. Embryonic growth requires carefully controlled mitosis.

**Question 308:**

Which of the following apply to Mendelian inheritance?

1. It only applies to plants.
2. It treats different traits as either dominant or recessive.
3. Heterozygotes have a 25% chance of expressing a recessive trait.

A. 1 only
B. 2 only
C. 3 only
D. 1 and 2
E. 1 and 3

**Question 309:**
Which of the following statements are correct?

A. Hormones are secreted into the blood stream and act over long distances at specific target organs.
B. Hormones are substances that almost always cause muscles to contract.
C. Hormones have no impact on the nervous or enteric systems.
D. Hormones are always derived from food and never synthesised.
E. Hormones act rapidly to restore homeostasis.

**Question 310:**
With regard to neuronal signalling in the body, which of the following are true?

1. Neuronal transmission can be caused by both electrical and chemical stimulation.
2. Synapses ultimately result in the production of an electrical current for signal transduction.
3. All synapses in humans are electrical and unidirectional.

A. 1 only      C. 3 only      E. 1 and 3
B. 2 only      D. 1 and 2

**Question 311:**
What is the **primary** reason that pH is controlled so tightly in the human body?

A. To allow rapid protein synthesis.
B. To allow for effective digestion throughout the GI tract.
C. To ensure ions can function properly in neural signalling.
D. To ensure enzymes are able to function properly.
E. To prevent changes in core body temperature.

**Question 312:**
Which of the following statements are correct regarding the bacterial cell wall?

1. It confers bacteria protection against external environmental stimuli.
2. It is an evolutionary remnant and now has little functional significance in most bacteria.
3. It is made up primarily of glucose in bacteria.

A. Only 1      C. Only 3      E. 2 and 3
B. Only 2      D. 1 and 2

**Question 313:**

Which of the following statements are correct regarding mitosis?

1. It is important in sexual reproduction.
2. A single round of mitosis results in the formation of 2 genetically distinct daughter cells.
3. Mitosis is vital for tissue growth, as it is the basis for cell multiplication.

A. Only 1          C. Only 3          E. 2 and 3
B. Only 2          D. 1 and 2

**Question 314:**

Which of the following is the best definition of a mutation?

A. A mutation is a permanent change in DNA.
B. A mutation is a permanent change in DNA that is harmful to an organism.
C. A mutation is a permanent change in the structure of intra-cellular organelles caused by changes in DNA/RNA.
D. A mutation is a permanent change in chromosomal structure caused by DNA/RNA changes.

**Question 315:**

In relation to mutations, which of the following statements are correct?

1. Mutations always lead to discernible changes in the phenotype of an organism.
2. Mutations are central to natural processes such as evolution.
3. Mutations play a role in cancer.

A. Only 1          C. Only 3          E. 2 and 3
B. Only 2          D. 1 and 2

**Question 316:**

Which of the following is the most accurate definition of an antibody?

A. An antibody is a molecule that protects red blood cells from changes in pH.
B. An antibody is a molecule produced only by humans and has a pivotal role in the immune system.
C. An antibody is a toxin produced by a pathogen to damage the host organism.
D. An antibody is a molecule that is used by the immune system to identify and neutralize foreign objects and molecules.
E. Antibodies are small proteins found in red blood cells that help increase oxygen carriage.

**Question 317:**

Which of the following statements about the kidney are correct?

1. The kidneys filter the blood and remove waste products from the body.
2. The kidneys are involved in the digestion of food.
3. In a healthy individual, the kidneys produce urine that contains high levels of glucose.

A. Only 1
B. Only 2
C. Only 3
D. 1 and 2
E. 2 and 3

**Question 318:**

Which of the following statements are correct?

1. Hormones are slower acting than nerves.
2. Hormones act for a very short time.
3. Hormones act more generally than nerves.
4. Hormones are released when you are frightened.

A. 1 only
B. 1 and 3 only
C. 2 and 4 only
D. 1, 3 and 4 only
E. 1, 2, 3 and 4

**Question 319:**

Which statements about homeostasis are correct?

1. Homeostasis is about ensuring the inputs within your body exceed the outputs to maintain a constant internal environment.
2. Homeostasis is about ensuring the inputs within your body are less than the outputs to maintain a constant internal environment.
3. Homeostasis is about balancing the inputs within your body with the outputs to ensure your body fluctuates with the needs of the external environment.
4. Homeostasis is about balancing the inputs within your body with the outputs to maintain a constant internal environment.

A. 1 only
B. 2 only
C. 3 only
D. 4 only
E. 1 and 3 only

**Question 320:**

Which of the following statements regarding the food chain is true?

A. There is more energy and biomass each time you move up a trophic level.
B. There is less energy and biomass each time you move up a trophic level.
C. There is more energy but less biomass each time you move up a trophic level.
D. There is less energy but more biomass each time you move up a trophic level.
E. There is no difference in the energy or biomass when you move up a trophic level.

**Question 321:**

Which of the following statements are true about asexual reproduction?

1. There is no fusion of gametes.
2. There are two parents.
3. There is no mixing of chromosomes.
4. Binary fission is an example of asexual reproduction.

A. 1, 3 and 4 only         C. 1 and 4 only         E. All are true
B. 1 and 3 only            D. 3 and 4 only

**Question 322:**

Put the following components of a stimulus-reponse arc in the order in which they are activated when Jonas sees a bowl of chicken and moves towards it.

1. Retina                  3. Sensory neuron        5. Muscle
2. Motor neuron            4. Brain

A. 1 - 3 - 4 - 5 - 2       C. 5 - 1 - 3 - 2 - 4      E. 1 - 3 - 4 - 2 - 5
B. 1 - 2 - 3 - 4 - 5       D. 1 - 3 - 2 - 4 - 5

**Question 323:**

The following statements relate to the flow of blood through the heart.

1. The right-hand side of the heart contains deoxygenated blood.
2. The aorta receives oxygenated blood from the left atrium.
3. The heart pumps deoxygenated blood into the pulmonary vein.
4. Valves are present to prevent flow of blood from the left ventricle to the right ventricle.

Which of these statements is / are correct?

A. 3 only
B. 1 and 3
C. 2 and 4
D. 1 only
E. None of the above

**Question 324:**
Which of the following statements are true about animal cloning?

1. Animals cloned from embryo transplants are genetically identical.
2. The genetic material is removed from an unfertilised egg during adult cell cloning.
3. Cloning can cause a reduced gene pool.
4. Cloning is only possible with mammals.

A. 1 only
B. 2 only
C. 1 and 2 only
D. 4 only
E. 1, 2 and 3 only

**Question 325:**
Which of the following statements are true with regards to evolution?

1. Individuals within a species show variation because of differences in their genes.
2. Beneficial mutations will accumulate within a population.
3. Gene differences are caused by sexual reproduction and mutations.
4. Species with similar characteristics never have similar genes.

A. 1 only
B. 1 and 4 only
C. 2 and 3 only
D. 2 and 4 only
E. 1, 2 and 3 only

**Question 326:**
Which of the following statements about genetics are correct?

1. Alleles are a similar version of different cells.
2. If you are homozygous for a trait, you have three alleles the same for that particular gene.
3. If you are heterozygous for a trait, you have two different alleles for that particular gene.
4. To show the characteristic that is caused by a recessive allele, both carried alleles for the gene have to be recessive.

A. 1 only
B. 2 only
C. 3 only
D. 4 only
E. 3 and 4 only

**Question 327:**
Which of the following statements are correct about meiosis?

1. The DNA content of a gamete is half that of a human red blood cell.
2. Meiosis requires ATP.
3. Meiosis only takes place in reproductive tissue.
4. In meiosis, a diploid cell divides in such a way so as to produce two haploid cells.

A. 1 only
B. 3 only
C. 1 and 2 only
D. 2 and 3 only
E. 2 and 4 only

**Question 328:**
Put the following statements in the correct order of events for when there is too little water in the blood.

1. Urine is more concentrated
2. Pituitary gland releases ADH
3. Blood water level returns to normal
4. Hypothalamus detects too little water in blood
5. Kidney affects water level

A. 1 - 2 - 3 - 4 - 5          C. 4 - 2 - 5 - 1 - 3          E. 5 - 2 - 3 - 4 - 1
B. 5 - 4 - 3 - 2 - 1          D. 3 - 2 - 4 - 1 - 5

**Question 329:**
The pH of venous blood is 7.35. Which of the following is the likely pH of arterial blood?

A. 5.2          B. 6.5          C. 7.0          D. 7.4          E. 8.0

**Question 330:**
Which of the following statements are true of the cytoplasm?

1. The vast majority of the cytoplasm is made up of water.
2. All contents of animal cells are contained in the cytoplasm.
3. The cytoplasm contains electrolytes and proteins.

A. 1 only          C. 3 only          E. 1 and 3 only
B. 2 only          D. 1 and 2 only

**Question 331:**
ATP is produced in which of the following organelles?

1. The cytoplasm
2. Plasmids
3. The mitochondria
4. The nucleus

A. 1 only          C. 3 only          E. 1 and 2
B. 2 only          D. 1 and 3

**Question 332:**
The cell membrane:

A. Is made up of a phospholipid bilayer which only allows active transport across it.
B. Is not found in bacteria.
C. Is a semi-permeable barrier to ions and organic molecules.
D. Consists purely of enzymes.

**Question 333:**

Cells of the *Polyommatus atlantica* butterfly of the Lycaenidae family have 446 chromosomes. Which of the following statements about a *P. atlantica* butterfly are correct?

1. Mitosis will produce 2 daughter cells each with 223 pairs of chromosomes
2. Meiosis will produce 4 daughter cells each with 223 chromosomes
3. Mitosis will produce 4 daughter cells each with 446 chromosomes
4. Meiosis will produce 2 daughter cells each with 223 pairs of chromosomes

A. 1 and 2 only        C. 2 and 3 only        E. 1, 2 and 3 only

B. 1 and 3 only        D. 3 and 4 only        F. 1, 2, 3 and 4

**Questions 334-336 are based on the following information:**

Assume that hair colour is determined by a single allele. The R allele is dominant and results in black hair. The r allele is recessive for red hair. Mary (red hair) and Bob (black hair) are having a baby girl.

**Question 334:**

What is the probability that the baby will have red hair?

A. 0% only        C. 50% only        E. 0% or 50%

B. 25% only        D. 0% or 25%        F. 25% or 50%

**Question 335:**

Mary and Bob have a second child, Tim, who is born with red hair. What does this confirm about Bob?

A. Bob is heterozygous for the red hair allele.
B. Bob is homozygous dominant for the red hair allele.
C. Bob is homozygous recessive for the red hair allele.
D. Bob does not have the red hair allele.

**Question 336:**

Mary and Bob go on to have a third child. What are the chances that this child will be born homozygous for black hair?

A. 0%        B. 25%        C. 50%        D. 75%        E. 100%

**Question 337:**

Why does air flow into the chest on inspiration?

1. Atmospheric pressure is less than intra-thoracic pressure during inspiration.
2. Atmospheric pressure is greater than intra-thoracic pressure during inspiration.
3. Anterior and lateral chest expansion decreases absolute intra-thoracic pressure.
4. Anterior and lateral chest expansion increases absolute intra-thoracic pressure.

A. 1 only        C. 2 and 3        E. 1 and 3

B. 2 only        D. 1 and 4

**Question 338:**
Which of the following components of a food chain represent the largest biomass?

A.  Producers
B.  Decomposers
C.  Primary consumers
D.  Secondary consumers
E.  Tertiary consumers

**Question 339:**
Concerning the nitrogen cycle, which of the following are true?

1.  The majority of the Earth's atmosphere is nitrogen.
2.  Most of the nitrogen in the Earth's atmosphere is inert.
3.  Bacteria are essential for nitrogen fixation.
4.  Nitrogen fixation occurs during lightning strikes.

A.  1 and 2
B.  1 and 3
C.  2 and 3
D.  2 and 4
E.  1, 2, 3 and 4

**Question 340:**
Which of the following statement are correct regarding mutations?

1.  Mutations always cause proteins to lose their function.
2.  Mutations always change the structure of the protein encoded by the affected gene.
3.  Mutations always result in cancer.

A.  Only 1
B.  Only 2
C.  Only 3
D.  1 and 2
E.  None of
    the above

**Question 341:**
Which of the following is not a function of the central nervous system?

A.  Coordination of movement
B.  Decision making and executive functions
C.  Control of heart rate
D.  Cognition
E.  Memory

**Question 342:**
Which of the following control mechanisms is / are involved in modulating the amount of blood that is pumped per unit time?

1.  Voluntary control.
2.  Sympathetic control to decrease heart rate.
3.  Parasympathetic control to increase heart rate.

A.  Only 1
B.  Only 2
C.  2 and 3
D.  1, 2 and 3
E.  None of
    the above

**Question 343:**

Vijay goes to see his GP with fatty, smelly stools that float in water. Which of the following enzymes is most likely to be malfunctioning?

A. Amylase
B. Lipase

C. Protease
D. Sucrase

E. Lactase

**Question 344:**

Which of the following statements concerning the cardiovascular system is correct?

A. Oxygenated blood from the lungs flows to the heart via the pulmonary artery.
B. All arteries carry oxygenated blood.
C. All animals have a double circulatory system.
D. The superior vena cava contains oxygenated blood
E. None of the above.

**Question 345:**

In which part of the GI tract is there the least enzymatic activity for digestion?

A. Mouth
B. Stomach

C. Small intestine
D. Large intestine

E. Rectum

**Question 346:**

Oge touches a hot stove and immediately moves her hand away. Which of the following components are **NOT** involved in this reflex reaction?

1. Thermo-receptor
2. Brain

3. Spinal Cord
4. Sensory nerve

5. Motor nerve
6. Muscle

A. 1 only
B. 2 only

C. 3 only
D. 1 and 2 only

E. 1, 2 and 3 only

**Question 347:**

Which of the following represents a scenario with an appropriate description of the mode of transport?

1. Osmosis = water moving from a hypotonic solution outside of a potato cell, across the cell wall and cell membrane and into the hypertonic cytoplasm of the potato cell.
2. Active transport = carbon dioxide moving across a respiring cell's membrane and dissolving in blood plasma.
3. Diffusion = reabsorption of amino acids against a concentration gradient in the glomeruluar apparatus.

A. 1 only
B. 2 only

C. 3 only
D. 1 and 2 only

E. 2 and 3 only

**Question 348:**

Which of the following equations represents anaerobic respiration in animal cells?

1. Carbohydrate + Oxygen → Energy + Carbon dioxide + Water
2. Carbohydrate → Energy + Lactic acid + Carbon dioxide
3. Carbohydrate → Energy + Lactic acid
4. Carbohydrate → Energy + Ethanol + Carbon dioxide

A. 1 only
B. 2 and 4

C. 3 and 4 only
D. 4 only

E. 3 only

**Question 349:**

Which of the following statements regarding respiration in animal cells are correct?

1. Mitochondria are the centres of both aerobic and anaerobic respiration.
2. The cytoplasm is the main site of anaerobic respiration.
3. In aerobic respiration, every two moles of glucose results in the liberation of 12 moles of $CO_2$.
4. Anaerobic respiration is more efficient than aerobic respiration.

A. 1 and 2
B. 1 and 4
C. 2 and 3
D. 2 and 4
E. 3 and 4

**Question 350:**

Which of the following statements are true?

1. The nucleus contains the cell's chromosomes.
2. The cytoplasm consists purely of water.
3. The plasma membrane is a single phospholipid layer.
4. The cell wall prevents plants cells from lysis due to osmotic pressure.

A. 1 and 2
B. 1 and 4

C. 1, 3 and 4
D. 1, 2 and 3

E. 1, 2 and 4

**Question 351:**

Which of the following statements are true about osmosis?

1. If a medium is more concentrated than the cell cytoplasm, the cell will gain water through osmosis.
2. If a medium is less concentrated than the cell cytoplasm, the cell will gain water through osmosis.
3. If a medium is less concentrated than the cell cytoplasm, the cell will lose water through osmosis.
4. If a medium is more concentrated than the cell cytoplasm, the cell will lose water through osmosis.
5. The medium's tonicity has no impact on the movement of water.

A. 1 only
B. 2 only
C. 1 and 3
D. 2 and 4
E. 5 only

**Question 352:**

Which of the following statements are true about stem cells?

1. Stem cells have the ability to differentiate into other mature types of cells.
2. Stem cells are unable to maintain their undifferentiated state.
3. Stem cells can be classified as embryonic stem cells or adult stem cells.
4. Stem cells are only found in embryos.

A. 1 and 3      B. 3 and 4      C. 2 and 3      D. 1 and 2      E. 2 and 4

**Question 353:**

Which of the following are **NOT** examples of natural selection?

1. Giraffes growing longer necks to eat taller plants.
2. Antibiotic resistance developed by certain strains of bacteria.
3. Pesticide resistance among locusts in farms.
4. Breeding of horses to make them run faster.

A. 1 only      B. 4 only      C. 1 and 3      D. 1 and 4      E. 2 and 4

**Question 354:**

Which of the following statements are true?

1. Enzymes stabilise the transition state and therefore lower the activation energy.
2. Enzymes distort substrates in order to lower activation energy.
3. Enzymes decrease temperature to slow down reactions and lower the activation energy.
4. Enzymes provide alternative pathways for reactions to occur.

A. 1 only      B. 1 and 3      C. 1 and 4      D. 2 and 4      E. 1, 2 and 4

**Question 355:**

Which of the following are examples of negative feedback?

1. Salivating whilst waiting for a meal.
2. Throwing a dart.
3. The regulation of blood pH.
4. The regulation of blood pressure.

A. 1 only      B. 1 and 2      C. 3 and 4      D. 2, 3, and 4      E. 1, 2, 3 and 4

**Question 356:**

Which of the following statements about the immune system are true?

1. White blood cells defend against bacterial and fungal infections.
2. Red blood cells are involved in the process of phagocytosis.
3. White blood cells use antibodies to fight pathogens.
4. Antibodies are produced by bone marrow stem cells.

A. 1 and 3     C. 2 and 3     E. 1, 2, and 3

B. 1 and 4     D. 2 and 4

**Question 357:**

The cardiovascular system does **NOT**:

A. Deliver vital nutrients to peripheral cells.
B. Oxygenate blood and transport it to peripheral cells.
C. Act as a mode of transportation for hormones to reach their target organ.
D. Facilitate thermoregulation.
E. Respond to exercise by increasing the heart rate.

**Question 358:**

Which of the following statements is correct?

A. Adrenaline can sometimes decrease heart rate.
B. Adrenaline is rarely released during flight or fight responses.
C. Adrenaline causes peripheral vasoconstriction.
D. Adrenaline only affects the cardiovascular system.
E. Adrenaline travels primarily in lymphatic vessels.
F. None of the above.

**Question 359:**

Which of the following statements is true?

A. Protein synthesis occurs solely in the nucleus.
B. Each amino acid is coded for by three DNA bases.
C. Each protein is coded for by three amino acids.
D. Red blood cells can create new proteins to prolong their lifespan.
E. Protein synthesis isn't necessary for mitosis to take place.

**Question 360:**

A solution of amylase and carbohydrate is present in a beaker, where the pH of the contents is 6.3. Assuming amylase is saturated, which of the following will increase the rate of production of the product?

1. Add sodium bicarbonate
2. Add carbohydrate
3. Add amylase
4. Increase the temperature to 100° C

A. 1 only      C. 1 and 3      E. 1 and 2
B. 2 only      D. 4 only

**Question 361:**

Celestial necrosis is a newly discovered autosomal recessive disorder. A female carrier and a male with the disease produce two sons. What is the probability that neither son's genotype contains the celestial necrosis allele?

A. 100%      B. 75%      C. 50%      D. 25%      E. 0%

**Question 362:**

Which of the following organs has **no** endocrine function?

A. The thyroid      C. The pancreas      E. None of the above.
B. The ovary      D. The testes

**Question 363:**

Which of the following statements are true?

1. Increasing levels of insulin cause a decrease in blood glucose levels.
2. Increasing levels of glycogen cause an increase in blood glucose levels.
3. Increasing levels of adrenaline decrease the heart rate.

A. 1 only
B. 2 only
C. 3 only
D. 1 and 2
E. 2 and 3

**Question 364:**

Which of the following rows is correct?

|  | **Oxygenated Blood** | | **Deoxygenated Blood** | |
|---|---|---|---|---|
| **A.** | Left atrium | Left ventricle | Right atrium | Right ventricle |
| **B.** | Left atrium | Right atrium | Left ventricle | Right ventricle |
| **C.** | Left atrium | Right ventricle | Right atrium | Right ventricle |
| **D.** | Right atrium | Right ventricle | Left atrium | Left ventricle |
| **E.** | Left ventricle | Right atrium | Left atrium | Right ventricle |

**Questions 365-367 are based on the following information:**

The pedigree below shows the inheritance of a newly discovered disease that affects connective tissue called Nafram syndrome.  Individual I is a normal homozygote (disease-free).

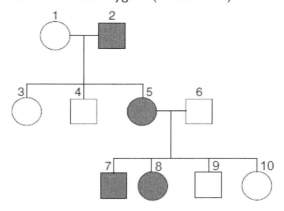

**Question 365:**

Based on the pedigree, what is the pattern of inheritance for Nafram syndrome?

A.  Autosomal dominant          C.  X-linked dominant          E.  Cannot be determined
B.  Autosomal recessive          D.  X-linked recessive

**Question 366:**

Which individuals in the pedigree must be heterozygous for Nafram syndrome?

A.  I and 2          C.  2 and 5          E.  6 and 8
B.  8 and 9          D.  5 and 6

## Question 367:

Taking N to denote a disease-conferring allele and n to denote a normal allele, which of the following are **NOT** possible genotypes for 6's parents?

1. NN x NN
2. NN x Nn
3. Nn x nn
4. Nn x Nn
5. nn x nn

A. 1 and 2
B. 1 and 3
C. 2 and 3
D. 2 and 5
E. 3 and 4

## Question 368:

Which of the following correctly describes the passage of urine through the body?

|   | 1st | 2nd | 3rd | 4th |
|---|-----|-----|-----|-----|
| A | Kidney | Ureter | Bladder | Urethra |
| B | Kidney | Urethra | Bladder | Ureter |
| C | Urethra | Bladder | Ureter | Kidney |
| D | Ureter | Kidney | Bladder | Urethra |

## Question 369:

Which of the following best describes the passage of blood from the body, through the heart, and back to the body?

A. Aorta → Left Ventricle → Left Atrium → Inferior Vena Cava → Right Atrium → Right Ventricle → Lungs → Aorta
B. Inferior vena cava → Left Atrium → Left Ventricle → Lungs → Right Atrium → Right Ventricle → Aorta
C. Inferior vena cava → Right Ventricle → Right Atrium → Lungs → Left Atrium → Left Ventricle → Aorta
D. Aorta → Left Atrium → Left Ventricle → Lungs → Right Atrium → Right Ventricle → Inferior Vena Cava
E. None of the above.

## Question 370:

Which of the following best describes the events during inspiration?

|   | Intrathoracic Pressure | Intercostal Muscles | Diaphragm |
|---|---|---|---|
| A | Increases | Contract | Contracts |
| B | Increases | Relax | Contracts |
| C | Increases | Contract | Relaxes |
| D | Increases | Relax | Relaxes |
| E | Decreases | Contract | Contracts |

**Questions 371-372 are based on the following information:**

DNA is made up of four nucleotide bases: adenine, cytosine, guanine and thymine. A triplet of bases (codon) is a sequence of three nucleotides which code for an amino acid. While there are only 20 amino acids there are 64 different combinations of the four DNA nucleotide bases. This means that more than one combination of 3 DNA nucleotide sequences code for the same amino acid.

**Question 371:**

Which property of the genetic code is described above?

A.  The code is unambiguous.
B.  The code is universal.
C.  The code is non-overlapping.
D.  The code is degenerate.
E.  The code is preserved.

**Question 372:**

Which type of mutation does the described property protect against the most?

A.  An insertion - where a single nucleotide is inserted.
B.  A point mutation - where a single nucleotide is replaced for another.
C.  A deletion - where a single nucleotide is deleted.
D.  A repeat expansion - where a repeated trinucleotide sequence is added.
E.  A duplication - where a piece of DNA is abnormally copied.

**Question 373:**

Which row of the table below describes what happens when the temperature decreases in the external environment?

| | Temperature Change Detected by | Sweat Gland Secretion | Cutaneous Blood Flow |
|---|---|---|---|
| **A** | Hypothalamus | Increases | Increases |
| **B** | Hypothalamus | Increases | Decreases |
| **C** | Hypothalamus | Decreases | Increases |
| **D** | Hypothalamus | Decreases | Decreases |
| **E** | Cerebral Cortex | Increases | Increases |

**Question 374:**

Which of the following processes involve active transport?

1.  Reabsorption of glucose in the kidney.
2.  Movement of carbon dioxide into the alveoli of the lungs.
3.  Movement of chemicals in a synapse.

A.  1 only
B.  2 only
C.  3 only
D.  1 and 2
E.  1 and 3

**Question 375:**

Which of the following statements is correct about enzymes?

A. All enzymes are made up of amino acids only.
B. Enzymes can sometimes slow the rate of reactions.
C. Enzymes are heat sensitive but resistant to changes in pH.
D. Enzymes are unspecific in their substrate use.
E. None of the above.

# SECTION 2: CHEMISTRY

Most students don't struggle with the content of BMAT chemistry as they'll be studying it at A level. However, there are certain questions that even very good students tend to find difficult under time pressure e.g. balancing equations and mass calculations. It is essential that you do enough practice so that you're able to do these questions quickly and accurately as they have the potential to really slow your progress through the Section 2 questions.

### *Balancing Equations*

For some reason, most students are rarely shown how to formally balance equations – including those studying it at A-level. Balancing equations intuitively or via trial and error will only get you so far in the BMAT as the equations you'll have to work with will be fairly complex. To avoid wasting valuable time, it is essential you learn a clear method that will allow you to consistently solve these in less than 60 seconds. The method shown below is the simplest way and requires you to be able to do quick mental arithmetic (which is something you should be aiming for anyway). The easiest way to do learn it is through an example:

The following equation shows the reaction between iodic acid ($HIO_3$), hydrochloric acid (HCl) and copper iodide ($CuI_2$):

$$\textbf{a } HIO_3 + \textbf{b } CuI_2 + \textbf{c } HCl \rightarrow \textbf{d } CuCl_3 + \textbf{e } ICl + \textbf{f } H_2O$$

What values of **a**, **b**, **c**, **d**, **e** and **f** are needed in order to balance the equation?

Step 1: Pick an element and see how many atoms there are on the left and right sides.

Step 2: Form an equation to represent this. For Cu: b = d

Step 3: See if any of the answer options given **don't** satisfy b=d. In this case, for option E, b is 8 and d is 10. This allows us to eliminate option E immediately.

|   | a | b | c | d | e | f |
|---|---|---|---|---|---|---|
| **A** | 5 | 4 | 25 | 4 | 13 | 15 |
| **B** | 5 | 4 | 20 | 4 | 8 | 15 |
| **C** | 5 | 6 | 20 | 6 | 8 | 15 |
| **D** | 2 | 8 | 10 | 8 | 8 | 15 |
| **E** | 6 | 8 | 24 | 10 | 16 | 15 |
| **F** | 6 | 10 | 22 | 10 | 16 | 15 |

Once you've eliminated as many options as possible using this method, go back to step 1 and pick another element.

For Hydrogen (H): a + c = 2. Then see if any of the answer options **don't** satisfy a + c = 2f.

- Option A: 5 + 25 is equal to 2 x 15
- Option B: 5 + 20 is not equal to 2 x 15
- Option C: 5 + 20 is not equal to 2 x 15
- Option D: 2 + 10 is not equal to 2 x 15

This allows us to eliminate option B, C and D. E has already been eliminated. Thus, the only solution possible is A.

This method works best when you get given a table above as this allows you to quickly eliminate options. However, it is still a viable method even if you don't get this information in the question. You might get given the equation with some numerical values present, so could apply the same method to that scenario.

## *Chemistry Calculations*

Equations you **MUST** know for Section 2:

- Atomic Mass = Mass/Moles
- Amount (mol) = Concentration (mol/dm³) x Volume (dm³)

## Avogadro's Constant:

One mole of anything contains $6 \times 10^{23}$ of it e.g. 5 Moles of water contain $5 \times 6 \times 10^{23}$ number of water molecules.

## Abundances:

The average atomic mass takes the abundances of all isotopes into account. Thus:

$A_r$ = (Abundance of Isotope 1) x (Mass of Isotope 1) + (Abundance of Isotope 2) x (Mass of Isotope 2) +...

## Converting between volumes:

It is useful to remember that $1 \text{ dm}^3 = 1000 \text{ cm}^3 = 1$ litre

# CHEMISTRY QUESTIONS

**Question 376:**
Which of the following most accurately defines an isotope?

A. An isotope is an atom of an element that has the same number of protons in the nucleus but a different number of neutrons orbiting the nucleus.
B. An isotope is an atom of an element that has the same number of neutrons in the nucleus but a different number of protons orbiting the nucleus.
C. An isotope is any atom of an element that can be split to produce nuclear energy.
D. An isotope is an atom of an element that has the same number of protons in the nucleus but a different number of neutrons in the nucleus.
E. An isotope is an atom of an element that has the same number of protons in the nucleus but a different number of electrons orbiting it.

**Question 377:**
Which of the following is an example of a displacement reaction?
1. $Fe + SnSO4 \rightarrow FeSO_4 + Sn$
2. $Cl_2 + 2KBr \rightarrow Br_2 + 2KCl$
3. $H_2SO_4 + Mg \rightarrow MgSO_4 + H_2$
4. $NaHCO_3 + HCl \rightarrow NaCl + CO_2 + H_2O$

A. 1 only
B. 1 and 2 only
C. 2 and 3 only
D. 3 and 4 only
E. 1, 2, 3 and 4

**Question 378:**
What values of **a**, **b** and **c** are needed to balance the equation below?

$$aCa(OH)_2 + bH_3PO_4 \rightarrow Ca_3(PO_4)_2 + cH_2O$$

A. $a = 3, b = 2, c = 6$
B. $a = 2, b = 2, c = 4$
C. $a = 3, b = 2, c = 1$
D. $a = 1, b = 2, c = 3$
E. $a = 4, b = 2, c = 6$

**Question 379:**
What values of **s**, **t** and **u** are needed to balance the equation below?

$$sAgNO_3 + tK_3PO_4 \rightarrow 3Ag_3PO_4 + uKNO_3$$

A. $s = 9, t = 3, u = 9$
B. $s = 6, t = 3, u = 9$
C. $s = 9, t = 3, u = 6$
D. $s = 9, t = 6, u = 9$
E. $s = 3, t = 3, u = 9$

**Question 380:**
Which of the following statements are true with regard to displacement?
1. A less reactive halogen can displace a more reactive halogen.
2. Chlorine cannot displace bromine or iodine from an aqueous solution of its salts.
3. Bromine can displace iodine according to the reactivity series.
4. Fluorine can displace chlorine as it is higher up the group.
5. Lithium can displace francium as it is higher up the group.

A. 3 only                     C. 1 and 2 only              E. 2, 3 and 5 only
B. 5 only                     D. 3 and 4 only

**Question 381:**
What mass of magnesium oxide is produced when 75g of magnesium is burned in excess oxygen?
Relative Atomic Masses: Mg = 24, O = 16

A. 80g          B. 100g          C. 125g          D. 145g          E. 175g

**Question 382:**
Hydrogen can combine with hydroxide ions to produce water.  Which process is involved in this?

A. Hydration                  C. Reduction                 E. Evaporation
B. Oxidation                  D. Dehydration

**Question 383:**
Which of the following statements about ammonia are correct?

1. It has a formula of $NH_3$.
2. Nitrogen contributes 82% to its mass.
3. It can be broken down again into nitrogen and hydrogen.
4. It is covalently bonded.
5. It is used to make fertilisers.

A. 1 and 2 only               C. 3, 4 and 5 only           E. 1, 2, 3, 4 and 5
B. 1 and 4 only               D. 1, 2 and 5 only

**Question 384:**
What colour will a universal indicator change to in a solution of whole milk (neutral pH) and lipase?

A. From green to orange.      C. From purple to green.     E. From yellow to purple.
B. From red to green.         D. From purple to orange.

**Question 385:**
Vitamin C [$C_6H_8O_6$] can be artificially synthesised from glucose [$C_6H_{12}O_6$]. What type of reaction is this likely to be?

A. Dehydration               C. Oxidation                 E. Displacement
B. Hydration                 D. Reduction

**Question 386:**

Which of the following statements are true?

1. $Cu^{64}$ will undergo oxidation faster than $Cu^{65}$.
2. $Cu^{65}$ will undergo reduction faster than $Cu^{64}$.
3. $Cu^{65}$ and $Cu^{64}$ have the same number of electrons.

A.  I only
B.  2 only
C.  3 only
D.  2 and 3 only
E.  I and 3 only
F.  I, 2 and 3

**Question 387:**

6g of $Mg^{24}$ is added to a solution containing 30g of dissolved sulguric acid ($H_2SO_4$). Which of the following statements are true?
Relative Atomic Masses: S = 32, Mg = 24, O = 16, H = 1

1.  In this reaction, the magnesium is the limiting reagent
2.  In this reaction, sulfuric acid is the limiting reagent
3.  The mass of salt produced equals the original mass of sulfuric acid

A.  I only
B.  2 only
C.  3 only
D.  I and 2 only
E.  I and 3 only

**Question 388:**

In which of the following mixtures will a displacement reaction occur?

1.  $Cu + 2AgNO_3$
2.  $Cu + Fe(NO_3)_2$
3.  $Ca + 2H_2O$
4.  $Fe + Ca(OH)_2$

A.  I only
B.  2 only
C.  3 only
D.  4 only
E.  I and 3 only

**Question 389:**

Which of the following statements is true about the following chain of metals?

$Na \rightarrow Ca \rightarrow Mg \rightarrow Al \rightarrow Zn$
Moving from left to right:
1.  The reactivity of the metals increases.
2.  The likelihood of corrosion of the metals increases.
3.  More energy is required to separate these metals from their ores.
4.  The metals lose electrons more readily to form positive ions.

A.  I and 2 only
B.  I and 3 only
C.  2 and 3 only
D.  I and 4 only
E.  None of the above

**Question 390:**

In which of the following mixtures will a displacement reaction occur?

1. $I_2 + 2KBr$
2. $Cl_2 + 2NaBr$
3. $Br_2 + 2KI$

A.  1 only
B.  2 only
C.  3 only
D.  1 and 2 only
E.  2 and 3 only

**Question 391:**

Which of the following statements about Al and Cu are true?

1. Al is used to build aircraft because it is lightweight and resists corrosion.
2. Cu is used to build electrical wires because it is a good insulator.
3. Both Al and Cu are good conductors of heat.
4. Al is commonly alloyed with other metals to make coins.
5. Al is resistant to corrosion because of a thin layer of aluminium hydroxide on its surface.

A.  1 and 3 only
B.  1 and 4 only
C.  1, 3 and 5 only
D.  1, 3, 4, 5 only
E.  2, 4 and 5 only

**Question 392:**

21g of $Li^7$ reacts completely with excess water.  Given that the molar gas volume is 24 dm³ under the conditions, what is the volume of hydrogen produced?

A.  12 dm³
B.  24 dm³
C.  36 dm³
D.  48 dm³
E.  72 dm³

**Question 393:**

Which of the following statements regarding bonding are true?

1. NaCl has stronger ionic bonds than $MgCl_2$.
2. Transition metals are able to lose varying numbers of electrons to form multiple stable positive ions.
3. All covalently bonded structures have lower melting points than ionically bonded compounds.
4. No covalently bonded structures conduct electricity.

A.  1 only
B.  2 only
C.  3 only
D.  4 only
E.  1 and 2 only

**Question 394:**

Consider the following two equations:

A.   $C + O_2 \rightarrow CO_2$          $\Delta H = -394$ kJ per mole
B.   $CaCO_3 \rightarrow CaO + CO_2$  $\Delta H = +178$ kJ per mole

Which of the following statements are true?

1.   Reaction **A** is exothermic and Reaction **B** is endothermic.
2.   $CO_2$ has less energy than C and $O_2$.
3.   CaO is more stable than $CaCO_3$.

A.  I only            C.  3 only            E.  I and 3
B.  2 only            D.  I and 2

**Question 395:**

Which of the following are true of regarding the oxides formed by Na, Mg and Al?

1.   All of the metals and their solid oxides conduct electricity.
2.   MgO has stronger bonds than $Na_2O$.
3.   Metals are extracted from their molten ores by fractional distillation.

A.  I only            C.  3 only            E.  2 and 3 only
B.  2 only            D.  I and 2 only

**Question 396:**

Which of the following pairs have the same electronic configuration?

1.   $Li^+$ and $Na^+$
2.   $Mg^{2+}$ and Ne
3.   $Na^{2+}$ and Ne
4.   $O^{2+}$ and a Carbon atom

A.  I only            C.  I and 3 only      E.  2 and 4 only
B.  I and 2 only      D.  2 and 3 only

**Question 397:**

In relation to the reactivity of elements in Groups I and 2, which of the following statements is correct?

1.   Reactivity decreases as you go down Group I.
2.   Reactivity increases as you go down Group 2.
3.   Group I metals are generally less reactive than Group 2 metals.

A.  Only I            C.  Only 3            E.  2 and 3
B.  Only 2            D.  I and 2

**Question 398:**

What role do catalysts fulfil in an endothermic reaction?

A.  They increase the temperature, causing the reaction to occur at a faster rate.
B.  They decrease the temperature, causing the reaction to occur at a faster rate.
C.  They reduce the energy of the reactants in order to trigger the reaction.
D.  They reduce the activation energy of the reaction.
E.  They increase the activation energy of the reaction.

**Question 399:**

Tritium $H^3$ is an isotope of hydrogen. Why is tritium commonly referred to as 'heavy hydrogen'?

A.  Because $H^3$ contains 3 protons making it heavier than $H^1$ that contains 1 proton.
B.  Because $H^3$ contains 3 neutrons making it heavier than $H^1$ that contains 1 neutron.
C.  Because $H^3$ contains 1 neutron and 2 protons making it heavier than $H^1$ that contains 1 neutron and 1 proton.
D.  Because $H^3$ contains 1 proton and 2 neutrons making it heavier than $H^1$ that contains 1 proton.
E.  Because $H^3$ contains 3 electrons making it heavier than $H^1$ that contains 1 electron.

**Question 400:**

In relation to redox reactions, which of the following statements are correct?

1.  Oxidation describes the loss of electrons.
2.  Reduction increases the electron density of an ion, atom or molecule.
3.  Halogens are powerful reducing agents.

A.  Only 1
B.  Only 2
C.  Only 3
D.  1 and 2
E.  2 and 3

**Question 401:**

Which one of the following statements is correct?

A.  At higher temperatures, gas molecules move at angles that cause them to collide with each other more frequently.
B.  Gas molecules have lower energy after colliding with each other.
C.  At higher temperatures, gas molecules attract each other resulting in more collisions.
D.  The average kinetic energy of gas molecules is the same for all gases at the same temperature.
E.  The momentum of gas molecules decreases as pressure increases.

**Question 402:**

Which of the following are exothermic reactions?

1. Burning magnesium in pure oxygen
2. The combustion of hydrogen
3. Aerobic respiration
4. Evaporation of water in the oceans
5. The reaction between a strong acid and a strong base

A. 1, 2 and 4        C. 1, 3 and 5        E. 1, 2, 3 and 5
B. 1, 2 and 5        D. 2, 3 and 4

**Question 403:**

Ethene reacts with oxygen to produce water and carbon dioxide. Which elements are oxidised/reduced?

A. Carbon is reduced and oxygen is oxidised.
B. Hydrogen is reduced and oxygen is oxidised.
C. Carbon is oxidised and hydrogen is reduced.
D. Hydrogen is oxidised and carbon is reduced.
E. Carbon is oxidised and oxygen is reduced.

**Question 404:**

In the reaction between zinc and copper (II) sulphate which elements act as oxidising + reducing agents?

A. Zinc is the reducing agent while sulfur is the oxidizing agent.
B. Zinc is the reducing agent while copper in $CuSO_4$ is the oxidizing agent.
C. Copper is the reducing agent while zinc is the oxidizing agent.
D. Oxygen is the reducing agent while copper in $CuSO_4$ is the oxidizing agent.
E. Sulfur is the reducing agent while oxygen is the oxidizing agent.

**Question 405:**

Which of the following statements is true?

A. Acids are compounds that act as proton acceptors in an aqueous solution.
B. Acids only exist in a liquid state.
C. Strong acids are partially ionized in a solution.
D. Weak acids generally have a pH of 6 to 7.
E. The reaction between a weak and strong acid produces water and salt.

## Question 406:

An unknown element, Z, has 3 isotopes: $Z^5$, $Z^6$ and $Z^8$. Given that the atomic mass of Z is 7, and the relative abundance of $Z^5$ is 20%, which of the following statements are correct?

1. $Z^5$ and $Z^6$ are present in the same abundance.
2. $Z^8$ is the most abundant of the isotopes.
3. $Z^8$ is more abundant than $Z^5$ and $Z^6$ combined.

A. 1 only
B. 2 only
C. 3 only
D. 1, 2 and 3
E. 2 and 3 only

## Question 407:

Which of following best describes the products when an acid reacts with a metal that is more reactive than hydrogen?

A. Salt and hydrogen
B. Salt and ammonia
C. Salt and water
D. A weak acid and a weak base
E. A strong acid and a strong base

## Question 408:

Choose an option from the table below to balance the following equation:
**a** $FeSO_4$ + **b** $K_2Cr_2O_7$ + **c** $H_2SO_4$ → **d** $(Fe)_2(SO_4)_3$ + **e** $Cr_2(SO_4)_3$ + **f** $K_2SO_4$ + **g** $H_2O$

|   | a | b | c | d | e | f | g |
|---|---|---|---|---|---|---|---|
| A | 6 | 1 | 8 | 3 | 1 | 1 | 7 |
| B | 6 | 1 | 7 | 3 | 1 | 1 | 7 |
| C | 2 | 1 | 6 | 2 | 1 | 1 | 6 |
| D | 12 | 1 | 14 | 4 | 1 | 1 | 14 |
| E | 4 | 1 | 12 | 4 | 1 | 1 | 12 |

## Question 409:

Which of the following statements is correct?

A. Matter consists of atoms that have a net electrical charge.
B. Atoms and ions of the same element have different numbers of protons and electrons but the same number of neutrons.
C. Over 80% of an atom's mass comes from its protons.
D. Atoms of the same element that have different numbers of neutrons react at significantly different rates.
E. Protons in the nucleus of atoms repel each other as they are positively charged.

**Question 410:**
Which of the following statements is correct?

A. The noble gases are chemically inert and therefore useless to man.
B. All of the noble gases have a full outer electron shell.
C. The majority of noble gases are brightly coloured.
D. The boiling point of the noble gases decreases as you progress down the Group.
E. Neon is the most abundant noble gas.

**Question 411:**
In relation to alkenes, which of the following statements is correct?
1. They all contain double bonds.
2. They can all be reduced to alkanes.
3. The equation 'alkene + hydrogen → alkane' is an example of a hydration reaction.

A. Only 1          C. Only 3          E. 2 and 3
B. Only 2          D. 1 and 2

**Question 412:**
Chlorine is made up of two isotopes, $Cl^{35}$ (atomic mass 34.969) and $Cl^{37}$ (atomic mass 36.966). Given that the atomic mass of chlorine is 35.453, which of the following statements is correct?

A. $Cl^{35}$ is about 3 times more abundant than $Cl^{37}$.
B. $Cl^{35}$ is about 10 times more abundant than $Cl^{37}$.
C. $Cl^{37}$ is about 3 times more abundant than $Cl^{35}$.
D. $Cl^{37}$ is about 10 times more abundant than $Cl^{35}$.
E. Both isotopes are equally abundant.

**Question 413:**
Which of the following statements regarding transition metals is correct?

A. Transition metals form ions that have multiple colours.
B. Transition metals usually form covalent bonds.
C. Transition metals cannot be used as catalysts as they are too reactive.
D. Transition metals are poor conductors of electricity.
E. Transition metals are found in group 2 of the periodic table.

**Question 414:**

20 g of impure $Na^{23}$ reacts completely with excess water to produce 8,000 cm³ of hydrogen gas under standard conditions. What is the percentage purity of sodium?

[Under standard conditions 1 mole of gas occupies 24 dm³]

A.  88.0%          B.  76.5%          C.  66.0%          D.  38.0%          E.  15.3%

**Question 415:**

An organic molecule contains 70.6% Carbon, 5.9% Hydrogen and 23.5% Oxygen. It has a molecular mass of 136. What is its chemical formula?

A.  $C_4H_4O$          B.  $C_5H_4O$          C.  $C_8H_8O_2$          D.  $C_{10}H_8O_2$          E.  $C_2H_2O$

**Question 416:**

Choose an option from the table below to balance the following equation:

$$aS + bHNO_3 \rightarrow cH_2SO_4 + dNO_2 + eH_2O$$

|   | a | b | c | d | e |
|---|---|---|---|---|---|
| **A** | 3 | 5 | 3 | 5 | 1 |
| **B** | 1 | 6 | 1 | 6 | 2 |
| **C** | 6 | 14 | 6 | 14 | 2 |
| **D** | 2 | 4 | 2 | 4 | 4 |
| **E** | 2 | 3 | 2 | 3 | 2 |

**Question 417:**

Which of the following statements is true?
1.  Ethane and ethene can both dissolve in organic solvents.
2.  Ethane and ethene can both be hydrogenated in the presence of nickel.
3.  Breaking C=C requires double the energy needed to break C-C.

A.  1 only                C.  3 only                E.  2 and 3 only
B.  2 only                D.  1 and 2 only

## Question 418:

Diamond, graphite, methane and ammonia all contain covalent bonds. Which row in the table adequately describes the properties associated with each compound?

| | Compound | Melting Point | Able to conduct electricity | Soluble in water |
|---|---|---|---|---|
| 1. | Diamond | High | Yes | No |
| 2. | Graphite | High | Yes | No |
| 3. | $CH_{4\,(g)}$ | Low | No | No |
| 4. | $NH_{3\,(g)}$ | Low | No | Yes |

A. 1 and 2 only
B. 2 and 3 only
C. 1 and 3 only
D. 1 and 4 only
E. 2, 3 and 4

## Question 419:

Which of the following statements about catalysts are true?
1. Catalysts reduce the energy required for a reaction to take place.
2. Catalysts are used up in reactions.
3. Catalysed reactions are almost always exothermic.

A. 1 only
B. 2 only
C. 1 and 2
D. 2 and 3
E. 1, 2 and 3

## Question 420:

What is the name of the molecule below?

A. But-1-ene
B. But-2-ene
C. Pent-3-ene
D. Pent-1-ene
E. Pent-2-ene
F. Pentane
G. Pentanoic acid

## Question 421:

Which of the following statements is correct regarding Group 1 elements? [Excluding hydrogen]

A. The oxidation number of Group 1 elements usually decreases in most reactions.
B. Reactivity decreases as you progress down Group 1.
C. Group 1 elements do not react with water.
D. All Group 1 elements react spontaneously with oxygen.
E. All of the above.
F. None of the above.

**Question 422:**

Which of the following statements about electrolysis are correct?

1. The cathode attracts negatively charged ions.
2. Atoms are reduced at the anode.
3. Electrolysis can be used to separate mixtures.

A. Only 1
B. Only 2
C. 2 and 3
D. Only 3
E. None of the above

**Question 423:**

Which of the following is **NOT** an isomer of pentane?

A. $CH_3CH_2CH_2CH_2CH_3$
B. $CH_3C(CH_3)CH_3CH_3$

C. $CH_3(CH_2)_3CH_3$
D. $CH_3C(CH_3)_2CH_3$

**Question 424:**

Choose an option to balance the following equation:
$Cu + HNO_3 \rightarrow Cu(NO_3)_2 + NO + H_2O$

A. $8\ Cu + 3\ HNO_3 \rightarrow 8\ Cu(NO_3)_2 + 4\ NO + 2\ H_2O$
B. $3\ Cu + 8\ HNO_3 \rightarrow 2\ Cu(NO_3)_2 + 3\ NO + 4\ H_2O$
C. $5Cu + 7HNO_3 \rightarrow 5\ Cu(NO_3)_2 + 4\ NO + 8\ H_2O$
D. $6\ Cu + 10\ HNO_3 \rightarrow 6\ Cu(NO_3)_2 + 3\ NO + 7\ H_2O$
E. $3\ Cu + 8\ HNO_3 \rightarrow 3\ Cu(NO_3)_2 + 2\ NO + 4\ H_2O$

**Question 425:**

Which of the following statements regarding alkenes is correct?

A. Alkenes are an inorganic homologous series.
B. Alkenes always have three times as many hydrogen atoms as they do carbon atoms.
C. Bromine water changes from clear to brown in the presence of an alkene.
D. Alkenes are more reactive than alkanes because they are unsaturated.
E. Alkenes frequently take part in subtraction reactions.

**Question 426:**

Which one of the following statements is correct regarding Group 17?

A. All Group 17 elements are electrophilic and therefore form negatively charged ions.
B. The reaction between sodium and fluorine is less vigorous than sodium and iodine.
C. Some Group 17 elements are found naturally as unbonded atoms.
D. All of the above.
E. None of the above.

**Question 427:**
Why does the electrolysis of NaCl solution (brine) require the strict separation of the products of anode and cathode?

A. To prevent the preferential discharge of ions.
B. In order to prevent spontaneous combustion.
C. In order to prevent production of $H_2$.
D. In order to prevent the formation of HCl.
E. In order to avoid CO poisoning.

**Question 428:**
In relation to the electrolysis of brine (NaCl), which of the following statements are correct?

1. Electrolysis results in the production of hydrogen and chlorine gas.
2. Electrolysis results in the production of sodium hydroxide.
3. Hydrogen gas is released at the anode and chlorine gas is released at the cathode.

A. Only 1        C. Only 3        E. 1 and 3
B. Only 2        D. 1 and 2

**Question 429:**
Which of the following statements is correct?

A. Alkanes consist of multiple C-H bonds that are very weak.
B. An alkane with 14 hydrogen atoms is called heptane.
C. All alkanes consist purely of hydrogen and carbon atoms.
D. Alkanes burn in excess oxygen to produce carbon monoxide and water.
E. Bromine water is decolourised in the presence of an alkane.

**Question 430:**
Which of the following statements are correct?

1. All alcohols contain a hydroxyl functional group.
2. Alcohols are highly soluble in water.
3. Alcohols are sometimes used as biofuels.

A. Only 1        C. Only 3        E. 1, 2 and 3
B. Only 2        D. 1 and 2

## Question 431:

Which row of the table below is correct?

| | | Non-Reducible Hydrocarbon | | | Reducible Hydrocarbon | |
|---|---|---|---|---|---|---|
| A | $C_nH_{2n}$ | $Br_{2(aq)}$ remains brown | Saturated | $C_nH_{2n+2}$ | Turns $Br_{2(aq)}$ colourless | Unsaturated |
| B | $C_nH_{2n+2}$ | Turns $Br_{2(aq)}$ colourless | Unsaturated | $C_nH_{2n}$ | $Br_{2(aq)}$ remains brown | Saturated |
| C | $C_nH_{2n}$ | $Br_{2(aq)}$ remains brown | Unsaturated | $C_nH_{2n+2}$ | Turns $Br_{2(aq)}$ colourless | Saturated |
| D | $C_nH_{2n+2}$ | Turns $Br_{2(aq)}$ colourless | Saturated | $C_nH_{2n}$ | $Br_{2(aq)}$ remains brown | Unsaturated |
| E | $C_nH_{2n+2}$ | $Br_{2(aq)}$ remains brown | Saturated | $C_nH_{2n}$ | Turns $Br_{2(aq)}$ colourless | Unsaturated |

## Question 432:

How many grams of magnesium chloride are formed when 10 grams of magnesium oxide are dissolved in excess hydrochloric acid? Relative atomic masses: Mg = 24, O = 16, H = 1, Cl = 35.5

A. 10.00
B. 14.95
C. 20.00
D. 23.75
E. 47.55

## Question 433:

Pentadecane has the molecular formula $C_{15}H_{32}$. Which one of the following statements is true?

A. Pentadecane has a lower boiling point than pentane.
B. Pentadecane is more flammable than pentane.
C. Pentadecane is more volatile than pentane.
D. Pentadecane is more viscous than pentane.
E. All of the above.

## Question 434:

The rate of reaction is normally dependent upon:

1. The temperature.
2. The concentration of reactants.
3. The concentration of the catalyst.
4. The surface area of the catalyst.

A. 1 and 2
B. 2 and 3
C. 2, 3 and 4
D. 1, 3 and 4
E. 1, 2, 3 and 4

**Question 435:**

The equation below shows the complete combustion of a sample of unknown hydrocarbon in excess oxygen.

$C_aH_b + O_2 \rightarrow cCO_2 + dH_2O$

The reaction yielded 176 grams of $CO_2$ and 108 grams of $H_2O$. What is the most likely formula of the unknown hydrocarbon? Relative atomic masses:

$H = 1, C = 12, O = 16$.

A. $CH_4$      B. $CH_3$      C. $C_2H_6$      D. $C_3H_9$      E. $C_2H_4$

**Question 436:**

What type of reaction must ethanol undergo in order to be converted to ethylene oxide ($C_2H_4O$)?

A. Oxidation      C. Dehydration      E. Redox

B. Reduction      D. Hydration

**Question 437:**

What values of *a*, *b* and *c* balance the equation below?

$$a\ Ba_3N_2 + 6H_2O \rightarrow b\ Ba(OH)_2 + c\ NH_3$$

|   | a | b | c |
|---|---|---|---|
| A | 1 | 2 | 3 |
| B | 1 | 3 | 2 |
| C | 2 | 1 | 3 |
| D | 2 | 3 | 1 |
| E | 3 | 1 | 2 |

**Question 438:**

What values of *a*, *b* and *c* balance the equation below?

$$a\ FeS + 7O_2 \rightarrow b\ Fe_2O_3 + c\ SO_2$$

|   | a | b | c |
|---|---|---|---|
| A | 3 | 2 | 2 |
| B | 2 | 4 | 1 |
| C | 3 | 1 | 5 |
| D | 4 | 1 | 3 |
| E | 4 | 2 | 4 |

**Question 439:**

Magnesium consists of 3 isotopes: $Mg^{23}$, $Mg^{25}$, and $Mg^{26}$ which are found naturally in a ratio of 80:10:10. Calculate the relative atomic mass of magnesium.

A. 23.3      C. 23.5      E. 24.6

B. 23.4      D. 23.6

**Question 440:**

Consider the three reactions:

1. $Cl_2 + 2Br^- \rightarrow 2Cl^- + Br_2$
2. $Cu^{2+} + Mg \rightarrow Cu + Mg^{2+}$
3. $Fe_2O_3 + 3CO \rightarrow 2Fe + 3CO_2$

Which of the following statements are correct?

A. $Cl_2$ and $Fe_2O_3$ are reducing agents.
B. CO and $Cu^{2+}$ are oxidising agents.
C. $Br_2$ is a stronger oxidising agent than $Cl_2$.
D. Mg is a stronger reducing agent than Cu.

**Question 441:**

Which row of the table below best describes the properties of NaCl?

| | Melting Point | Solubility in Water | Conducts electricity? | |
| | | | As a solid | In solution |
|---|---|---|---|---|
| A | High | Yes | Yes | Yes |
| B | High | No | Yes | No |
| C | High | Yes | No | Yes |
| D | High | No | No | No |
| E | Low | Yes | Yes | Yes |

**Question 442:**

80g of sodium hydroxide reacts with excess zinc nitrate to produce zinc hydroxide. Calculate the mass of zinc hydroxide produced. Relative atomic mass: N = 14, Zn = 65, O = 16, Na = 23.

A. 49g          C. 99g          E. 198g
B. 95g          D. 100g

**Question 443:**

Which of the following statements is correct?

A. The reaction between all Group 1 metals and water is exothermic.
B. Sodium reacts less vigorously with water than potassium does.
C. All Group 1 metals react with water to produce elemental hydrogen.
D. All Group 1 metals react with water to produce a metal hydroxide.
E. All of the above.

**Question 444:**
Which one of the following statements is correct?

A. NaCl can be separated using sieves.
B. $CO_2$ can be separated using electrolysis.
C. Dyes in a sample of ink can be separated using chromatography.
D. Oil and water can be separated using fractional distillation.
E. Methane and diesel can be separated using a separating funnel.

**Question 445:**
Which of the following statements about the reaction between caesium and fluoride are correct?

1. It is an exothermic reaction and therefore requires catalysts.
2. It results in the formation of a salt.
3. The addition of water will make the reaction safer.

A. Only 1       C. Only 3       E. 2 and 3
B. Only 2       D. 1 and 2

**Question 446:**
Which of the following statements is generally true about stable isotopes?

1. The nucleus contains an equal number of neutrons and protons.
2. The nuclear charge is equal and opposite to the peripheral charge due to the orbiting electrons.
3. They can all undergo radioactive decay into more stable isotopes.

A. Only 1       C. Only 3       E. 2 and 3
B. Only 2       D. 1 and 2

**Question 447:**
Why do most salts have very high melting points?

A. Their surface is able to radiate away a significant portion of the heat to their environment.
B. The ionic bonds holding them together are very strong.
C. The covalent bonds holding them together are very strong.
D. They tend to form large macromolecules as each salt molecule bonds with multiple other molecules.
E. All of the above.

**Question 448:**
A bottle of water contains 306ml of pure deionised water. How many protons are in the bottle from the water?
[Avogadro Constant = $6 \times 10^{23}$ mol$^{-1}$]

A. $1 \times 10^{22}$       B. $1 \times 10^{23}$       C. $1 \times 10^{24}$       D. $1 \times 10^{25}$       E. $1 \times 10^{26}$

**Question 449:**

On analysis, an organic substance is found to contain 41.4% carbon, 55.2% oxygen and 3.45% hydrogen by mass. Which of the following could be the empirical formula of this substance?

A. $C_3O_3H_6$

B. $C_3O_3H_{12}$

C. $C_4O_2H_4$

D. $C_4O_4H_4$

E. More information needed

**Question 450:**

A is a Group 2 element and B is a Group 17 element. Which row best describes what happens when A reacts with B?

| | B is | Formula |
|---|---|---|
| **A** | Reduced | AB |
| **B** | Reduced | $A_2B$ |
| **C** | Reduced | $AB_2$ |
| **D** | Oxidised | AB |
| **E** | Oxidised | $A_2B$ |

# SECTION 2: PHYSICS

If you haven't done physics at AS level then you'll have to ensure that you are confident with commonly examined topics like Newtonian mechanics, electrical circuits and radioactive decay as you may not have covered these at GCSE level depending on the specification you did.

The first step to improving in this section of the BMAT is to memorise by rote all the equations listed on the next page, and build up an understanding of their relationship to the concepts listed on the BMAT specification.

The majority of the physics questions involve a fair bit of maths – this means you need to be comfortable with converting between units and also powers of 10. Manipulating numbers at speed without using a calculator is the key to success in this section, alongside memorising the equations listed. **Most BMAT physics questions require two-step calculations**. Consider the example:

A metal ball is released from the roof of a 20-metre building. Assuming air resistance is negligible; calculate the velocity at which the ball hits the ground. [$g = 10ms^{-2}$]

A.   5 ms⁻ˡ              B.   10 ms⁻ˡ              C.   15 ms⁻ˡ              D.   20 ms⁻ˡ              E.   25 ms⁻ˡ

When the ball hits the ground, all of its gravitational potential energy has been converted to kinetic energy.

Thus, $E_p = E_k$:
$$mg\Delta h = \frac{mv^2}{2}$$
Thus, $v = \sqrt{2gh} = \sqrt{2 \text{ x } 10 \text{ x } 20}$
$$= \sqrt{400} = 20ms^{-1}$$

Here, you were required to not only recall two equations but apply and rearrange them very quickly to get the answer - all in under 60 seconds. Thus, it is easy to understand why the physics questions are generally much harder to complete in the time given than the biology and some of the chemistry questions.

Note that if you were comfortable with basic Newtonian mechanics, you could have also solved this using a single suvat equation: $v^2 = u^2 + 2as$
$$v = \sqrt{2 \text{ x } 10 \text{ x } 20} = 20ms^{-1}$$

This is why you're **strongly advised to learn the 'suvat' equations** on the next page even if they're technically not on the syllabus for the BMAT.

### SI Units
Remember that in order to get the correct answer you must always work in SI units i.e. do your calculations in terms of metres (not centimetres) and kilograms (not grams), etc.

*Top tip!* Knowing SI units is extremely useful because they allow you to **'work out' equations** if you ever forget them e.g. the units for density are $kg/m^3$. Since kg is the SI unit for mass, and $m^3$ is represented by volume –the equation for density must be = Mass/Volume.

This can also work the other way, for example we know that the unit for pressure is pascal (Pa). But based on the fact that Pressure = Force/Area, a pascal must be equivalent to $N/m^2$. Some physics questions will test your ability to manipulate units like this so it's important you are comfortable converting between them.

## FORMULAE YOU MUST KNOW:

### Equations of Motion:

- $s = ut + 0.5at^2$
- $v = u + at$
- $a = (v-u)/t$
- $v^2 = u^2 + 2as$

### Equations relating to Force:

- Force = mass x acceleration
- Force = Momentum/Time
- Pressure = Force / Area
- Moment of a Force = Force x Distance
- Work done = Force x Displacement

### For objects in equilibrium:

- Sum of clockwise moments = Sum of anti-clockwise moments
- Sum of all resultant forces = 0

### Equations relating to Energy:

- Kinetic Energy = $0.5 \, mv^2$
- $\Delta$ in Gravitational Potential Energy = $mg\Delta h$
- Energy Efficiency = (Useful energy/ Total energy) x 100%

### Equations relating to Power:

- Power = Work done / time
- Power = Energy transferred / time
- Power = Force x velocity

## Electrical Equations:

- $Q = It$
- $V = IR$
- $P = IV = I^2R = V^2/R$
- V = Potential difference (V, Volts)
- R = Resistance (Ohms)
- P = Power (W, Watts)
- Q = Charge (C, Coulombs)
- t= Time (s, seconds)

| Factor | Text | Symbol |
|--------|------|--------|
| $10^{12}$ | Tera | T |
| $10^{9}$ | Giga | G |
| $10^{6}$ | Mega | M |
| $10^{3}$ | Kilo | k |
| $10^{2}$ | Hecto | h |
| $10^{-1}$ | Deci | d |
| $10^{-2}$ | Centi | c |
| $10^{-3}$ | Milli | m |
| $10^{-6}$ | Micro | $\mu$ |
| $10^{-9}$ | Nano | n |
| $10^{-12}$ | Pico | p |

For Transformers: $\frac{V_p}{V_s} = \frac{n_p}{n_s}$ where:

- V: Potential difference
- n: Number of turns (on coil)
- p: Primary
- s: Secondary

## Other:

- Weight = mass x $g$
- Density = Mass / Volume
- Momentum = Mass x Velocity
- $g = 9.81$ ms$^{-2}$ (unless otherwise stated)

# PHYSICS QUESTIONS

### Question 451:
Which one of the following statements is **FALSE**?

A. Electromagnetic waves cause things to heat up.
B. X-rays and gamma rays can knock electrons out of their orbits.
C. Loud sounds can make objects vibrate.
D. Wave power can be used to generate electricity.
E. The amplitude of a wave determines its mass.

### Question 452:
A spacecraft is analysing a newly discovered exoplanet. A rock of unknown mass falls on the planet from a height of 30 m. Given that $g = 5.4$ ms$^{-2}$ on the planet, calculate the speed of the rock when it hits the ground and the time it took to fall.

| | Speed (ms⁻¹) | Time (s) |
|---|---|---|
| A | 18 | 3.3 |
| B | 18 | 3.1 |
| C | 12 | 3.3 |
| D | 10 | 3.7 |
| E | 9 | 2.3 |

### Question 453:
A canoe floating on the sea rises and falls 7 times in 49 seconds. The waves pass it at a speed of 5 ms⁻¹. How long are the waves?

A. 12 m        B. 22 m        C. 25 m        D. 35 m        E. 57 m

### Question 454:
Miss Orrell lifts her 37.5 kg bike for a distance of 1.3 m in 5 s. The acceleration of free fall is 10 ms⁻². What is the average power that she generates?

A. 9.8 W
B. 12.9 W
C. 57.9 W
D. 79.5 W
E. 97.5W

**Question 455:**

A truck accelerates at 5.6 ms$^{-2}$ from rest for 8 seconds. Calculate the final speed and the distance travelled in 8 seconds.

| | Final Speed (ms$^{-1}$) | Distance (m) |
|---|---|---|
| **A** | 40.8 | 119.2 |
| **B** | 40.8 | 129.6 |
| **C** | 42.8 | 179.2 |
| **D** | 44.1 | 139.2 |
| **E** | 44.8 | 179.2 |

**Question 456:**

Which of the following statements is true when a skydiver jumps out of a plane?

A. The skydiver leaves the plane and will accelerate until the air resistance is greater than their weight.
B. The skydiver leaves the plane and will accelerate until the air resistance is less than their weight.
C. The skydiver leaves the plane and will accelerate until the air resistance equals their weight.
D. The skydiver leaves the plane and will accelerate until the air resistance equals their weight squared.
E. The skydiver will travel at a constant velocity after leaving the plane.

**Question 457:**

A 100 g apple falls on Isaac's head from a height of 20 m. Calculate the apple's momentum before the point of impact.
Take g = 10 ms$^{-2}$

A.  0.1 kgms$^{-1}$          C.  1 kgms$^{-1}$          E.  10 kgms$^{-1}$
B.  0.2 kgms$^{-1}$          D.  2 kgms$^{-1}$

**Question 458:**

Which of the following characteristics do all electromagnetic waves all have in common?

1.  They can travel through a vacuum.
2.  They can be reflected.
3.  They are the same length.
4.  They have the same amount of energy.

A.  1, 2 and 3 only          C.  4 and 5 only          E.  1 and 2 only
B.  1, 2, 3 and 4 only          D.  3 and 4 only

**Question 459:**

A battery with an internal resistance of 0.8 Ω and e.m.f of 36 V is used to power a drill with resistance 1 Ω. What is the current in the circuit when the drill is connected to the power supply?

A.  5 A          B.  10 A          C.  15 A          D.  20 A          E.  25 A          F.  30 A

**Question 460:**
Officer Bailey throws a 20 g dart at a speed of 100 ms$^{-1}$. It strikes the dartboard and is brought to rest in 10 milliseconds. Calculate the average force exerted on the dart by the dartboard.

A. 0.2 N                    C. 20 N                    E. 2,000 N
B. 2 N                      D. 200 N                   F. 20,000 N

**Question 461:**
Professor Huang lifts a 50 kg bag through a distance of 0.7 m in 3 s. What average power does she generate to 3 significant figures? Take $g = 10$ms$^{-2}$

A. 113 W                    C. 115 W                   E. 117 W
B. 114 W                    D. 116 W

**Question 462:**
An electric scooter is travelling at a speed of 30 ms$^{-1}$ and is kept going at a constant speed against a 50 N frictional force by a driving force of 300 N in the direction of motion. Given that the engine runs at 200 V, calculate the current in the scooter.

A. 4.5 A                    C. 450 A                   E. 45,000 A
B. 45 A                     D. 4,500 A

**Question 463:**
Which of the following statements about the physical definition of work are correct?

1. $Work\ done = \frac{Force}{distance}$
2. The unit of work is equivalent to kgms$^{-2}$.
3. Work is defined as a force causing displacement of the body upon which it acts.

A. Only 1                   C. Only 3                  E. 2 and 3
B. Only 2                   D. 1 and 2

**Question 464:**
Which of the following statements about kinetic energy are correct?
1. It is defined as $E_k = \frac{mv^2}{2}$
2. The unit of kinetic energy is equivalent to Pa x m$^3$.
3. Kinetic energy is equal to the amount of energy needed to decelerate the body in question from its current speed.

A. Only 1              C. 2 and 3         E. 1, 2 and 3
B. Only 2              D. 1 and 3

**Question 465:**

In relation to radiation, which of the following statements is **FALSE**?

A. Radiation is the emission of energy from a substance in the form of waves or particles.
B. Radiation can be either ionizing or non-ionizing.
C. Gamma radiation has very high energy.
D. Alpha radiation is of higher energy than beta radiation.
E. X-rays are an example of wave radiation.

**Question 466:**

In relation to the physical definition of half-life, which of the following statements are correct?

1. In radioactive decay, the half-life is independent of atom type and isotope.
2. Half-life is defined as the time required for exactly half of the entities to decay.
3. Half-life applies to situations of both exponential and non-exponential decay.

A. Only 1
B. Only 2
C. Only 3
D. 1 and 2
E. 2 and 3
F. 1 and 3

**Question 467:**

A radioactive element has a half life of 24 days. After 192 days, it has a count rate of 56.
What was the original count rate?

A. 7,168
B. 14,280
C. 14,336
D. 28,672
E. 43,008

**Question 468:**

Which of the following statements concerning radioactive decay is / are true?

1. As a material decays, the rate of decay decreases.
2. All nuclei of the same element will have the same half-life, as it is an innate quality of an element.
3. Radioactive decay is a highly predictable process

A. Only 1
B. Only 2
C. Only 3
D. 1 and 2
E. 2 and 3

**Question 469:**

Two identical resistors ($R_a$ and $R_b$) are connected in a series circuit. Which of the following statements are true?

1. The current through both resistors is the same.
2. The voltage through both resistors is the same.
3. The voltage across the two resistors is given by Ohm's Law.

A. Only 1          C. Only 3          E. 1, 2 and 3
B. Only 2          D. 1 and 2

**Question 470:**

The sun is 8 light-minutes away from the earth. Estimate the circumference of the earth's orbit around the sun. Assume that the earth is in a circular orbit around the sun. Speed of light = $3 \times 10^8$ ms$^{-1}$

A.  $10^{24}$ m                    C.  $10^{18}$ m                    E.  $10^{12}$ m
B.  $10^{21}$ m                    D.  $10^{15}$ m

**Question 471:**

Which of the following statements about calculating speed are true?

1.  Speed is the same as velocity.
2.  The internationally standardised unit for speed is ms$^{-2}$.
3.  Velocity = distance/time.

A.  Only 1          C.  Only 2          E.  None of
B.  1 and 2        D.  Only 3                the above

**Question 472:**

Which of the following statements best defines Ohm's Law?

A. The current passing through an insulator between two points is indirectly proportional to the potential difference across the two points.
B. The current passing through an insulator between two points is directly proportional to the potential difference across the two points.
C. The current passing through a conductor between two points is inversely proportional to the potential difference across the two points.
D. The current passing through a conductor between two points is proportional to the square of the potential difference across the two points.
E. The current passing through a conductor between two points is directly proportional to the potential difference across the two points.

**Question 473:**

Which of the following statements regarding Newton's Second Law are correct?

1. For objects at rest, the resultant force must be 0 Newtons
2. Force = Mass x Acceleration
3. Force = Rate of change of Momentum

A. Only 1    C. 1 and 3    E. 1, 2 and 3
B. 2 and 3   D. 1 and 2

**Question 474:**

Which of the following equations concerning electrical circuits are correct?

1. $Charge = \frac{Voltage \; x \; time}{Resistance}$

2. $Charge = \frac{Power \; x \; time}{Voltage}$

3. $Charge = \frac{Current \; x \; time}{Resistance}$

A. Only 1    C. Only 3    E. 2 and 3
B. Only 2    D. 1 and 2

**Question 475:**

An elevator has a mass of 1,600 kg and is carrying passengers that have a combined mass of 200 kg. A constant frictional force of 4,000 N retards its motion upward. What force must the motor provide for the elevator to move with an upward acceleration of 1 ms$^{-2}$? Assume: $g = 10$ ms$^{-2}$

A. 1,190 N    B. 11,900 N    C. 18,000 N    D. 22,000 N    E. 23,800 N

**Question 476:**

A 1,000 kg car accelerates from rest at 5 ms$^{-2}$ for 10 s. Then, a braking force is applied to bring it to rest within 20 seconds. What is the total distance travelled by the car?

A. 125 m    C. 650 m
B. 250 m    D. 750 m    E. More information needed

**Question 477:**

An electric heater is connected to 120 V mains by a copper wire that has a resistance of 8 ohms. What is the power of the heater?

A. 90W    B. 180W    C. 900W    D. 1800W    E. More information needed

**Question 478:**

In a particle accelerator, electrons are accelerated through a potential difference of 40 MV and emerge with an energy of 40MeV ($1$ MeV $= 1.60 \times 10^{-13}$ J). Each pulse contains 5,000 electrons. The current is zero between pulses. Assuming that the electrons have zero energy prior to being accelerated what is the power delivered by the electron beam?

A. 1 kW        C. 100 kW        E. More information needed

B. 10 kW        D. 1,000 kW

**Question 479:**

Which **one** of the following statements is **true**?

A. When an object is in equilibrium with its surroundings, there is no energy transferred to or from the object and so its temperature remains constant.

B. When an object is in equilibrium with its surroundings, it radiates and absorbs energy at the same rate and so its temperature remains constant.

C. Radiation is faster than convection but slower than conduction.

D. Radiation is faster than conduction but slower than convection.

E. None of the above.

**Question 480:**

A 6kg block is pulled from rest along a horizontal frictionless surface by a constant horizontal force of 12 N. Calculate the speed of the block after it has moved 300 cm.

A. $2\sqrt{3}\,ms^{-1}$        C. $4\sqrt{3}\,ms^{-1}$        E. $\sqrt{\frac{3}{2}}\,ms^{-1}$

B. $4\sqrt{3}\,ms^{-1}$        D. $12\,ms^{-1}$

**Question 481:**

A 100 V heater heats 1.5 litres of pure water from 10°C to 50°C in 50 minutes. Given that 1 kg of pure water requires 4,000 J to raise its temperature by 1°C, calculate the resistance of the heater.

A. 12.5 ohms        C. 125 ohms        E. 500 ohms

B. 25 ohms        D. 250 ohms

**Question 482:**

Which of the following statements are **true**?

1. The half life of a radioactive substance is equal to half the time taken for its nuclei to decay.
2. When a nucleus emits a beta particle, it is converted to a new element.
3. When a nucleus emits an alpha particle, one of its neutrons becomes a proton and an electron.

A. Only 1        C. 2 only        E. None of

B. 2 and 3        D. 1 and 2          the above

**Question 483:**

Which of the following statements are **true**? Assume $g = 10$ ms$^{-2}$.

1. Gravitational potential energy is defined as $\Delta E_p = m \times g \times \Delta h$.
2. Gravitational potential energy is a measure of the work done against gravity.
3. A reservoir situated 1 km above ground level with $10^6$ litres of water has a potential energy of 1 Giga Joule.

A. Only 1          C. Only 3          E. 1, 2 and 3
B. Only 2          D. 1 and 3

**Question 484:**

Which of the following statements are correct in relation to Newton's 3rd law?

1. For every action there is an equal and opposite reaction.
2. According to Newton's 3rd law, there are no isolated forces.
3. When a rifle recoils as a bullet is fired from it, according to Newton's third law of motion, the acceleration of the recoiling rifle is the same size as the acceleration of the bullet.

A. Only 1          C. 2 and 3          E. 1, 2 and 3
B. Only 2          D. 1 and 2

**Question 485:**

Which of the following statements are correct?
1. Positively charged objects have gained electrons.
2. Electrical charge in a circuit over a period of time can be calculated if the voltage and resistance are known.
3. Objects can be charged by friction.

A. Only 1          C. Only 3          E. 2 and 3          G. 1, 2 and 3
B. Only 2          D. 1 and 2          F. 1 and 3

**Question 486:**

Which of the following statements is true?

A. The gravitational force between two objects is independent of their mass.
B. Each planet in the solar system exerts a gravitational force on the Earth.
C. Two objects dropped from the Eiffel tower will always land on the ground at the same time if they have the same mass.
D. All of the above.
E. None of the above.

**Question 487:**

Which of the following best defines an electrical conductor?

A.  Conductors are usually made from metals, and they conduct electrical charge in multiple directions.
B.  Conductors are usually made from non-metals, and they conduct electrical charge in multiple directions.
C.  Conductors are usually made from metals, and they conduct electrical charge in one fixed direction.
D.  Conductors are usually made from non-metals, and they conduct electrical charge in one fixed direction.
E.  Conductors allow the passage of electrical charge with zero resistance because they contain freely mobile charged particles.

**Question 488:**

An 800 kg compact car delivers 20% of its power output to its wheels. If the car has a mileage of 30 miles/gallon and travels at a speed of 60 miles/hour, how much power is delivered to the wheels?  I gallon of petrol contains $9 \times 10^8$ J.

A.  10 kW          B.  20 kW          C.  40 kW          D.  50 kW          E.  100 kW

**Question 489:**

Which of the following statements about beta radiation are true?

1.  After a beta particle is emitted, the atomic mass number is unchanged.
2.  Beta radiation can penetrate paper but not aluminium foil.
3.  A beta particle is emitted from the nucleus of the atom when an electron transforms to a neutron.

A.  I only                    C.  I and 3                    E.  2 and 3
B.  2 only                    D.  I and 2                    F.  I, 2 and 3

**Question 490:**

A car with a weight of 15,000 N is travelling at a speed of 15 ms$^{-1}$ when it crashes into a wall and is brought to rest in 10 milliseconds. Calculate the average braking force exerted on the car by the wall. Take g = 10 ms$^{-2}$

A.  $1.25 \times 10^4 N$              C.  $1.25 \times 10^6 N$              E.  $2.25 \times 10^6 N$
B.  $1.25 \times 10^5 N$              D.  $2.25 \times 10^4 N$

**Question 491:**

Which of the following statements are correct?

1.  Electrical insulators are usually metals e.g. copper.
2.  The flow of charge through electrical insulators is extremely low.
3.  Electrical insulators can be charged by rubbing them together.

A.  Only I                    C.  Only 3                    E.  2 and 3
B.  Only 2                    D.  I and 2

**The following information is needed for Questions 492 and 493:**

This graph represents a car's movement. At t=0 the car's displacement was 0 m.

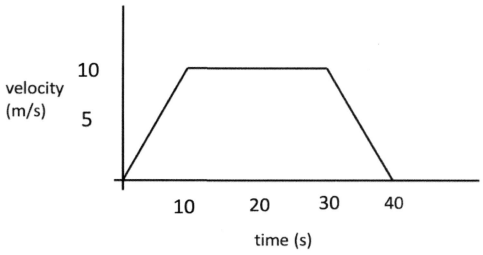

**Question 492:**

Which of the following statements are **NOT true**?

1. The car is reversing after t = 30.
2. The car moves with constant acceleration from t = 0 to t = 10.
3. The car moves with constant speed from t = 10 to t = 30.

A. 1 only      C. 3 only      E. 1 and 2

B. 2 only      D. 1 and 3

**Question 493:**

Calculate the distance travelled by the car.

A. 200 m      C. 350 m      E. More information needed

B. 300 m      D. 400 m

**Question 494:**

A 1,000 kg rocket is launched during a thunderstorm and reaches a constant velocity 30 seconds after launch. Suddenly, a strong gust of wind acts on the rocket for 5 seconds with a force of 10,000 N in the direction of movement.
What is the resulting change in velocity?

A. 0.5 ms⁻¹      C. 50 ms⁻¹      E. More information needed

B. 5 ms⁻¹      D. 500 ms⁻¹

**Question 495:**
A 0.5 tonne crane lifts a 0.01 tonne wardrobe by 100 cm in 5,000 milliseconds.
Calculate the average power generated by the crane. Take $g = 10$ ms$^{-2}$.

A.  0.2 W
B.  2 W

C.  5 W
D.  20 W

E.  More information needed

**Question 496:**
A 20 V battery is connected to a circuit consisting of a 1 Ω and 2 Ω resistor in parallel. Calculate the overall current of the circuit.

A.  6.67 A
B.  8 A

C.  12 A
D.  20 A

E.  30 A

**Question 497:**
Which **one** of the following statements is correct?

A.  The speed of light changes when it enters water.
B.  The speed of light changes when it leaves water.
C.  The direction of light changes when it enters water.
D.  The direction of light changes when it leaves water.
E.  All of the above.
F.  None of the above.

**Question 498:**
In a parallel circuit, a 60 V battery is connected to two branches. Branch *A* contains 6 identical 5 Ω resistors and branch *B* contains 2 identical 10 Ω resistors.

Calculate the current in branches *A* and *B*.

| | $I_A$ (A) | $I_B$ (A) |
|---|---|---|
| **A** | 0 | 6 |
| **B** | 6 | 0 |
| **C** | 2 | 3 |
| **D** | 3 | 2 |
| **E** | 1 | 5 |

**Question 499:**
Calculate the voltage of an electrical circuit that has a power output of 50,000,000,000 nW and a current of 0.000000004 GA.

A. 0.0125 GV
B. 0.0125 MV
C. 0.0125 kV
D. 0.0125 nV
E. 0.0125 mV

**Question 500:**
Which of the following statements about radioactive decay is correct?

A. Radioactive decay is highly predictable.
B. An unstable element will continue to decay until it reaches a stable nuclear configuration.
C. All forms of radioactive decay release gamma rays.
D. All forms of radioactive decay release X-rays.
E. None of the above.

**Question 501:**
A circuit contains three identical resistors of unknown resistance connected in series with a 15 V battery. The power output of the circuit is 60 W.
Calculate the overall resistance of the circuit when two further identical resistors are added to it.

A. 0.125 $\Omega$
B. 1.25 $\Omega$
C. 3.75 $\Omega$
D. 6.25 $\Omega$
E. 18.75 $\Omega$

**Question 502:**
The engine in a 5,000 kg tractor uses 1 litre of fuel to move 0.1 km. 1 ml of the fuel contains 20 kJ of energy. Calculate the engine's efficiency. Take $g = 10$ ms$^{-2}$

A. 2.5 %
B. 25 %
C. 38 %
D. 50 %
E. More information needed.

**Question 503:**
Which of the following statements are correct?

1. Electromagnetic induction occurs when a wire moves relative to a magnet.
2. Electromagnetic induction occurs when a magnetic field changes.
3. An electrical current is generated when a coil rotates in a magnetic field.

A. Only 1
B. 1 and 3
C. 2 and 3
D. 1 and 2
E. 1, 2 and 3

**Question 504:**

Which of the following statements are correct regarding parallel circuits?

1. The current flowing through a branch is dependent on the resistance of that branch.
2. The total current flowing into the branches is equal to the total current flowing out of the branches.
3. An ammeter will always give the same reading regardless of its location in the circuit.

A. Only I
B. Only 2
C. 2 and 3
D. I and 2
E. All of the above

**Question 505:**

Which of the following statements regarding series circuits are true?

1. The overall resistance of a circuit is given by the sum of all resistors in the circuit.
2. Electrical current moves from the positive terminal to the negative terminal.
3. Electrons move from the positive terminal to the negative terminal.

A. Only I
B. Only 2
C. Only 3
D. I and 2
E. I and 3

**Question 506:**

The graphs below show current vs. voltage plots for 4 different electrical components.

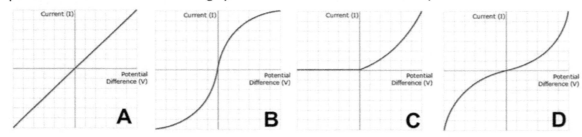

Which of the following graphs represents a resistor at constant temperature, and which represents a filament lamp?

|   | Fixed Resistor | Filament Lamp |
|---|----------------|---------------|
| A | A              | B             |
| B | A              | C             |
| C | D              | D             |
| D | C              | A             |
| E | C              | C             |

~ 176 ~

**Question 507:**

Which of the following statements are true about vectors?

A. Vectors can be added or subtracted.
B. All vector quantities have a defined magnitude.
C. All vector quantities have a defined direction.
D. All of the above.
E. None of the above.

**Question 508:**

The acceleration due to gravity on the Earth is six times greater than that on the moon. Dr Tyson records the weight of a rock as 250 N on the moon.

Calculate the density of the rock given that it has a volume of 250 cm³. Take $g_{Earth}$ = 10 ms⁻²

A. 0.2 kg/cm³          C. 0.6 kg/cm³          E. More information needed.
B. 0.5 kg/cm³          D. 0.7 kg/cm³

**Question 509:**

A radioactive element $X^{225}_{78}$ undergoes alpha decay. What is the atomic mass and atomic number after 5 alpha particles have been released?

|   | Mass Number | Atomic Number |
|---|---|---|
| A | 200 | 56 |
| B | 200 | 58 |
| C | 215 | 64 |
| D | 205 | 68 |
| E | 215 | 58 |

**Question 510:**

A 20 A current passes through a circuit with resistance of 10 Ω. The circuit is connected to a transformer that contains a primary coil with 5 turns and a secondary coil with 10 turns. Calculate the potential difference exiting the transformer.

A. 100 V          C. 400 V          E. 2,000 V
B. 200 V          D. 500 V

**Question 511:**

A metal ball of unknown mass is dropped from an altitude of 1 km and reaches terminal velocity 300 m before it hits the ground. Given that resistive forces do a total of 10 kJ of work for the last 100 m before the ball hits the ground, calculate the mass of the ball. Take $g$ = 10ms⁻².

A. 1 kg          C. 5 kg          E. More information needed.
B. 2 kg          D. 10 kg

**Question 512:**

Which of the following statements about the electromagnetic spectrum is correct?

A. The wavelength of ultraviolet waves is shorter than that of x-rays.
B. For waves in the electromagnetic spectrum, wavelength is directly proportional to frequency.
C. Waves in the electromagnetic spectrum travel at the speed of sound.
D. Humans are able to visualise the majority of the electromagnetic spectrum.
E. None of the above.

**Question 513:**

In relation to the Doppler effect, which of the following statements are true?
1. If an object emitting a wave moves towards the sensor, the wavelength increases and frequency decreases.
2. An object that originally emitted a wave of a wavelength of 20 mm followed by a second reading delivering a wavelength of 15 mm is moving towards the sensor.
3. The faster the object is moving away from the sensor, the greater the increase in frequency.

A. Only 1          C. Only 3          E. 2 and 3
B. Only 2          D. 1 and 2

**Question 514:**

A 5 g bullet travels at 1 km/s and hits a brick wall. It penetrates 50 cm before being brought to rest 100 ms after impact. Calculate the average braking force exerted by the wall on the bullet.

A. 50 N             C. 5,000 N         E. More information needed.
B. 500 N            D. 50,000 N

**Question 515:**

Polonium (Po) is a highly radioactive element that has no known stable isotope. $Po^{210}$ undergoes radioactive decay to $Pb^{206}$ and Y. Calculate the number of protons in 10 moles of Y. [Avogadro's Constant = $6 \times 10^{23}$ mol$^{-1}$]

A. 0                     C. $1.2 \times 10^{25}$      E. $2.4 \times 10^{25}$
B. $1.2 \times 10^{24}$      D. $2.4 \times 10^{24}$

**Question 516:**

Dr Sale measures the background radiation in a nuclear wasteland to be 1,000 Bq. He then detects a spike of 16,000 Bq from a nuclear rod made up of an unknown material. 300 days later, he visits and can no longer detect a reading higher than 1,000 Bq from the rod, even though it hasn't been disturbed.
What is the longest possible half-life of the nuclear rod?

A. 25 days          C. 75 days          E. More information needed
B. 50 days          D. 100 days

## Question 517:

A radioactive element $Y_{89}^{200}$ undergoes several stages of beta ($\beta^-$) and gamma decay. What are the numbers of protons and neutrons in the element after the emission of 5 beta particles and 2 gamma waves?

|   | Protons | Neutrons |
|---|---------|----------|
| A | 79      | 101      |
| B | 84      | 116      |
| C | 89      | 111      |
| D | 94      | 111      |
| E | 94      | 106      |

## Question 518:

Most symphony orchestras tune to 'standard pitch' (frequency = 440 Hz). When they are tuning, sound directly from the orchestra reaches audience members that are 500 m away in 1.5 seconds.
**Estimate** the wavelength of 'standard pitch'.

A. 0.05 m          C. 0.75 m          E.  More information needed
B. 0.5 m           D. 1.5 m

## Question 519:

A 1 kg cylindrical artillery shell with a radius of 50 mm is fired at a speed of 200 ms$^{-1}$. It strikes an armour-plated wall and is brought to rest in 500 μs.

Calculate the average pressure exerted on the artillery shell by the wall at the time of impact.

A. $5 \times 10^6$ Pa          C. $5 \times 10^8$ Pa          E.  More information needed
B. $5 \times 10^7$ Pa          D. $5 \times 10^9$ Pa

## Question 520:

A 1,000 W display fountain launches 120 litres of water straight up every minute. Given that the fountain is 10% efficient, calculate the maximum possible height that the stream of water could reach.
Assume that there is negligible air resistance and $g = 10$ ms$^{-2}$.

A. 1 m          C. 10 m          E.  50m
B. 5 m          D. 20 m

## Question 521

In relation to transformers, which of the following is true?
1.  Step up transformers increase the voltage leaving the transformer.
2.  In step down transformers, the number of turns in the primary coil is smaller than in the secondary coil.
3.  For transformers that are 100% efficient: $I_p V_p = I_s V_s$

A. Only 1          C. Only 3          E.  1 and 3
B. Only 2          D. 2 and 3

**Question 522:**

The half-life of Carbon-14 is 5,730 years. A bone is found that contains 6.25% of the amount of $C^{14}$ that would be found in a modern-day bone. How old is the bone?

A.  11,460 years
B.  17,190 years

C.  22,920 years
D.  28,650 years

E.  34,380 years

**Question 523:**

A wave has a velocity of 2,000 mm/s and a wavelength of 250 cm. What is its frequency in MHz?

A.  $8 \times 10^{-3}$ MHz
B.  $8 \times 10^{-4}$ MHz

C.  $8 \times 10^{-5}$ MHz
D.  $8 \times 10^{-6}$ MHz

E.  $8 \times 10^{-7}$ MHz

**Question 524:**

A radioactive element has a half-life of 25 days. After 350 days it has a count rate of 50. What was its original count rate?

A.  102,400
B.  162,240

C.  204,800
D.  409,600

E.  819,200

**Question 525:**

Which of the following units is **NOT** equivalent to a Volt (V)?

A.  $JA^{-1}s^{-1}$
B.  $WA^{-1}$

C.  $Nms^{-1}A^{-1}$
D.  $NmC$

E.  $JC^{-1}$

# SECTION 2: MATHS

BMAT maths questions are designed to be time-consuming, and a lack of proper exam technique can really trip up some candidates. During your question practice, you will have the opportunity to assess how quickly you are able to complete the calculations. If you find yourself consistently not finishing, it might be worth leaving the maths (and probably physics) questions until the very end of the paper, so you are able to complete as many of the other questions as possible under timed conditions. Good students sometimes have a habit of making easy questions difficult; remember that the BMAT only tests GCSE level knowledge so you are not expected to know or use calculus or trigonometry in any part of the exam.

Formulae you **MUST** know:

| 2D Shapes | | 3D Shapes | | |
|---|---|---|---|---|
| **Area** | | | **Surface Area** | **Volume** |
| **Circle** | πr² | **Cuboid** | Sum of all 6 faces | Length x width x height |
| **Parallelogram** | Base x Vertical height | **Cylinder** | 2 πr² + 2πrl | πr² x l |
| **Trapezium** | 0.5 x h x (a+b) | **Cone** | πr² + πrl | πr² x (h/3) |
| **Triangle** | 0.5 x base x height | **Sphere** | 4 πr² | (4/3) πr³ |

Even good students who are studying maths at A2 level can struggle with certain BMAT maths topics because they're usually glossed over at school. These include:

### Quadratic Formula

The solutions for a quadratic equation in the form $ax^2 + bx + c = 0$ are given by: $x = \frac{-b \pm \sqrt{b^2 - 4ac}}{2a}$

Remember that you can also use the discriminant to quickly see if a quadratic equation has any solutions:

$$If\ b^2 - 4ac < 0: No\ solutions$$
$$If\ b^2 - 4ac = 0: One\ solution$$
$$If\ b^2 - 4ac > 2: Two\ solutions$$

### Completing the Square

If a quadratic equation cannot be factorised easily and is in the format $ax^2 + bx + c = 0$ then you can rearrange it into the form $a\left(x + \frac{b}{2a}\right)^2 + \left[c - \frac{b^2}{4a}\right] = 0$

This looks more complicated than it is – remember that in the BMAT, you're extremely unlikely to get quadratic equations where $a > 1$ and an equation that doesn't have any easy factors. This gives you an easier equation: $\left(x + \frac{b}{2}\right)^2 + \left[c - \frac{b^2}{4}\right] = 0$ and is best understood with an example.

Consider: $x^2 + 6x + 10 = 0$

This equation cannot be factorised easily but note that: $x^2 + 6x - 10 = (x + 3)^2 - 19 = 0$

Therefore, $x = -3 \pm \sqrt{19}$. Completing the square is an important skill – make sure you're comfortable with it.

### Difference between 2 Squares

If you are asked to simplify expressions and find that there are no common factors but find that the expressions involve square numbers – you might be able to factorise by using the 'difference between two squares'.

For example, $x^2 - 25$ can also be expressed as $(x + 5)(x - 5)$.

# MATHS QUESTIONS

**Question 526:**

Robert has a box of building blocks. The box contains 8 yellow blocks and 12 red blocks. He picks three blocks from the box and stacks them up high. Calculate the probability that he stacks two red building blocks and one yellow building block, in **any** order.

A. $\dfrac{8}{20}$ 　　　 B. $\dfrac{44}{95}$ 　　　 C. $\dfrac{11}{18}$ 　　　 D. $\dfrac{8}{19}$ 　　　 E. $\dfrac{12}{20}$

**Question 527:**

Solve $\dfrac{3x+5}{5} + \dfrac{2x-2}{3} = 18$

A. 12.11 　　　 B. 13.21 　　　 C. 13.95 　　　 D. 15.2 　　　 E. 19

**Question 528:**

Solve $3x^2 + 11x - 20 = 0$

A. 0.75 and $-\dfrac{4}{3}$ 　　　　　　 C. -5 and $\dfrac{4}{3}$ 　　　　　　 E. 12 only

B. -0.75 and $\dfrac{4}{3}$ 　　　　　　 D. 5 and $\dfrac{4}{3}$

**Question 529:**

Express $\dfrac{5}{x+2} + \dfrac{3}{x-4}$ as a single fraction.

A. $\dfrac{15x-120}{(x+2)(x-4)}$ 　　　　　　 C. $\dfrac{8x-14}{(x+2)(x-4)}$ 　　　　　　 E. 24

B. $\dfrac{8x-26}{(x+2)(x-4)}$ 　　　　　　 D. $\dfrac{15}{8x}$

**Question 530:**

The value of p is directly proportional to the cube root of q. When p = 12, q = 27. Find the value of q when p = 24.

A. 32 　　　 B. 64 　　　 C. 124 　　　 D. 128 　　　 E. 216

**Question 531:**

Which of the following is equivalent to $(\sqrt{7} - 2)^4$?

A. $233 - 88\sqrt{7}$
B. $233 + 88\sqrt{7}$
C. $49 - 16$
D. $121 - 44\sqrt{7}$
E. $49 - 2$

**Question 532:**

Calculate: $\dfrac{2.302 \; x \; 10^5 + 2.302 \; 10^2}{1.151 \; x \; 10^{10}}$

A. 0.0000202
B. 0.00020002
C. 0.00002002
D. 0.00000002
E. 0.000002002

**Question 533:**

Given that $y^2 + \mathbf{a}y + \mathbf{b} = (y + 2)^2 - 5$, find the values of **a** and **b**.

|   | a  | b  |
|---|----|----|
| A | -1 | 4  |
| B | 1  | 9  |
| C | -1 | -9 |
| D | -9 | 1  |
| E | 4  | -1 |

**Question 534:**

Express $\dfrac{4}{5} + \dfrac{m-2n}{m+4n}$ as a single fraction in its simplest form:

A. $\dfrac{6m+6n}{5(m+4n)}$

B. $\dfrac{9m+26n}{5(m+4n)}$

C. $\dfrac{20m+6n}{5(m+4n)}$

D. $\dfrac{3m+9n}{5(m+4n)}$

E. $\dfrac{3(3m+2n)}{5(m+4n)}$

**Question 535:**

A is inversely proportional to the square root of B. When A = 4, B = 25.
Calculate the value of A when B = 16.

A. 0.8    B. 4    C. 5    D. 6    E. 10

**Question 536:**
S, T, U and V are points on the circumference of a circle, and O is the centre of the circle.

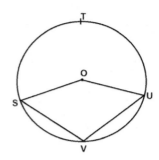

Given that angle SVU = 89°, calculate the size of the smaller angle SOU.

A. 89°          C. 102°          E. 182°
B. 91°          D. 178°

**Question 537:**
Open cylinder A has a surface area of 8π cm² and a volume of 2π cm³. Open cylinder B is an enlargement of A and has a surface area of 32π cm². Calculate the volume of cylinder B.

A. 2π cm³                    C. 10π cm³                    E. 16π cm³
B. 8π cm³                    D. 14π cm³

**Question 538:**
Express $\frac{8}{x(3-x)} - \frac{6}{x}$ in its simplest form.

A. $\frac{3x-10}{x(3-x)}$          C. $\frac{6x-10}{x(3-2x)}$          E. $\frac{6x-10}{x(3-x)}$

B. $\frac{3x+10}{x(3-x)}$          D. $\frac{6x-10}{x(3+2x)}$

**Question 539:**
A bag contains 10 balls. 9 of the balls are white and 1 is black. What is the probability that the black ball is drawn in the tenth and final draw if the drawn balls are not replaced?

A. 0          B. $\frac{1}{10}$          C. $\frac{1}{100}$          D. $\frac{1}{10^{10}}$          E. $\frac{1}{362,880}$

**Question 540:**
Gambit has an ordinary deck of 52 cards. What is the probability of Gambit drawing 2 Kings (without replacement)?

A. 0          B. $\frac{1}{169}$          C. $\frac{1}{221}$          D. $\frac{4}{663}$          E. None of the above

**Question 541:**
I have two identical unfair dice. The probability of rolling a 6 is twice as high as the probability of rolling any other number.
What is the probability that when I roll both dice the total will be 12?

A. 0          B. $\frac{4}{49}$          C. $\frac{1}{9}$          D. $\frac{2}{7}$          E. None of the above

**Question 542:**

A roulette wheel consists of 36 numbered spots and 1 zero spot (i.e. 37 spots in total).
What is the probability that the ball will stop in a spot either divisible by 3 or 2?

A. 0

B. $\frac{25}{37}$

C. $\frac{25}{36}$

D. $\frac{18}{37}$

E. $\frac{24}{37}$

**Question 543:**

I have a fair coin that I flip 4 times. What is the probability I get 2 heads and 2 tails?

A. $\frac{1}{16}$

B. $\frac{3}{16}$

C. $\frac{3}{8}$

D. $\frac{9}{16}$

E. None of the above

**Question 544:**

Shivun rolls two fair dice. What is the probability that he gets a total of 5, 6 or 7?

A. $\frac{9}{36}$

B. $\frac{7}{12}$

C. $\frac{1}{6}$

D. $\frac{5}{12}$

E. None of the above

**Question 545:**

Dr Savary has a bag that contains x red balls, y blue balls and z green balls (and no others). He pulls out a ball, replaces it, and then pulls out another. What is the probability that he picks one red ball and one green ball?

A. $\frac{2(x+y)}{x+y+z}$

B. $\frac{xz}{(x+y+z)^2}$

C. $\frac{2xz}{(x+y+z)^2}$

D. $\frac{(x+z)}{(x+y+z)^2}$

E. $\frac{4xz}{(x+y+z)^4}$

**Question 546:**

Mr Kilbane has a bag that contains x red balls, y blue balls and z green balls (and no others). He pulls out a ball, does **NOT** replace it, and then pulls out another. What is the probability that he picks one red ball and one blue ball?

A. $\frac{2xy}{(x+y+z)^2}$

B. $\frac{2xy}{(x+y+z)(x+y+z-1)}$

C. $\frac{2xy}{(x+y+z)^2}$

D. $\frac{xy}{(x+y+z)(x+y+z-1)}$

E. $\frac{4xy}{(x+y+z-1)^2}$

**Question 547:**

There are two tennis players. The first player wins the point with probability p, and the second player wins the point with probability 1-p. The rules of tennis say that the first player to score four points wins the game, unless the score is 4-3. At this point the first player to be two points ahead wins the game.

What is the probability that the first player wins in exactly 5 rounds?

A. $4p^4(1-p)$
B. $p^4(1-p)$
C. $4p(1-p)$
D. $4p(1-p)^4$
E. $4p^5(1-p)$

**Question 548:**

The equation below gives $y$ in terms of $x$.

$$y = 2(\frac{x}{4} - 7)^2 - 5$$

Rearrange the equation to give an expression for $x$ in terms of $y$.

A. $x = 28 \pm 4\sqrt{\frac{y+5}{2}}$

B. $x = 7 \pm 4\sqrt{\frac{y+5}{2}}$

C. $x = 28 \pm 4\sqrt{\frac{y-5}{2}}$

D. $x = 7 \pm 4\sqrt{\frac{y-5}{2}}$

E. $x = 28 \pm 4\sqrt{\frac{y\pm5}{2}}$

**Question 549:**

The volume of a sphere is $V = \frac{4}{3}\pi r^3$, and the surface area of a sphere is $S = 4\pi r^2$. Express S in terms of V

A. $S = (4\pi)^{2/3}(3V)^{2/3}$
B. $S = (8\pi)^{1/3}(3V)^{2/3}$
C. $S = (4\pi)^{1/3}(9V)^{2/3}$
D. $S = (4\pi)^{1/3}(3V)^{2/3}$
E. $S = (16\pi)^{1/3}(9V)^{2/3}$

**Question 550:**

Express the volume of a cube, $V$, in terms of its surface area, $S$.

A. $V = (S/6)^{3/2}$
B. $V = S^{3/2}$
C. $V = (6/S)^{3/2}$
D. $V = (S/6)^{1/2}$
E. $V = (S/36)^{1/2}$

**Question 551:**
Solve the equations $4 + 3y = 7$ and $2x + 8y = 12$

A. $(x, y) = \left(\frac{17}{13}, \frac{10}{13}\right)$

B. $(x, y) = \left(\frac{10}{13}, \frac{17}{13}\right)$

C. $(x, y) = (1, 2)$

D. $(x, y) = (2, 1)$

E. $(x, y) = (6, 3)$

**Question 552:**
Rearrange $\frac{(7x+10)}{(9x+5)} = 3y^2 + 2$, to make x the subject.

A. $x = \frac{15\,y^2}{7 - 9(3y^2+2)}$

B. $x = \frac{15\,y^2}{7 + 9(3y^2+2)}$

C. $x = -\frac{15\,y^2}{7 - 9(3y^2+2)}$

D. $x = -\frac{15\,y^2}{7 + 9(3y^2+2)}$

E. $x = -\frac{5\,y^2}{7 + 9(3y^2+2)}$

F. $x = \frac{5\,y^2}{7 + 9(3y^2+2)}$

**Question 553:**
Simplify $3x\left(\frac{3x^7}{x^{\frac{1}{3}}}\right)^3$

A. $27\,x^{20}$

B. $87\,x^{20}$

C. $9\,x^{21}$

D. $27\,x^{21}$

E. $81\,x^{21}$

**Question 554:**
Simplify $2x[(2x)^7]^{\frac{1}{14}}$

A. $2x\sqrt{2\,x^4}$

B. $2x\sqrt{2x^3}$

C. $2\sqrt{2\,x^4}$

D. $2\sqrt{2x^3}$

E. $8\,x^3$

**Question 555:**
What is the circumference of a circle with an area of $10\pi$?

A. $2\pi\sqrt{10}$

B. $\pi\sqrt{10}$

C. $10\pi$

D. $20\pi$

E. $\sqrt{10}$

**Question 556:**
If $a.b = (ab) + (a + b)$, then calculate the value of $(3.4).5$

A. 19

B. 54

C. 100

D. 119

E. 132

**Question 557:**
If $a.b = \frac{a^b}{a}$, calculate $(2.3).2$

A. $\frac{16}{3}$

B. 1

C. 2

D. 4

E. 8

**Question 558:**

Solve $x^2 + 3x - 5 = 0$

A. $x = -\frac{3}{2} \pm \frac{\sqrt{11}}{2}$

B. $x = \frac{3}{2} \pm \frac{\sqrt{11}}{2}$

C. $x = -\frac{3}{2} \pm \frac{\sqrt{11}}{4}$

D. $x = \frac{3}{2} \pm \frac{\sqrt{29}}{2}$

E. $x = -\frac{3}{2} \pm \frac{\sqrt{29}}{2}$

**Question 559:**

How many times do the curves $y = x^3$ and $y = x^2 + 4x + 14$ intersect?

A.  0          B.  I          C.  2          D.  3          E.  4

**Question 560:**

Which of the following graphs **do not** intersect?

1.  y = x          2.  y = x²          3.  y = 1-x²          4.  y = 2

A.  I and 2          C.  3 and 4          E.  I and 4

B.  2 and 3          D.  I and 3

**Question 561:**

Calculate the product of 897,653 and 0.009764.

A.  87646.8          C.  876.468          E.  8.76468

B.  8764.68          D.  87.6468

**Question 562:**

Solve for x:  $\frac{7x+3}{10} + \frac{3x+1}{7} = 14$

A. $x = \frac{929}{51}$          B. $x = \frac{949}{47}$          C. $x = \frac{949}{79}$          D. $x = \frac{980}{79}$

**Question 563:**

What is the area of an equilateral triangle with side length $x$.

A. $\frac{x^2\sqrt{3}}{4}$          B. $\frac{x\sqrt{3}}{4}$          C. $\frac{x^2}{2}$          D. $\frac{x}{2}$          E. $x^2$

**Question 564:**

Simplify $3 - \frac{7x(25x^2 - 1)}{49x^2(5x+1)}$

A. $3 - \frac{5x-1}{7x}$          C. $3 + \frac{5x-1}{7x}$          E. $3 - \frac{5x^2}{49}$

B. $3 - \frac{5x+1}{7x}$          D. $3 + \frac{5x+1}{7x}$

**Question 565:**
Solve the equation $x^2 - 10x - 100 = 0$

A. $-5 \pm 5\sqrt{5}$

B. $-5 \pm \sqrt{5}$

C. $5 \pm 5\sqrt{5}$

D. $5 \pm \sqrt{5}$

E. $5 \pm 5\sqrt{125}$

F. $-5 \pm \sqrt{125}$

**Question 566:**
Rearrange $x^2 - 4x + 7 = y^3 + 2$ to make x the subject.

A. $x = 2 \pm \sqrt{y^3 + 1}$

B. $x = 2 \pm \sqrt{y^3 - 1}$

C. $x = -2 \pm \sqrt{y^3 - 1}$

D. $x = -2 \pm \sqrt{y^3 + 1}$

E. $x$ cannot be made the subject of this equation.

**Question 567:**
Rearrange $3x + 2 = \sqrt{7x^2 + 2x + y}$ to make y the subject.

A. $y = 4x^2 + 8x + 2$

B. $y = 4x^2 + 8x + 4$

C. $y = 2x^2 + 10x + 2$

D. $y = 2x^2 + 10x + 4$

E. $y = x^2 + 10x + 2$

F. $y = x^2 + 10x + 4$

**Question 568:**
Jane has a bag containing 12 sweets. She has 4 bonbons, 6 gobstoppers and 2 toffees.

Calculate the probability that she picks out 2 bonbons and 1 toffee in any order when she removes 3 sweets from the bag.

A. $\dfrac{24}{1728}$

B. $\dfrac{24}{1320}$

C. $\dfrac{72}{1320}$

D. $\dfrac{72}{1728}$

E. $\dfrac{9}{12}$

**Question 569:**
The aspect ratio of my television screen is 4:3 and the diagonal is 50 inches. What is the area of my television screen?

A. 1,200 inches

B. 1,000 inches²

C. 120 inches²

D. 100 inches²

E. More information needed.

**Question 570:**
Rearrange the equation $\sqrt{1 + 3x^{-2}} = y^5 + 1$ to make x the subject.

A. $x = \dfrac{(y^{10} + 2y^5)}{3}$

B. $x = \dfrac{3}{(y^{10} + 2y^5)}$

C. $x = \sqrt{\dfrac{3}{y^{10} + 2y^5}}$

D. $x = \sqrt{\dfrac{y^{10} + 2y^5}{3}}$

E. $x = \sqrt{\dfrac{y^{10} + 2y^5 + 2}{3}}$

**Question 571:**
Solve $3x - 5y = 10$ and $2x + 2y = 13$.

A. $(x, y) = (\frac{19}{16}, \frac{85}{16})$

B. $(x, y) = (\frac{85}{16}, -\frac{19}{16})$

C. $(x, y) = (\frac{85}{16}, \frac{19}{16})$

D. $(x, y) = (-\frac{85}{16}, -\frac{19}{16})$

E. No solutions possible.

**Question 572:**
The two inequalities $x + y \leq 3$ and $x^3 - y^2 < 3$ define a region on a plane. Which of the following points lies inside the region?

A. $(2, 1)$

B. $(2.5, 1)$

C. $(1, 2)$

D. $(3, 5)$

E. $(1, 2.5)$

F. None of the above.

**Question 573:**
How many times do $y = x + 4$ and $y = 4x^2 + 5x + 5$ intersect?

A. 0      B. 1      C. 2      D. 3      E. 4

**Question 574:**
How many times do $y = \quad^3$ and $y = x$ intersect?

A. 0      B. 1      C. 2      D. 3      E. 4

**Question 575:**
A cube has unit length sides. What is the length of a line joining a vertex to the midpoint of the opposite side?

A. $\sqrt{2}$

B. $\sqrt{\frac{3}{2}}$

C. $\sqrt{3}$

D. $\sqrt{5}$

E. $\frac{\sqrt{5}}{2}$

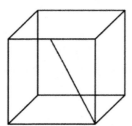

**Question 576:**
Simplify the following:

$$5x(2x^{-\frac{1}{3}})^3$$

A. $10x^{\frac{26}{27}}$

B. $40x^{\frac{26}{27}}$

C. $40x$

D. $40$

E. $10$

**Question 577:**
Fully factorise: $3a^3 - 30a^2 + 75a$

A. $3a(a - 3)^3$
B. $a(3a - 5)^2$

C. $3a(a^2 - 10a + 25)$
D. $3a(a - 5)^2$

E. $3a(a + 5)^2$

**Question 578:**
Solve for x and y:

$$4x + 3y = 48$$
$$3x + 2y = 34$$

|   | x | y |
|---|---|---|
| A | 8 | 6 |
| B | 6 | 8 |
| C | 3 | 4 |
| D | 4 | 3 |
| E | 30 | 12 |
| F | 12 | 30 |
| G | No solutions possible | |

**Question 579:**
Evaluate: $\dfrac{-\left(5^2 - 4 \times 7\right)^2}{-6^2 + 2 \times 7}$

A. $-\dfrac{3}{50}$
B. $\dfrac{11}{22}$
C. $-\dfrac{3}{22}$
D. $\dfrac{9}{50}$
E. $\dfrac{9}{22}$

**Question 580:**
All license plates are 6 characters long. The first 3 characters are letters, and the next 3 characters are numbers. If all letters and numbers can be used, how many unique license plates are possible?

A. 676,000
B. 6,760,000

C. 67,600,000
D. 1,757,600

E. 17,576,000
F. 175,760,000

**Question 581:**
How many solutions are there for the following equation: $2(2(x^2 - 3x)) = -9$

A. 0
B. 1
C. 2
D. 3
E. Infinite solutions.

**Question 582:**
Evaluate: $\left(x^{\frac{1}{2}} y^{-3}\right)^{\frac{1}{2}}$

A. $\dfrac{x^{\frac{1}{2}}}{y}$
B. $\dfrac{x}{y^{\frac{3}{2}}}$
C. $\dfrac{x^{\frac{1}{4}}}{y^{\frac{3}{2}}}$
D. $\dfrac{y^{\frac{1}{4}}}{x^{\frac{3}{2}}}$

**Question 583:**

Given that:

$4^x \times 16^y = 2^z$

Express $z$ in terms of $x$ and $y$.

A. $z = 2x + 4y$

B. $z = x + y + 6$

C. $z = \frac{x}{2} \times \frac{y}{4}$

D. $z = \frac{2}{x} + \frac{4}{y}$

E. $z = 2x \times 4y$

**Question 584:**

Evaluate: $5\,[5(6^2 - 5 \times 3) + 400^{\frac{1}{2}}]^{1/3} + 7$

A.  0          B.  25          C.  32          D.  49          E.  56          F.  200

**Question 585:**

What is the area of a regular hexagon with side length 1 unit?

A. $3\sqrt{3}$          C. $\sqrt{3}$          E.  6

B. $\frac{3\sqrt{3}}{2}$          D. $\frac{\sqrt{3}}{2}$          F.  More information needed

**Question 586:**

Dexter moves into a new rectangular room that is 19 metres longer than it is wide, and its total area is 780 square metres. What are the dimensions of this room?

A.  Width = 20 m; Length = -39 m          D.  Width = -39 m; Length = 20 m

B.  Width = 20 m; Length = 39 m          E.  Width = -20 m; Length = 39 m

C.  Width = 39 m; Length = 20 m

**Question 587:**

Tom uses 34 meters of fencing to enclose his rectangular plot. He measured the diagonals to 13 metres long. What is the length and width of the plot?

A.  3 m by 4 m          C.  6 m by 12 m          E.  9 m by 15 m

B.  5 m by 12 m          D.  8 m by 15 m          F.  10 m by 10 m

**Question 588:**

Solve $\frac{3x-5}{2} + \frac{x+5}{4} = x+1$

A. 1

B. 1.5

C. 3

D. 3.5

E. 4.5

F. None of the above

**Question 589:**

Calculate: $\frac{5.226 \times 10^6 + 5.226 \times 10^5}{1.742 \times 10^{10}}$

A. 0.033

B. 0.0033

C. 0.00033

D. 0.000033

E. 0.0000033

**Question 590:**

Calculate the area of the triangle shown to the right:

A. $3 + \sqrt{2}$

B. $\frac{2 + 2\sqrt{2}}{2}$

C. $2 + 5\sqrt{2}$

D. $3 - \sqrt{2}$

E. $3$

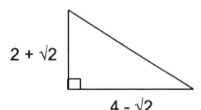

$2 + \sqrt{2}$

$4 - \sqrt{2}$

**Question 591:**

Rearrange $\sqrt{\frac{4}{x} + 9} = y - 2$ to make x the subject.

A. $x = \frac{11}{(y-2)^2}$

B. $x = \frac{9}{(y-2)^2}$

C. $x = \frac{4}{(y+1)(y-5)}$

D. $x = \frac{4}{(y-1)(y+5)}$

E. $x = \frac{4}{(y+1)(y+5)}$

**Question 592:**
When 5 is subtracted from 5x the result is half the sum of 2 and 6x. What is the value of x?

A. 0　　　　　　B. 1　　　　　　C. 2　　　　　　D. 3　　　　　　E. 4

**Question 593:**
Estimate $\dfrac{54.98 + 2.25^2}{\sqrt{905}}$

A. 0　　　　　　B. 1　　　　　　C. 2　　　　　　D. 3　　　　　　E. 4

**Question 594:**
At a restaurant called Pizza Parlour, you can order single, double or triple cheese in the crust. You also have the option to include ham, olives, pepperoni, bell pepper, meatballs, tomato slices, and pineapple.  How many different types of pizza are available at Pizza Parlour?

A. 10　　　　　　　　　C. 192　　　　　　　　　E.  768
B. 96　　　　　　　　　D. 384

**Question 595:**
Solve the simultaneous equations $x^2 + y^2 = 1$ and $x + y = \sqrt{2}$, for x, y > 0

A.  $(x,y) = (\frac{\sqrt{2}}{2}, \frac{\sqrt{2}}{2})$

B.  $(x,y) = (½, \frac{\sqrt{3}}{2})$

C.  $(x,y) = (\sqrt{2} - 1, 1)$
D.  $(x,y) = (\sqrt{2}, ½)$
E.  $(x,y) = (2, 2)$

**Question 596:**
Which of the following statements is **FALSE**?

A.  Congruent objects always have the same dimensions and shape.
B.  Congruent objects can be mirror images of each other.
C.  Congruent objects do not always have the same angles.
D.  Congruent objects can be rotations of each other.
E.  Two triangles are congruent if they have two sides and one angle of the same magnitude.

**Question 597:**
Solve the inequality $x2 \geq 6 - x$

A. $x \leq -3$ and $x \leq 2$
B. $x \leq -3$ and $x \geq 2$
C. $x \geq -3$ and $x \leq 2$
D. $x \geq 2$ only
E. $x \geq -3$ only

**Question 598:**
The hypotenuse of an isosceles right-angled triangle is $x$ cm. What is the area of the triangle in terms of $x$?

A. $\frac{\sqrt{x}}{2}$
B. $\frac{x^2}{4}$
C. $\frac{x}{4}$
D. $\frac{3x^2}{4}$
E. $\frac{x^2}{10}$

**Question 599:**
Mr Heard derives a formula: $Q=\frac{(X+Y)^2 A}{3B}$. He doubles the values of X and Y, halves the value of A and triples the value of B. What happens to the value of Q?

A. Decreases by $\frac{1}{3}$
B. Increases by $\frac{1}{3}$
C. Decreases by $\frac{2}{3}$
D. Increases by $\frac{2}{3}$
E. Increases by $\frac{4}{3}$

**Question 600:**
Consider the graphs $y = x^2 - 2x + 3$, and $y = x^2 - 6x - 10$. Which of the following is true?

A. Both equations intersect the x-axis.
B. Neither equation intersects the x-axis.
C. The first equation does not intersect the x-axis; the second equation intersects the x-axis.
D. The first equation intersects the x-axis; the second equation does not intersect the x-axis.
E. More information is required to determine if the equations intersect the x-axis.

# SECTION 3

### *The Basics*

In BMAT Section 3, you have to write a short essay in response to one of three questions. The essay must not exceed one side of A4 and is a test of your ability to communicate clearly and concisely. The essay questions can span a wide variety of topics and thus demand different levels of comprehension and knowledge, but it is important to realise that one of the major skills being tested is actually your ability to construct a logical and coherent argument- and to convey it to the lay-reader.

Section 3 of the BMAT is frequently neglected by lots of students, who choose to spend their time on sections 1 & 2 instead due to the large amount of content on the specification. However, it's important to put in the work for Section 3 as it's testing skills directly relevant to medicine, and your essay will frequently be discussed at interview. Happily, our experience shows that Section 3 has the highest returns per hour of work out of all three sections, so it is well worth putting time into.

The aim of Section 3 is not to write as much as you can to fill the space available.  Rather, the examiner is looking for you to make interesting and well-supported points to construct tight arguments, and for you to tie everything neatly together for a strong conclusion.  Make sure you're writing critically and concisely; rambling costs you precious space and time. **Irrelevant material can actually lower your score.** You only get one side of A4 for your BMAT essay, so make it count!

### *Essay Structure*

Most BMAT essay questions require you to address 3 main areas:

1)   Explain what a quote or a statement means.
2)   Argue for or against the statement.
3)   Ask you "to what extent" you agree with the statement.

Part 1 should be the smallest portion of the essay (no more than 4 lines) and be used to provide a smooth introduction into the rather more demanding "argue for/against" part of the question. This is the main body of the essay and requires you to demonstrate a firm grasp of the concept being discussed and the ability to strengthen and support the argument with a wide variety of examples from multiple fields. This section should present a balanced response to the essay question, exploring **at least two distinct ideas**. Supporting evidence should be provided throughout the essay, with examples referred to when possible.

The third and final part effectively asks for your personal opinion and is a chance for you to shine - be brave and make an **innovative yet firmly grounded conclusion** for an exquisite mark. The conclusion should bring together all sides of the argument, in order to reach a clear and concise answer to the question. In short, this final section of the essay is your opportunity to demonstrate a unique perspective. It is important not to get too carried away here; ensure that your conclusion is an obvious or logical next step from the overall structure of your essay, which reflects careful planning and preparation.

## Paragraphs

Paragraphs are an important formatting tool which show that you have thought through your arguments and are able to structure your ideas clearly. A new paragraph should be used every time a new idea is introduced. There is no single correct way to arrange paragraphs, but it's important that each paragraph flows smoothly from the last using connecting words and phrases. Examples of useful phrases to connect adjacent paragraphs might be "as a result of this", "in addition to", "in contrast to" etc.  A slick, interconnected essay shows that you have the ability to communicate and organise your ideas effectively.

Given that you only have a limit of one A4 page to write in, **you shouldn't have more than 5 paragraphs. To save space,** use indents to inidicate individual paragraphs – don't leave empty lines! In general, 2 of these 5 paragraphs will be taken up by the introduction and conclusion respectively, leaving you with 3 larger paragraphs in which to make the main arguments of your essay.

Remember- the emphasis should remain on the quality and not quantity of writing. An essay with fewer paragraphs, but with well-developed ideas, is much more effective than a number of short, unsubstantial paragraphs that fail to fully address the question at hand, or an essay that isn't sufficiently focused.

### *Approaching the Essay*

Section 3 can be broken down into 3 components; selecting your essay title, planning and writing it.

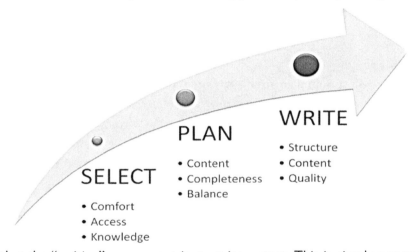

WRITE
- Structure
- Content
- Quality

PLAN
- Content
- Completeness
- Balance

SELECT
- Comfort
- Access
- Knowledge

Most students think that the "writing" component is most important. This is simply not true.

The vast **majority of problems are caused by a lack of planning and a poor choice of essay title -** usually because students just want to get writing as quickly as possible since they are worried about finishing on time. Thirty minutes is long enough to be able to plan your essay well and *still* have time to write it so don't feel pressured to immediately start writing. Investing time in the planning process will make the writing much more efficient.

### Step 1: Selecting

Making the right choice of essay titles is crucial to your success in Section 3. It is imperative that you are comfortable with the topic and that you fully understand the question being asked - it sounds silly but about 25% of essays that we mark score poorly because they don't actually answer the question!

**Take two minutes to read all the questions at the start of Section 3.** While one essay might initially stand out as being the easiest, if you haven't invested time to carefully think through it you might quickly find yourself running out of ideas. Likewise, a seemingly difficult essay might actually offer you a good opportunity to make interesting points and feel more accessible after spending a few moments working through the facets of the question.

Use this time to carefully select which question you will answer by gauging how comfortable you are with it given your background knowledge and suitable examples. Remember that Section 3 is not primarily a test of knowledge but rather a test of how well you are able to argue, so you will need to use relevant examples to support your points.

It's surprisingly easy to change a question into something similar, but with a different meaning. Thus, you may end up answering a completely different essay title by misconstruing the original question. Once you've decided which question you're going to do, read it very carefully a few times to make sure you fully understand what is being raised by the question, and ensure you can answer all aspects of the question. Keep reading it as you answer to ensure you stay on track!

### Step 2: Planning

**Why should I plan my essay?**

There are multiple reasons you should plan your essay for the first 5-10 minutes of section 3:

- Section 3 is a test of communication – your writing will be clearer and more effective if you plan
- You don't have much space to write – make the most of it by writing a very well organised essay.
- Planning enables you to organise your thoughts and change the order before you start writing
- You run the risk of missing the point of the essay or only answering part of it if you don't plan adequately
- Section 3 is time pressured – you'll write the essay faster if you have a clear plan

**How much time should I spend planning?**

As a rough guide, it is **worth spending about 5-10 minutes to plan** and the remaining time to write the essay. However, this is not a strict rule, and you are advised to tailor your time management to suit your individual style. The planning process should enable you to write the essay more efficiently, as you will not have to spend time thinking up your next argument or example once you are writing it. However, it is important to strike a balance between developing a robust plan and leaving adequate time to write the essay in full. Completing past papers under timed conditions will enable you to find a ratio of time spent planning vs writing that works for you.

**How should I go about the planning process?**

There are a variety of methods that can be employed in order to plan essays (e.g. bullet-points, mind-maps etc). If you don't already know what works best for you, it's a good idea to experiment with different methods using past BMAT questions as examples.

Generally, the first step is to gather ideas relevant to the question, which will form the basic arguments around which the essay can be composed. You can then begin to structure your essay, including the way that points will be linked. At this stage it is worth considering the balance of your argument, and confirming that you have included arguments to support both sides of the debate. Once this general structure has been established, you must plan the examples or real world information you can use to help to support your arguments. Finally, you should assess the plan as a whole, and establish what your conclusion will be based on your arguments.

### Step 3: Writing
#### Introduction

### Why are introductions important?
An introduction provides the examiner with their first opportunity to evaluate your work. The introduction is where first impressions are formed of both your writing style and the strength of the arguments you present throughout your essay. A well-constructed introduction shows that you have really thought about the question in a logical way, and gives an indication of the arguments that will follow. It should leave the reader in no doubt as to what to expect from your essay.

.

### What should an introduction do?
A good introduction should **briefly explain the statement or quote** in the essay question and give any relevant background information in a concise manner. However, don't fall into the trap of just repeating the statement in a different way. The introduction is the first opportunity to suggest an answer to the question posed, and the main body of your essay is effectively your chance to justify your answer.

### Main Body
### How do I go about making a convincing point?
Each idea that you propose should be supported and justified, in order to build a convincing overall argument. A point can be solidified through a basic Point → Evidence → Evaluation structure. This is a useful framework to ensure that each sentence within a paragraph builds upon the last, and that all the ideas presented are well developed.

### How do I achieve a logical flow between ideas?
One of the most effective ways to display a good understanding of the question is to keep a logical flow throughout your essay. This means linking points effectively between paragraphs, and creating a congruent train of thought for the examiner as the argument develops. A good way to generate this flow of ideas is to provide ongoing comparisons of arguments, and discussing whether points support or dispute one another as you progress through the essay.

### Should I use examples?
In short – yes! Examples can help boost the validity of arguments, and can help display high quality writing skills. Examples can add a lot of weight to your argument and make an essay much more relevant to the reader by demonstrating real-world representations of your points. When using examples, you should ensure that they are relevant and supportive of the point being made, in order to bolster your overall argument.

Some questions will provide more opportunities to include examples than others so don't worry if you aren't able to use as many examples as you would have liked. There is no set rule about how many examples should be included!

*Top tip!* Remember that there is no single correct answer to these questions and you're not expected to be able to fit everything onto one page. Instead it's better to pick a few key points to produce a focused essay.

### Conclusion

The conclusion provides an opportunity to emphasise the **overall position of your essay,** and package it into a neat summary for readers to take away. The conclusion serves two key purposes: firstly, it should summarise what has been discussed during the main body of the essay and secondly it should give a definitive answer to the question.

Some students use the conclusion to **introduce a new idea that hasn't been discussed**. This can be an interesting addition to an essay, and can help make you stand out. However, adopting this approach takes some considerable skill and our advice to the majority of students would be to present a well-organised, 'standard' conclusion since it is likely to be more effective than an adventurous but poorly executed one. It's worth bearing in mind throughout the whole process that the BMAT essay is a test of clear communication rather than literary style, so it's important to ensure you are doing the basics well rather than taking too many stylistic risks.

### Medical Ethics

Usually there is a medical ethics question in the BMAT section 3, so it's well worth knowing the basics. There are huge ethics textbooks available, and indeed it's possible to study medical ethics at PhD level, however for the purposes of the BMAT you really only need to be familiar with the basic principles.

**These ethical principles can be applied to all cases** regardless of the social/ethnic background the healthcare professional or patient is from. In addition to being helpful in the BMAT, you'll need to know them for the interview stage of the application process so they're well worth learning now. The principles are:

**Beneficence:** The wellbeing of the patient should be the doctor's first priority. In medicine this means that one must act in the patient's best interests to ensure the best outcome is achieved for them i.e. 'Do Good'.

**Non-Maleficence**: This is the principle of avoiding harm to the patient (i.e. do no harm). There can be a danger that in a willingness to treat, doctors can sometimes cause more harm to the patient than good. This can especially be the case with major interventions, such as chemotherapy or surgery. Where a course of action has both potential harms and potential benefits, non-maleficence must be balanced against beneficence.

**Autonomy:** The patient has the right to decide about the treatment they receive. This principle requires the doctor to be a good communicator, so that the patient has sufficient information to make a meaningful decision. 'Informed consent' is thus a vital precursor to any treatment. A doctor must respect a patient's refusal of treatment even if they think it is not the correct choice. Note that patients cannot <u>demand</u> treatment – only refuse it, e.g. an alcoholic patient can refuse rehabilitation but cannot demand a liver transplant.

There are many situations where the application of autonomy can be quite complex, for example:

- **Treating children**: consent is required from the parents, although the autonomy of the child is taken into account increasingly as they get older.

- **Treating adults without the capacity** to make important decisions. The first challenge with this is in assessing whether or not a patient has the capacity to make the decisions. Just because a patient has a mental illness does not necessarily mean that they lack the capacity to make decisions about their health care. Where patients do lack capacity, the power to make decisions is transferred to the next of kin (or Legal Power of Attorney, if one has been set up).

**Justice**: This principle deals with the fair distribution and allocation of healthcare resources for the population.

**Consent**: This is an extension of the principle of autonomy - patients must agree to a procedure or intervention. For consent to be valid, it must be **voluntary informed consent.** This means that the patient must have sufficient mental capacity to make the decision and must be presented with all the relevant information (benefits, side effects and the likely complications) in a way they can understand.

**Confidentiality**: Patients expect that the information they reveal to doctors will be kept private- this is a key component in maintaining the trust between patients and doctors. You must ensure that patient details are kept confidential. Confidentiality can be broken if you suspect that a patient is a risk to themselves or to others e.g. where a doctor reasonably believes a patient might be involved in terrorism or has plans to complete suicide.

When answering a question on medical ethics, you need to ensure that you show an appreciation for two (or more) approaches to the ethical problem. Where appropriate, you should outline each point of view and how it pertains to the main principles of medical ethics before coming to a reasoned judgement to give a conclusion to the essay.

### Common Mistakes
### Ignoring the other side of the argument
Although you're normally required to support one side of the debate, it's important to **consider arguments against your judgement** in order to get higher marks. A good way to do this is to propose an argument that might be used against you, and then to argue why it doesn't hold true. You may use the format: *"some may say that…but this doesn't seem to be important because…"* in order to dispel opposition arguments, whilst still displaying that you have considered them. For example, *"some say that fox hunting shouldn't be banned because it is a tradition. However, witch hunting was also once a tradition – we must move with the times".*

### Answering the topic/Answering only part of the question
One of the most common mistakes is to only answer a part of the question whilst ignoring the rest of it as it feels inaccessible. According to the official mark scheme, **in order to get a score of 3 or more, you must write "…an answer that addresses ALL aspects of the question".** This should be your minimum standard- anything else that you write should then point you towards achieving 4/5.

## Long Introductions

A key mistake to avoid is an excessively long, rambling introduction. Not only will it take up valuable space on your answer sheet, but it will also signal to the examiner that your answer is not clearly focused. Although background information about the topic can be useful, it is normally not necessary. Instead, the **emphasis should be placed on responding to the question**. Some students also just **rephrase the question** rather than actually explaining it. The examiner knows what the question is, and repeating it in the introduction is simply a waste of space in an essay where you are limited to just one A4 side.

## Not including a Conclusion

An essay that lacks a conclusion is incomplete. This is easily avoided by ensuring you plan your essay carefully and stick to strict time-keeping while writing to allow yourself a few minutes at the end to construct a conclusion. Practising under timed conditions is therefore essential to avoid this costly mistake – an essay without a conclusion demonstrates to the examiner that you have not fully considered the question, and worse, that your organisational and planning skills are lacking. **The conclusion should be a distinct paragraph** in its own right and not just a couple of rushed lines at the end of the essay – you should invest time planning your conclusion at the beginning.

## Sitting on the Fence

Students sometimes don't reach a clear conclusion. Although this is generally acceptable in a longer piece of writing, the BMAT requires you to **give a decisive answer to the question** and clearly explain how you've reached this judgement. Essays that do not come to a clear conclusion generally have a smaller impact and score lower. Remember, it is a test of communicating complex ideas clearly, so the reader must be provided with an obvious take-home message. When planning, keep this in mind, and ensure you are clear about the message before you write.

## Exceeding the one page limit

The page limit is there for a reason – don't exceed it under any circumstances as any material over the limit won't be marked and it will appear that you haven't read the instructions.

## Not using all the available space

Remember that you only have one A4 side to write on so ensure you make the maximum use of the space available to you. Don't leave lines to show paragraphs – instead, you should use indents. Similarly, you should also use the top-most line in the response sheet and avoid crossing entire sentences out unless in a dire emergency! Investing time in planning your essay and practising under timed conditions will make it easier to maximise your use of the space.

### Marking your Essays

Practising section 3 can be tricky because most students don't know how to mark their essay. However, if you have a willing friend/family member, it is possible to get useful feedback and mark your work. You can use the diagram below to get an idea of your score. Keep in mind that this is just a very rough guide – examiners will look at several other factors when deciding on your overall score.

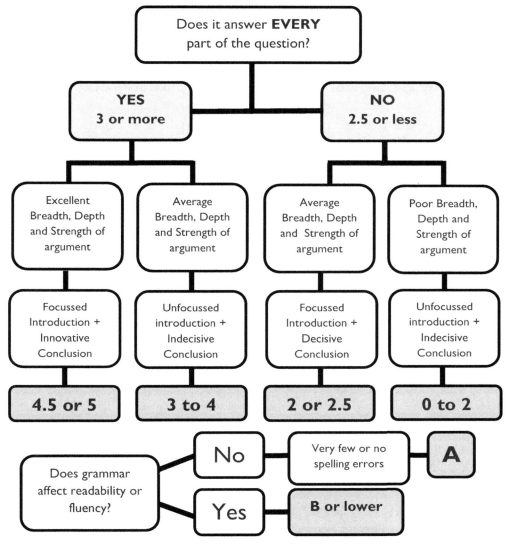

# ANNOTATED ESSAYS

*Example Essay 1:*

## "A doctor should never disclose medical information about his patients"

What does this statement mean? Argue to the contrary using examples to strengthen your response.

To what extent do you agree with this statement?

*The statement suggests that one of a doctor's most vital qualities is maintaining confidentiality of a patient's medical record. This involves all doctors with various specialities in different work places such as the clinics.*

*Disclosing medical informations regarding to their patients by doctors is considered as an unacceptable act within the medical society. For Example, by informing unrelated people about the patient might result in the individual's most embarrased health situation to be exposed. For example, suffering pain from their private parts and this may disgust other. This situation would inevitably upset the patient as their health privacy has been breached by others without consent leading to a sence of distrust towards doctors.*

*However, disclosing such matters to certain suitable people such as family and relatives may be crucial. For example, if the patient is the head of the family or the guardian to the children. As these individuals are in charge of leading and taking are of the family, they need to be able to perform mundane task (such as providing good support to the children) at their optimum. Also, to ensure that the members realise that the patient should not over exert him or herself despite their health conditions. Also, a sudden collapse will reduce shock when the family is to rush the patient back to the hospital knowing that the illness is related to the situation.*

*Overall, a patient's confidentially should not be disclosed without consent or any importance by all means. This is to respect their health privacy and to avoid any inconvenience within the medical society.*

## Examiner's Comments:

**Introduction:** The student appears to have an understanding of the topic but frequently makes statements that don't add much to the argument e.g. the second sentence of the first paragraph. The introduction would be better used to set up the counter arguments that will form the bulk of the main body.

**Main Body:**  The first paragraph actually supports the statement and is therefore not actually answering the question (argue to the contrary). The example doesn't really add much either. The key issue that needed to be discussed was a doctor's duty to the patient – not about "disgusting others". The last sentence of the first paragraph is good and starts to address the question but it comes far too late. By that point the examiner will have already formed an opinion on the quality of writing and content of the essay, which could be hard to reverse.

The second paragraph is better but misses key points of the essay that needed discussion i.e. when can patient confidentiality be broken? Examples would include suspected terrorism, notifiable diseases, criminal activity, suicides etc, and you would be expected to be able to include and expand on at least a few of these points.

**Conclusion:** The conclusion doesn't really address the counter-arguments for breaking confidentiality. It gives a clear position but it is unclear how this has been arrived at and doesn't link well to the main essay. It also contains confusing terminology e.g. one discloses confidential information, not 'confidentiality'. The sentence concerning "inconvenience within the medical community" is also somewhat ambiguous.

**Language:** The poor grammar hinders the points that the student is trying to make throughout the essay e.g. "suffering pain from their private parts and this may disgust other". There are also frequent spelling mistakes like "embarrased" and "sence" that reduce the fluency significantly.  Writing clearly is crucial in BMAT essays.

**Score: D2**

### *Example Essay 2*

#### "A doctor should never disclose medical information about his patients"
What does this statement mean? Argue to the contrary using examples to strengthen your response.
To what extent do you agree with this statement?

*This statement is one of the duties set out by the General Medical Council for doctors to comply with, which is to respect patient's autonomy. It means that a doctor cannot share patient's medical information with other parties unless the patients, themselves, have granted permission to do so.*

*The ethical principle of respecting patients' autonomy cannot be applied in all cases, as some cases require doctors to disclose medical information about patients. First, when it involves a criminal act that has been comitted by a patient, a doctor has to report to an appropriate authority, such as the police. This is because the patient may potentially cause even more harm to others and as doctors, they have to prevent that from happening. An example of a case would be if a patient has a gunshot wound and he told his doctor that he had killed someone in the fight.*

*Next, another incident when a doctor has no choice but to disclose patients' medical information is when it may affect the health of society and could potentially cause an epidemic. Such patients might have an infectious disease and do not wish to let other people know about it. For instance, there has been many cases in West Africa where people who have Ebola are afraid to let their neighbours or friends find out because they do not want to be stigmatised and ostrilised from the society. However, these patients could spread the disease and so a doctor must not withold the information. Last of all, if a patient is underage, then he/ she is still not competent enough to make her own decision. Therefore, any medical information must be shared with his/ her legal guardian.*

*Respecting patient's autonomy by never disclosing their information is also important because patients have the right to chose who gets to know about it. It is his own body. He is the only person who knows the consequences of sharing this sensitive information. In conclusion, I believe that never disclosing patients' medical information cannot be complied in every incident. Respecting their autonomy is important but we have to treat each case separately.*

**Examiner's Comments:**
**Introduction:** The introduction is well written but could be improved by making it explicitly clear that confidentiality can be breached in certain circumstances. This would then set up the main body nicely as the student would then be able to go straight into giving examples.

**Main Body:** The first sentence of the second paragraph is well written but should have gone in the introduction. There is a good breadth of argument with the important points being covered like a doctor's duty to prevent harm to others, 'public good' and the issue of 'capacity'. However, there is unnecessary padding that doesn't add much e.g. there was no need to expand on your example of infectious diseases. The extra space from avoiding this would have allowed the student to write about the fact that although confidentiality must sometimes be breached, a doctor has certain professional duties. For example, informing the patient both before and after and explaining why they have disclosed what they have to try and mitigate any damage to the doctor-patient relationship. In this way, public trust in medical professionals would be maintained.

**Conclusion:** The conclusion concisely summarises the arguments put forth in the main body and offers a nice resolution by saying that each case is different.

**Language:** Whilst it is clear that the student understands the question, there is some confusion as to the difference between "autonomy" and "confidentiality" (It's important to know the basics of medical ethics as they'll be helpful for the interview stage as well). Furthermore, there are minor spelling & grammar mistakes like "comitted" and "withold". In the conclusion, they assume that patients are male – "it is his own body" vs. "it is their own body".

**Score: B3.5**

*Example Essay 3*

**"A doctor should never disclose medical information about his patients"**
What does this statement mean? Argue to the contrary using examples to strengthen your response.
To what extent do you agree with this statement?

*Confidentiality is a basic patient right. The patient provides information to the doctor not to be unnecessarily shared with others without their knowledge or permission. On this basis, the statement argues that a doctor should never reveal medical data, such as results from tests or prescriptions given.*

*However, it can be argued that there are many circumstances whereby it is necesary to breach patient confidentiality and disclose medical information. More specifically, if the patient poses a threat to the public health, their medical situation should be disclosed immediately so that actions can be taken to prevent the spread. For instance, under the Public Health Act 1988, if a patient is suspected of communicable diseases such as tuberculosis, the doctor is required to inform the local health authorities immediately so that they can make precautions to protect the other citizens. In addition, a doctor should also disclose medical information if the patient has broken the law. For instance, the doctor should reveal medical data to the detectives and other relevant professionals if they request for it, to enable them to come to a conclusion of the case more quickly and accurately.*

*However, I agree with this statement to a large extent. After all, the patient should have the right over what happens to his medical documents and information. Revealing information about the patient unnecessarily will take this basic right away, and it is extremely unfair for the patient. Furthermore, this unprofessional decision may undermine the confidence between the patient and doctor. The patient may be less willing to reveal vital personal information to the doctor in the future, in fear that he might release this information as well. This would be extremely detrimental to the diagnoses and treatment for the patient or the doctor might not be able to gain sufficient information to make a more informed decision.*

*In conclusion, a doctor should never disclose medical information about his patients unless there are other external circumstances that oblige the doctor to do so. Breaking this confidentiality will cause the patient-doctor relationship to collapse, compromising the trust between them. However, in some cases, the decision to disclose is not that clear-cut; if a patient had sexually-transmitted infections, should the doctor disclose this information to his spouse? Such situations have to be decided on a case-by-case basis.*

**Examiner's Comments:**

**Introduction:** This is a bold introduction that catches one's attention and gets straight to the point. The student however does make a rather generalised statement - "confidentiality is a basic patient right". A pedantic examiner could easily challenge this so it's important to be careful with wording statements like this to avoid tripping up.

**Main Body:** There is a good level of breadth and depth of argument here. However, there are again some generalised statements that are incorrect e.g. doctors don't need to break confidentiality if a patient has broken ANY law – just serious ones e.g. committed or intend to commit murder/terrorism etc. There is however, excellent discussion of the consequences of breaking confidentiality and a good level of detail (e.g. Public Health Act 1988).

**Conclusion:** this is an excellent conclusion that not only summarises the main arguments from both sides but also builds upon these to offer a solution as to when to break confidentiality by treating it on a case-by-case basis.

**Language:** There is only one spelling mistake ("*necessry*") and although the somewhat general phrases stop this from scoring a perfect A5, it is still an excellent essay that displays good insight. As a general point, it's important to spend time making sure that you write exactly what you mean, and ensure you don't overcomplicate sentences or make over-ambitious arguments such that the overall meaning becomes unclear.

**Score: A4.5**

*Example Essay 4*

**"Medicine is a science; not an art."**
Explain what this statement means. Argue to the contrary that medicine is in fact an art using examples to illustrate your answer.  To what extent, if any, is medicine a science?

*I will explain the following statement "Medicine is a science, not an art" and argue that medicine is in fact an art with supports and to what extent is medicine a science.*

*I will talk about medicine and art in my opinion why, I think medicine is in fact an art and argue with the above statement. I think medicine is an art because of the human body its like a piece of artwork with creations and it is fascinating even more than a artwork of Picccasso or Van Gough's painting. It's like the artries and vessels ressemble the brushstroke of a painting and the heart is the meaning of the painting. To study about that and become a Doctor is like studying art to become and artist. Both Medicine and Art depend on passion if you don't have the passion you will not enjoy saving lives and will not create beautiful paintings. Medicine and Art are the most fascinating majors. They are completely different but at the sane time completely the same. Emotionally the same.*

*Now I will talk about the what extent is medicine a science. It depends on what course you are choosing in medicine For e.g. Biomedical it all counts as science it includes chemistry and maths which makes you a Biochemist or Phisyology, these are some interesting courses. Medicine is science because it depends on knowledge the years to study to become a doctor and save lives which is not an easy opprotunity to get.*

*In my essay I wrote about why I think that medicine is in face not all about sciene but about art too and argued with the above essay. I think Medicine is as fascinating and breathtaking as Art is with all the colours and bueatiful creations made my artists and saved by doctors.*

**Examiner's Comments:**

**Introduction:** Although it is sometimes useful to outline what you are going to discuss when writing academic essays – you simply do not have enough space to do this in the BMAT. The introduction should be a clear and concise explanation of the statement, which isn't really done in this essay. Repeating the statement in the essay should also be avoided as it simply wastes valuable space and time.

**Main Body:** The student doesn't really have a good grasp of what the question is asking and as a result, the argument is off topic and slightly incoherent. The question requires the student to discuss things like medicine is a science because doctors put into practice medical principles that have an empirical factual basis. Whilst the third paragraph does this to a certain extent, the message is diluted somewhat because of a lack of focus. Medicine is also an 'art' because doctors also need to be able to communicate well with patients, to interpret clinical signs etc. The student seems have interpreted the question to literally mean "medicine is art" vs. "medicine is an art".

**Conclusion:** When writing a conclusion it is good practice to just make your point, as opposed to telling the reader you are making it. Thus, meta-writing is again not necessary in the conclusion. The final sentence, although interesting, is again off-topic.

**Language:** There are frequent spelling mistakes e.g. "sane time", "ressemble" and "*bueatiful*". The phrasing and grammatical errors are more serious and significantly affect the essay's fluency e.g. "talk about the what extent".

**Score: D1**

### *Example Essay 5*

**"Medicine is a science; not an art."**
Explain what this statement means. Argue to the contrary that medicine is in fact an art using examples to illustrate your answer. To what extent, if any, is medicine a science?

*Medicine. Arguably one of the most advancing fields in today's society. As a result, many of us have often thought about what medicine actually encompasses. The statement, "medicine is a science; not an art." is one that is constantly the subject of debate today. It questions to what extent that medicine may be considered an art, and to what extent a science. I feel that the statement does not suggest that medicine is an art form but instead, is well and truly a science, and is well within the definition of one.*

*An art form is usually something which is viewed as being expressive and emotional, as well as also being delicate. One can argue that the notion of caring for patients can be viewed as the non-scientific aspect of medicine, and therefore could be considered art as it requires one to be emotional and expressive. In order for a patient's rehabilitation process to be complete and succesful, the care directed at the patient should be tailored for them as the recovery of the psychological side of the human body is just as important as the physiological aspect. In order to be truly effective, the doctor should be able to be empathetic and try and understand the patient's pain when comforting them. This aspect of medicine does not involve the science of the human body or the knowledge of the intricate metabolic reactants which allow the human body to function so effectively.*

*However, another side of the debate could be that medicine is very much a science. This is due to the fact that medicine involves the analysis of a human body, for example, when diagnosing a patient or maybe understanding the effects a drug could bring to specific situations in the human body, something that is viewed with the utmost importance when administering a drug. The fact that in order to succesfully become a medical practitioner, one has to understand the physiology of the human body and have an immense and thorough knowledge of the anatomy of the human body, is the reason that medicine is associated with mainly being a science. This stems back to the days when we used to learn biology and chemistry back in school, and because medicine is largely based on those two core subjects, medicine, as a result, is widely regarded as solely being a science.*

**Examiner's Comments:**

**Introduction:** The opening is catchy although unnecessarily long-winded. Thus, whilst the first sentence grabs the attention, the rest of it does little to keep it the next few sentences are very wordy and don't actually say very much. This is a prime example of just rephrasing the statement rather than explaining it, which wastes time and space.

**Main Body:** There are a good range of examples in the second paragraph - especially those about the rehabilitation process and empathy. Whilst the pro-science arguments are also well made, they are a bit one-dimensional. It would be better to discuss how trials are done to ensure safety rather than just concentrating on human anatomy and physiology. The last sentence also doesn't really add anything and if anything detracts from the final paragraph.

**Conclusion:** The essay is badly let down by a lack of a conclusion. This title required a critical analysis of the strengths of the two sides of the arguments in order to produce a well-constructed conclusion that answered the question, and this was not done effectively in this essay.

**Language:** There are some very elegant turns of phrase here however this sometimes results in a loss of focus. This doesn't affect the essay's readability (and therefore the language score) but indirectly affects the strength of the argument quite substantially. Nevertheless, as all parts of the question are answered to a sufficient level, it still scores a solid 3 for content/argument.

**Score: A3**

*Example Essay 6*

**"Medicine is a science; not an art."**
Explain what this statement means. Argue to the contrary that medicine is in fact an art using examples to illustrate your answer. To what extent, if any, is medicine a science?

*This statement argues that medicine is more deeply rooted with the facts and set observations associated with scientific principles, and that no aspect of medicine is in itself open to interpretation; or art.*

*However many of the facets of medicine could very well be regarded as art. The manual dexterity and presision required by surgeons; particularly the visually aesthetic finish reconstructive or plastic surgery aims towards has a deep basis in artistic ability. Medicine as a career has a hugely important social aspect too; healthcare proffessionals are expected to be involved with communication and, when it comes to patients, even dealing with emotions has an interpretative aspect, and as such could be viewed as art. There is not one set approach to these situations; rather the outcome is reliant on a doctor's own personal judgement and choices as to the best course of action.*

*Theoretical medicine, too, in terms of research may find success in new, recently discovered techniques; the development of which requires thinking 'outside of the box'. The clinical aspect of diagnostic medicine too is subject to unique approached, particularly when introducing extremely complex cases.*

*On the other hand, of course medicine involves most of the main scientific discplines. It is involved with biological structures, chemical processes and even principles of physics- generally all empirical; based on evidence and set in stone. In many cases there is a clear distinction between the right interpretation and thus course of action and the wrong one; for example when prescribing- for many patients (such as when allergies are involved) there are a whole host of drugs and courses of action that are unnacceptable. Therefore, the understanding of the human body and its inner workings that is so crucial for appropriate and successful medicine could well be argued to be science. Yet its application; its uses by doctors and other healthcare proffessionals is less impirical, more open to interpretation, and therefore more so an art. I feel that despite the fact medicine involves understanding and knowledge of the physiology and anatomy of the human body, it also involves the integral of caring for others, which is definitely more of an art form than a science, showing us that despite all the debates, medicine manages to combine art and science together resulting in the formation of a wondrous profession.*

### Examiner's Comments:

**Introduction:** An efficient introduction that explains the statement well. It could be improved by setting up the counter-argument.

**Main Body:** This is a good effort at a tricky essay – there is good breadth of argument with lots of examples like surgical precision and communication. There is also good consideration of the counter-arguments for why medicine is a science with good depth of argument e.g. drug prescriptions.

**Conclusion:** A strong conclusion that addresses the question well and summarises arguments from both sides concisely. It uses unnecessarily romantic language "wondrous profession" but nevertheless is an effective closing paragraph.

**Language:** Although there are a noticeable number of spelling mistakes ("*proffessionals*" and "*impirical*"), they do not detract from the flow of the essay, which is otherwise well written and fairly clear.

### Score: B4.5

*Example Essay 7*

### "The primary duty of a doctor is to prolong life as much as possible"

What does this statement mean? Argue to the contrary, that the primary duty of a doctor is not to prolong life. To what extent do you agree with this statement?

*The most important responsibility of doctor is to cure diseases and extend a life of patients at his most ability acquired. The statement also states that doctors should try their best to prolong life of the sufferers as the first principle to consider. However, some might argue with this.*

*It is true to say that doctors are responsible for improving the conditions of diseases and alleviate the symptoms. This does not necessarily mean that is a major factor to tackle with each disease. Preventive care should be introduced at an early stage, and therefore the primary duty of medical professions, especially doctors should adopt this principle to be their main concern. For example, doctors should be aware of other health conditions of his or her patients that might be developed in the future regarding to patient's lifestyle or eating habits. To only address the present problems, relating to particular disease is not enough. Hence, prolonging life of patients is not the primary concern of doctors but to improve quality of life of the sufferers. By preventing the possible disease and acknowledging the patients are a proper most important role of a doctor.*

*Some people might argue with the statement as there have been a very controversial issue raised in recent years, euthanasia. Nowadays it is evidently seen that some patients in Switzerland and some other countries have their right to urge a doctor to help end their lives peacefully. Doctor may put an emphasis on methods or alternative ways to help prolong life of patient. Their prime concern is also finding the best beneficial treatment in order to fight with the disease unless there is a possible way. Therefore, putting patients at ease by ending their lives is also a primary concern to a doctor in some countries.*

*To some extent, I agree and support this statement as doctors have to delegate roles as healer to those who are in pain. Although it is illegal in some regions of the world to allow doctors taking life of a patient with their consent, it does mean that this method apart from prolonging life is one of the main duty for doctors to be well aware.*

**Examiner's Comments:**

**Introduction:** This is a concise introduction that effectively just rephrases the statement rather than developing on it much – effectively not advancing an argument and thus wasting valuable space. A discussion of what a doctor's <u>primary</u> duty actually is would have been more appropriate here and would have set up the main body far better.

**Main Body:**  This is a rather confusing and muddled answer The second paragraph is difficult to follow and strays from the real topic at hand. The student correctly identifies that a doctor's job is to improve quality of life and not duration. However, this isn't expressed with any degree of clarity or any examples. The third paragraph regarding euthanasia is better but again it is difficult to assess what point the student is trying to make.

**Conclusion:** Although the aim is to reach a clear conclusion supporting one side of the argument, you must consider and reflect on the counter arguments. Thus, it was necessary here to consider that both quality of life <u>and</u> duration are important. In addition, the euthanasia part is somewhat misguided – it is not necessarily true that doctors who do not prioritise duration of life are in favour of euthanasia.

**Language:** There are frequent grammatical errors e.g. "as there have been a very" which reduce the essay's fluency. The sentence phrasing also impacts the essay's overall readability, ultimately leading to a poor language score.

**Score: C2**

*Example Essay 8*

## "The primary duty of a doctor is to prolong life as much as possible"

What does this statement mean? Argue to the contrary, that the primary duty of a doctor is not to prolong life. To what extent do you agree with this statement?

*A doctors' job is to cure disease through medical treatment to extend the life of the patient as much as possible. However, there is a certain limit to which doctors can go in order to prolong life as often quality of life is equally (if not more) important as quantity of life.*

*Doctors provide treatments to patients to help them overcome their disease so that they can live longer. This is also what the patients want. For example, for patients with kidney diseases, doctors will suggest them to have dialysis in order to remove the toxic substance in their body, which will kill them. Through dialysis, the patient's life will be extended and as this is the patient's will; a doctor's primary duty is to prolong life. People take preventative method, such as endoscopy of large intestine for symptoms of cancer, to avoid late discovery of disease, which will lead to a high chance of death. Therefore as a doctor has the skills to help people to extend their life, they should do as much as they can to fulfil the patient's wish, which is prolonging life.*

*However, doctors should also respect the patient's autonomy. If a patient doesn't want a treatment, even if the treatment is effective, doctors should not carry the treatment out, as everyone has the right to control their own life. Even when doctors want to help their patients, doctors should not over-ride the will of the patients.*

*Although one of a doctor's duties is to prolong life – this shouldn't be at the expense of quality of life. A doctor's primary duty is to offer the best possible medical advice and minimise suffering. Although the impact of this is usually to prolong life, in some cases, it may result in maximising quality of life.*

## Examiner's Comments:

**Introduction:** An excellent introduction that sets the scene very nicely for the main body and immediately conveys to the examiner that the student understands the essay of the essay.

**Main Body:** There are good points made throughout e.g. dialysis and the inclusion of preventative treatment shows a good insight into medicine. However, the student is not able to put together a substantial enough argument against prolonging life as they spend too much space discussing the reasons for prolonging life (which are less important). This is a perfect example of an unbalanced essay. In general, there is limited focus on the question and as a result, weak depth of argument.

**Conclusion:** A satisfactory conclusion that expresses the sentiments of the conclusion nicely and addresses the question well. It gives a clear position but also demonstrates insight into alternative points of view.

**Language:** The introduction and conclusion rescue this essay – as they convey a high degree of understanding in only a couple of sentences. The essay itself reads well and there are no obvious errors that reduce its fluency.

## Score: A3.5

*Example Essay 9*

**Animal euthanasia should be made illegal.**

Explain what this statement means. Argue to the contrary that animal euthanasia should remain legal. To what extent do you agree with the statement?

*The statement refers to the ethical dilemma of euthanasia. Euthanasia, synonymous of mercy killing, is the ending of someone's life because of a particular situation in which this living creature's future will be painful, sometimes short or it will ultimately be better to end it soon. The first argument for this statement is the fact that we as humans are generally kind hearted and benevolent: we see pain as a thing to be eradicated if not suppressed, and hence euthanasia could be seen as merciful, given this nature of ours. However, the natural argument against this is the undeniable fact that in the eyes of many, euthanasia is glorified murder, which goes against most people's morals since killing is seen as a negative thing in most societies nowadays. Another argument in favour of this process could be the fact that killing is not only condemned but also morally wrong since it involves us "removing" an otherwise healthy living being. The counter-argument illustrated by this statement is the fact that most people would look upon this as a grateful act of mercy, where although the consequences are taken into account, it is, morally, for some, the best thing to do, particularly if an animal, a source of fondness for some, is involved. The last argument to put forth is that animals are intelligent creatures capable of feeling pain like us and should hence receive the same mercy as is sometimes shown to humans. Naturally, people would say that in some cases this would be murder rather than mercy killing, eg the killing of old horses for glue rather than because of old age. I conclude this should remain legal since animals cannot voice their own opinion and hence give more weight to a decision.*

**Examiner's Comments:**

**Introduction:** This is a good albeit somewhat long introduction. The student has defined euthanasia well and then established that there is an ethical dilemma surrounding it. However, the very long sentences make it needlessly difficult to follow.

**Main Body:** Whilst the writing style is excellent, there is a limited amount of content here. The student presents arguments for both sides simultaneously which sometimes makes it difficult to follow. This is made more confusing by the lack of paragraphs which means that the essay doesn't flow as well.

There are also some long and rambling sentences that detract from the clarity of the argument. The essay would benefit from a more focussed approach in which the student gets to the point. The point about killing horses for glue is also not as relevant to euthanasia outside a slippery slope argument (which isn't expanded upon).

**Conclusion:** The conclusion does not really build upon any of the arguments from the main body. This gives the impression that it was rushed with little planning.

**Language:** There are no obvious spelling errors but colloquialisms like 'nowadays' should be avoided. Overall, the student clearly understands the topic – but the essay is let down by a limited focus on the question and poor structure due to very long sentences and a lack of paragraphs.

**Score: A3**

*Example Essay 10*

**Animal euthanasia should be made illegal.**

Explain what this statement means. Argue to the contrary that animal euthanasia should remain legal. To what extent do you agree with the statement?

*This statement means that the purposeful act of killing animals, carried out by veterinary practitioners, should be made against the law. Currently, human euthanasia is illegal and the introduction of legal euthanasia brings with it many potentially harmful implications such as the 'putting down' of healthy animals.*

*An ethical pillar of medicine is non-maleficence. By making animal euthanasia illegal we uphold this pillar and avoiding causing harm to potentially healthy animals. If animal euthanasia were to be legalised then some people may think it justified to slaughter animals for less than noble purposes.*

*However, there are many cases in which euthanasia may be the best way of progression in the medical treatment of animals. For example: if an injured or terminally ill animal has no chance of recovery and is suffering then euthanasia may be the most kind and compassionate thing to do e.g. if a horse has broken its leg and will never be able to walk again. In addition, if the quality of life of an animal is very low e.g. they have no home, are starving and there is nowhere for them to live, then euthanasia may also be the most compassionate course of action. This may be especially the case where an area is overpopulated with stray cats and dogs.*

*Another case where euthanasia seems the most beneficial course of action is if an animal has become infected with a disease that could spread to other animals and humans potentially causing widespread and significant harm e.g. if a dog becomes infected with rabies or a cow becomes infected with foot and mouth disease.*

*To conclude, I disagree with the statement as I think animal euthanasia should remain legal. It should however, only be carried out by a veterinary professional and only when the animal is undergoing significant suffering.*

**Examiner's Comments:**

**Introduction:** A concise and focussed introduction that answers the first part of the question well and sets up the main body nicely.

**Main Body:** The student presents a sophisticated argument that addresses all the aspects of the question and uses good examples to back up their points. The arguments are well thought out and naturally follow on from each other. It would be better to argue why euthanasia should remain legal **before** giving reasons for it to be made illegal. This would help improve the flow.

**Conclusion:** A succinct and well-supported conclusion that ties together the major arguments in the main body. It also introduces a new idea —only vets should be allowed to perform euthanasia. This is a good point but should have been developed somewhat more.

**Language:** The student clearly understands the essay and puts together a strong essay. There are no glaring spelling or grammatical errors and it is easy to read and follow.

**Score: A4.5**

*Summary*

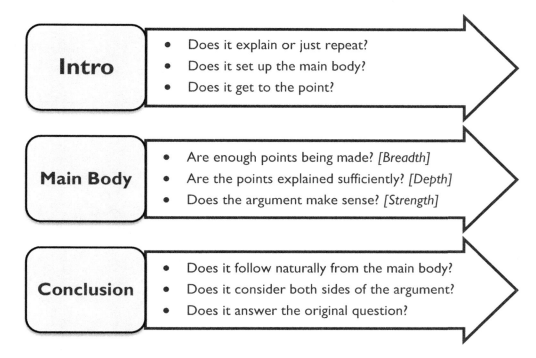

**Intro**
- Does it explain or just repeat?
- Does it set up the main body?
- Does it get to the point?

**Main Body**
- Are enough points being made? *[Breadth]*
- Are the points explained sufficiently? *[Depth]*
- Does the argument make sense? *[Strength]*

**Conclusion**
- Does it follow naturally from the main body?
- Does it consider both sides of the argument?
- Does it answer the original question?

*General Advice*

✓ Always answer the question clearly – this is the key thing examiners look for in an essay.

✓ Analyse each argument made, justifying or dismissing with logical reasoning.

✓ Keep an eye on the time/space available – an incomplete essay may be taken as a sign of a candidate with poor organisational or planning skills.

✓ Use pre-existing knowledge when possible – examples and real world data can be a great way to strengthen an argument- but don't make up statistics!

✓ Present ideas in a neat, logical fashion (easier for an examiner to absorb).

✓ Complete some practise papers in advance, in order to best establish your personal approach to the paper (particularly timings, how you plan etc.).


✗ Attempt to answer a question that you don't fully understand, or ignore part of a question.

✗ Rush or attempt to use too many arguments – it is much better to have fewer, more substantial points.

✗ Attempt to be too clever, or make up examples to support an argument – a tutor may call out incorrect facts etc.

✗ Panic if you don't know the answer the examiner wants – there is no right answer, the essay is not a test of knowledge but a chance to display reasoning and communication skills.

✗ Leave an essay unfinished – if time/space is short, wrap up the essay early in order to provide a conclusive response to the question.

# ANSWERS

# ANSWER KEY

| Question | Answer | Question | Answer | Question | Answer | Question | Answer |
|---|---|---|---|---|---|---|---|
| 1 | A | 39 | D | 77 | B | 115 | C |
| 2 | C | 40 | A | 78 | D | 116 | B |
| 3 | A | 41 | B | 79 | A | 117 | C |
| 4 | A | 42 | B | 80 | B | 118 | D |
| 5 | C | 43 | E | 81 | E | 119 | A |
| 6 | D | 44 | B | 82 | B | 120 | B |
| 7 | D | 45 | D | 83 | C | 121 | D |
| 8 | A | 46 | E | 84 | C | 122 | C |
| 9 | A | 47 | B | 85 | D | 123 | D |
| 10 | B | 48 | D | 86 | C | 124 | B |
| 11 | D | 49 | B | 87 | C | 125 | A |
| 12 | C | 50 | D | 88 | A | 126 | C |
| 13 | D | 51 | A | 89 | C | 127 | E |
| 14 | A | 52 | B | 90 | C | 128 | C |
| 15 | D | 53 | D | 91 | A | 129 | E |
| 16 | A | 54 | A | 92 | A | 130 | C |
| 17 | B | 55 | C | 93 | D | 131 | C |
| 18 | B | 56 | D | 94 | D | 132 | A |
| 19 | A | 57 | C | 95 | C | 133 | B |
| 20 | B | 58 | A | 96 | B | 134 | B |
| 21 | A | 59 | D | 97 | D | 135 | C |
| 22 | C | 60 | D | 98 | E | 136 | D |
| 23 | C | 61 | D | 99 | D | 137 | D |
| 24 | A | 62 | B | 100 | B | 138 | C |
| 25 | B | 63 | C | 101 | D | 139 | C |
| 26 | A | 64 | B | 102 | B | 140 | B |
| 27 | D | 65 | B | 103 | E | 141 | C |
| 28 | A | 66 | D | 104 | E | 142 | E |
| 29 | A | 67 | E | 105 | B | 143 | B |
| 30 | B | 68 | C | 106 | C | 144 | D |
| 31 | A | 69 | E | 107 | E | 145 | B |
| 32 | C & E | 70 | D | 108 | A | 146 | D |
| 33 | B | 71 | F | 109 | A | 147 | E |
| 34 | B | 72 | B | 110 | D | 148 | C |
| 35 | D | 73 | A | 111 | A | 149 | E |
| 36 | A | 74 | C | 112 | C | 150 | C |
| 37 | A | 75 | D | 113 | D | | |
| 38 | B | 76 | A | 114 | D | | |

| Question | Answer | Question | Answer | Question | Answer | Question | Answer |
|---|---|---|---|---|---|---|---|
| 151 | D | 189 | D | 227 | C | 265 | C |
| 152 | B | 190 | C | 228 | E | 266 | C |
| 153 | E | 191 | C | 229 | D | 267 | A |
| 154 | E | 192 | B | 230 | C | 268 | C |
| 155 | D | 193 | C | 231 | B | 269 | B |
| 156 | E | 194 | C | 232 | E | 270 | E |
| 157 | E | 195 | C | 233 | D | 271 | D |
| 158 | A | 196 | D | 234 | A | 272 | C |
| 159 | C | 197 | C | 235 | C | 273 | B |
| 160 | D | 198 | E | 236 | A | 274 | E |
| 161 | C | 199 | D | 237 | B | 275 | C |
| 162 | C & E | 200 | C | 238 | C | 276 | C |
| 163 | D | 201 | A | 239 | A | 277 | E |
| 164 | C | 202 | A | 240 | B | 278 | B |
| 165 | B | 203 | C & E | 241 | E | 279 | D |
| 166 | A | 204 | D | 242 | C | 280 | C |
| 167 | C | 205 | D | 243 | E | 281 | D |
| 168 | B | 206 | B | 244 | B | 282 | E |
| 169 | C | 207 | D | 245 | B | 283 | B |
| 170 | D | 208 | A | 246 | C | 284 | C |
| 171 | B & C | 209 | B | 247 | C | 285 | C |
| 172 | B | 210 | C | 248 | C | 286 | D |
| 173 | B & D | 211 | B | 249 | E | 287 | B |
| 174 | D | 212 | C | 250 | C | 288 | E |
| 175 | E | 213 | D | 251 | A | 289 | C |
| 176 | D | 214 | D | 252 | C | 290 | A |
| 177 | D | 215 | C | 253 | A | 291 | C |
| 178 | B & D | 216 | C | 254 | B | 292 | C |
| 179 | B | 217 | C | 255 | B | 293 | D |
| 180 | C | 218 | A | 256 | E | 294 | A |
| 181 | C | 219 | C | 257 | E | 295 | D |
| 182 | D | 220 | A | 258 | C | 296 | D |
| 183 | B | 221 | E | 259 | B | 297 | C |
| 184 | C | 222 | C | 260 | C | 298 | C |
| 185 | B | 223 | B | 261 | D | 299 | C |
| 186 | E | 224 | B | 262 | C | 300 | E |
| 187 | B | 225 | C | 263 | B | | |
| 188 | D | 226 | B | 264 | D | | |

| Question | Answer | Question | Answer | Question | Answer | Question | Answer |
|----------|--------|----------|--------|----------|--------|----------|--------|
| 301 | A | 339 | E | 377 | E | 415 | C |
| 302 | D | 340 | E | 378 | A | 416 | B |
| 303 | B | 341 | C | 379 | A | 417 | A |
| 304 | A | 342 | E | 380 | D | 418 | E |
| 305 | C | 343 | B | 381 | C | 419 | A |
| 306 | C | 344 | E | 382 | B | 420 | E |
| 307 | D | 345 | E | 383 | E | 421 | D |
| 308 | B | 346 | B | 384 | A | 422 | E |
| 309 | A | 347 | A | 385 | C | 423 | B |
| 310 | D | 348 | C | 386 | C | 424 | E |
| 311 | D | 349 | C | 387 | E | 425 | D |
| 312 | A | 350 | B | 388 | E | 426 | A |
| 313 | C | 351 | D | 389 | E | 427 | D |
| 314 | A | 352 | A | 390 | E | 428 | D |
| 315 | E | 353 | B | 391 | A | 429 | C |
| 316 | D | 354 | C | 392 | C | 430 | E |
| 317 | A | 355 | C | 393 | B | 431 | E |
| 318 | D | 356 | A | 394 | D | 432 | D |
| 319 | D | 357 | B | 395 | B | 433 | D |
| 320 | B | 358 | C | 396 | E | 434 | E |
| 321 | A | 359 | B | 397 | B | 435 | C |
| 322 | E | 360 | C | 398 | D | 436 | A |
| 323 | D | 361 | E | 399 | D | 437 | B |
| 324 | E | 362 | F | 400 | D | 438 | E |
| 325 | E | 363 | A | 401 | D | 439 | C |
| 326 | E | 364 | A | 402 | E | 440 | D |
| 327 | D | 365 | A | 403 | E | 441 | C |
| 328 | C | 366 | C | 404 | B | 442 | C |
| 329 | E | 367 | A | 405 | B | 443 | E |
| 330 | E | 368 | A | 406 | D | 444 | C |
| 331 | D | 369 | E | 407 | A | 445 | B |
| 332 | C | 370 | E | 408 | B | 446 | B |
| 333 | A | 371 | D | 409 | E | 447 | B |
| 334 | E | 372 | B | 410 | B | 448 | E |
| 335 | A | 373 | D | 411 | D | 449 | D |
| 336 | A | 374 | A | 412 | A | 450 | C |
| 337 | C | 375 | E | 413 | A | | |
| 338 | A | 376 | D | 414 | B | | |

| Question | Answer | Question | Answer | Question | Answer | Question | Answer |
|---|---|---|---|---|---|---|---|
| 451 | E | 489 | D | 527 | C | 565 | C |
| 452 | A | 490 | E | 528 | C | 566 | B |
| 453 | D | 491 | E | 529 | C | 567 | D |
| 454 | E | 492 | A | 530 | E | 568 | C |
| 455 | E | 493 | B | 531 | A | 569 | A |
| 456 | C | 494 | C | 532 | C | 570 | C |
| 457 | D | 495 | D | 533 | E | 571 | C |
| 458 | E | 496 | E | 534 | E | 572 | C |
| 459 | D | 497 | E | 535 | C | 573 | B |
| 460 | D | 498 | C | 536 | D | 574 | D |
| 461 | E | 499 | C | 537 | E | 575 | E |
| 462 | B | 500 | B | 538 | E | 576 | D |
| 463 | C | 501 | D | 539 | B | 577 | D |
| 464 | E | 502 | E | 540 | C | 578 | B |
| 465 | D | 503 | E | 541 | B | 579 | E |
| 466 | E | 504 | D | 542 | B | 580 | E |
| 467 | C | 505 | D | 543 | C | 581 | B |
| 468 | A | 506 | A | 544 | D | 582 | C |
| 469 | E | 507 | D | 545 | C | 583 | A |
| 470 | E | 508 | C | 546 | B | 584 | C |
| 471 | E | 509 | D | 547 | A | 585 | B |
| 472 | E | 510 | C | 548 | A | 586 | B |
| 473 | E | 511 | D | 549 | D | 587 | B |
| 474 | D | 512 | E | 550 | A | 588 | C |
| 475 | E | 513 | B | 551 | B | 589 | C |
| 476 | D | 514 | A | 552 | A | 590 | A |
| 477 | E | 515 | C | 553 | E | 591 | C |
| 478 | E | 516 | C | 554 | D | 592 | D |
| 479 | B | 517 | E | 555 | A | 593 | C |
| 480 | A | 518 | C | 556 | D | 594 | D |
| 481 | C | 519 | B | 557 | D | 595 | A |
| 482 | C | 520 | B | 558 | E | 596 | C |
| 483 | D | 521 | E | 559 | B | 597 | B |
| 484 | D | 522 | C | 560 | C | 598 | B |
| 485 | E | 523 | E | 561 | B | 599 | A |
| 486 | B | 524 | E | 562 | C | 600 | C |
| 487 | A | 525 | D | 563 | A | | |
| 488 | E | 526 | B | 564 | A | | |

# WORKED ANSWERS

**Question 1: A**
Whilst **B**, **C** and **D** may be true, they are not completely stated in the passage. **A** is clearly stated and so is the correct answer.

**Question 2: C**
The main argument of the first paragraph is to propose the point that society controls gender behaviour more than genetics. **A** and **D** do not indicate either as they only allude to the end result of gendered behaviour and so are incorrect. Hormonal effects are not mentioned in the first paragraph and so **B** is incorrect. **C** would undermine the argument that society *predominately* controls gender, and so is correct.

**Question 3: A**
**B**, **C** and **D** are not stated and so are incorrect. **A** is directly stated in the passage and so is correct.

**Question 4: A**
**B** and **D** are contradicted by the statement and so are incorrect. **C** could be true but implies children always like the same thing as their same-gendered parent irrespective of how they are treated as a child, which is contrary to the statement and so is not correct. **A** is correct as it is the overall message conveyed by the passage.

**Question 5: C**
**D** may help prevent problems with sexual identity but does not prevent stereotyping and so is incorrect. **A** is not stated, and **B** is implied but not stated and so are incorrect. **C** is the end message of how to prevent gender stereotyping and so is correct.

**Question 6: D**
**A**, **B** and **C** may be true but are not mentioned in the statement and so are incorrect. The statement implies that children born with different external organs to those that their sex chromosomes would ordinarily give rise to may find it difficult to accept this difference and be uncomfortable.

**Question 7: D**
The text states that 'Those who regularly took 30-minute naps were more than twice as likely to remember simple words such as those of new toys.' Which means those who napped were twice as likely to remember teddy's name than the 5% who did not, 5% x 2 = 10%, which would be twice as likely, ruling out **A** and **B**. But being 'more than twice', the only possible answer is **D**.

**Question 8: A**
The answer requires you to work out 10% (the percentage of napping toddlers more likely to suffer night disturbances) of 75% (the percentage of toddlers who regularly nap). Hence the answer is A: 10 % of 75% is 7.5%.

**Question 9: A**
**B**, **C** and **D** may be true but there is nothing in the text to support the statements. **A** is suggested, as the passage states 'non-napping counterparts, who also had higher incidences of memory impairment, behavioural problems and learning difficulties'. If the impaired memory were the cause, as opposed to the result, of irregular sleeping then it would offer an alternative reason why those who nap less remember less.

## Question 10: B

**A** and **C** are possible implications of the passage but are not stated and so are incorrect. It is said that parents credit napping as having 'the benefits of their child having a regular routine' so **B** is more correct than **D** as it refers to the benefit to the toddlers' rather than the parents.

## Question 11: D

**B**, if true, would contradict the conclusion by implying that the study is skewed. The same is true of **C**, which if true, would imply unreliable results, as the toddlers sampled are all the same age within a year, but not within a few weeks. **A**, if true, would not provide any additional support to the conclusion and so is incorrect. **D**, if true, would provide the most support for the conclusion, as it proposes using groups with a higher incidence of napping in comparison to those with a lower incidence.

## Question 12: C

Although it can be argued that **A, B, D** and **E** are true, they are not the best answer to demonstrate a flaw in Tom's father's argument. **C** is the best answer, because it accounts for other factors determining success for the Geography A-level exam, such as aptitude for the subject.

## Question 13: D

**A** is never stated and is incorrect. **B** and **C** are referred to being 'many people's' beliefs – these options present others' opinions not an argument supported by evidence in the passage, and so are not valid conclusions. It is implied by the passage that the NHS may have to reduce its services in the future, some of which could be fertility treatments, so **D** is the correct answer.

## Question 14: A

**C** does not severely affect the strength of the argument, as it is only relevant to the length of the time taken for the effects of the argument to come into place.

**D** is incorrect, as people breaking speed limits already would not negate the argument that speed limits should be removed, but could even be seen as supporting it. These people may count as the 'dangerous drivers' who would be ultimately weeded out of the population.

**B** may affect part of the argument's logic (as it undermines the idea that dangerous drivers are born to dangerous drivers), but the final conclusion that dangerous drivers will end up killing only themselves still stands, and so the ultimate population of only safe drivers may be obtained. The fact that one dead dangerous driver could have produced a safe one does not necessarily challenge the main point of this argument.

**A** if true would most weaken the argument as it states that a fast driver is more likely to harm others and not harm the driver themselves, which would negate the whole argument.

## Question 15: D

Whilst is it stated that the government assesses risk, it is not described as an obligation, hence **A** is incorrect. The overall conclusion of the statement is that, on balance, the government was justified in not spending money on flooding preparation, as it was unlikely to occur, so **C, B** and **E** are incorrect, and **D** is correct.

## Question 16: A

**C** is incorrect and **D** is a possible course of action rather than a conclusion. **B** and **E** are possible inferences but not the conclusion of the statement. The overall conclusion of the statement is that the way that children interact and play has changed over time to now mainly involve the solitary act of playing computer games.

## Question 17: B
The passage does state that in this case the £473 million could have been put to better use, however, there is no mention that no drug should ever be stockpiled for a similar possible pandemic. The passage discusses the lack of evidence behind Tamiflu and therefore is stating that in a situation where there is a lack of evidence, there may not be justification for stockpiling millions of pounds worth of the drug. Stockpiling in the case of drugs with high effectiveness is not discussed so we should not assume this is a generic argument against preparation for any pandemic and stockpiling of any drug.

## Question 18: B
The passage discusses the fact that unhealthy eating is associated with other aspects of an unhealthy lifestyle so the argument that tackling <u>only</u> the unhealthy eating aspect does not logically follow. The other statements are all possible reasons why the solution given may not be optimal, but are not directly referred to in the passage.

## Question 19: A
This is a tricky question in which **A**, **B**, **C** and **D** are all true. However, the question asks for the conclusion of the passage, which is best represented by **A**.
**B** is a premise (upon which the rest of the argument rests) that gives justification for why the elderly should take care of themselves and **C** provides a justification for why they may not.
**D** is implied in the text, but statement **A** is explicitly stated.
**E** is incorrect as the passage implies that people should spend the money that they have in old age, not stop saving altogether.

## Question 20: B
The passage states stem cell research is an area where there are possible high financial and personal gains, however there is no mention of these being the main driving factors in either this area of research or others. Although rivalry between groups may be a reason driving publishing, this is not mentioned in the passage. The image discrepancies were in only one paper, but the passage implies the protocol and replication problems were in both papers.

## Question 21: A
**D** actually weakens the argument and is therefore not a conclusion. **C** is simply a fact stated to introduce the argument and is not a conclusion. **B** is a reason given in the passage to support the main conclusion. If we accept **B** as being true, it helps support the statement in **A**. **E** is not discussed in the passage. **A** is the main conclusion of this passage

## Question 22: C
The passage describes improved safety features and better brakes in cars, and concludes that this means the road speed limit could be increased to 80mph without causing more fatalities. However, if **C** is not true, this conclusion no longer follows on from this reasoning. At no point is it stated that **C** is true, so **C** is therefore the assumption in the passage. The statements in **B** and **D** are not *required* to be true for the argument's conclusion to lead on from its reasoning. **A** is a statement which is strengthened by this passage, and is not an assumption from the passage. **E** is not relevant to the conclusion or mentioned in the passage.

**Question 23: C**
Answers **A** and **D** are both reasons given to explain fingerprints under the theory of evolution, and contribute towards the notion given in **C**, that they do not offer support to intelligent design. Thus, **A** and **D** are reasons given in the passage, and **C** is the main conclusion. **B** is simply a fact stated to introduce the passage, whilst **E** actually contradicts something mentioned in the argument (namely that intelligent design is religious-based, and scientifically discredited). Neither of these options are conclusions.

**Question 24: A**
Answers **C**, **D** and **E** obviously present ways in which the conclusions drawn from the study could be wrong without any mistakes being made by those carrying out the study, and thus are potential reasons. **B** is also a potential reason, because those with a low alcohol consumption could have many other risk factors for cancer, and thus may end up with a higher *overall* risk. If the study does not take account of these, it could produce erroneous conclusions. **A** cannot be a valid reason because the passage *states* that it is *'proven'* that alcohol increases the risk of cancer. Thus, we must accept this as true, so **A** is not a potential reason.

**Question 25: B**
The passage states that the average speed *including* time spent stood still at stations was 115mph. Thus, **A** is incorrect, as the stopping points have already been included in the calculations of journey time. Similarly, the passage states that the train completes its journey at Kings cross, so **D** is incorrect. **C** is not correct because we have been given the total length of the journey. Whether it took the most direct route is irrelevant. **E** is completely irrelevant and does not affect the answer. **B** is an assumption, because we have only been given the *scheduled* time of departure. If the train was delayed in leaving, it would not have left at 3:30, and so would have arrived *after* 5:30.

**Question 26: A**
The argument discusses healthcare spending in England and Scotland, and whether this means the population in Scotland will be healthier. It says nothing about whether this system is fair, and does not mention the expenditure in Wales. Thus, **C** and **D** are incorrect. Similarly, the argument makes no reference to whether healthcare spending should be increased, so **B** is incorrect. **E** is true but not the main message of the passage. The passage does suggest that the higher healthcare expenditure per person in Scotland does not necessarily mean that the Scottish population will be healthier, so **A** is the conclusion from this passage.

**Question 27: D**
**C** is an incorrect statement, as the passage says that Polio *hasn't* been eradicated yet. **A** and **B** are reasons given to support the conclusion, which is that given in **D**. **E**, meanwhile, is an opinion given in the passage, and is not relevant to the conclusion.

**Question 28: A**
This passage provides various positive points of the Y chromosome, before describing how all of this means it is a fantastic tool for genetic analysis. Thus, the conclusion is clearly that given in **A**. The statement in **B** is a further point given to provide evidence of its utility, as stated in the passage. Thus, **B** is not a conclusion in itself, but further evidence to support the main conclusion, given in **A**. **C** is also a reason given to support the conclusion in **A**, whilst **D** is simply a fact stated to introduce the passage. As for **E**, there is no mention of Genghis Khan's children (only his descendants).

**Question 29: A**

Answers **C** and **E** are not valid assumptions because the argument has *stated* that a patient *must* be treated with antibiotics for a bacterial infection to clear. **B** is not a flaw, because this does not affect whether the antibiotics would clear the infection if it were bacterial. **D** is an irrelevant statement, and also contradicts a phrase in the passage (that antibiotics are required to clear a bacterial infection). **A** is a valid flaw, because the passage does not say that antibiotics are *sufficient* or *guaranteed* to clear a bacterial infection, simply that they are *necessary*. Thus, it is possible that the infection *is* bacterial, but the antibiotics failed to clear it.

**Question 30: B**

**A**, **C** and **D**, if accepted as true, all contribute towards supporting the statement given in **B**, which is a valid conclusion given in this passage. Thus, **A**, **C** and **D** are all reasons given to support the main conclusion, which is the statement given in **B**. **E** is not a valid conclusion, as the passage makes no reference to action that should be taken relating to smoking, it simply discusses its position as the main risk factor for lung cancer.

**Question 31: A**

**D** is only given as a method, with no mention of its effectiveness. We do not know if **C** is true because it is not stated. **B** is not discussed in the passage. Whilst statement **E** is true, it is supporting evidence for the conclusion, not the conclusion itself.

**Question 32: C & E**

Whilst **A** and **B** may be true, cost is not mentioned as a deterring factor and we are only concerned with use in the UK, so they are irrelevant. Whether cannabis was the only class C drug is not important to the argument, so **D** is not correct. **C** and **E** are the correct answers because the statement concerns the use of cannabis in the UK, directly stating its use will decrease if people know it has been upgraded to a more dangerous category, due to fear of being given a longer prison sentences from use of high-class drugs.

**Question 33: B**

Whilst **A** and **C** may be true, they are not part of the argument. **D** is a possible but cannot be logically proposed from the information above. **E** would be a flaw if the argument were 'all levels of sports teams reduce bullying' but the passage explicitly states 'well-performing' teams. Hence **B** is correct as it undermines the whole argument, reversing the cause and effect.

**Question 34: B**

Options **A**, **C** and **D** do not directly weaken the argument as if any 16-year-olds were buying/drinking alcohol (whether the minority or majority), police would still be spending time catching them. The suggested benefit to reduce police time spent catching underage drinkers would be negated if **B** were true, hence it is the correct answer.

**Question 35: D**

**A** is an interpretation of the last sentence and doesn't accurately summarise the argument in the passage. **B** is untrue as there is no mention of if the government can afford to give grants or not. **C** and **E** are incorrect as the passage only talks about small businesses. **D** is correct as it best summarises the change in government policy regarding small businesses.

**Question 36: A**

The statement discusses a case that was reported but aims to argue that there may be important errors occurring every day in medicine that go unreported. Option **A**, if true, would significantly weaken this argument as it would negate it being a possibility. **B, C, D** and **E** may be true, but they do not negate the argument – if doctors are trained, accidents like the above may still occur. Operations that are successful do not affect those that are not, nor do unavoidable errors have any relation to avoidable ones. That the patient may have died if these errors had not occurred does not mean that they should not be considered errors.

**Question 37: A**

The main point of the statement is to highlight that although there are numerous safety precautions in place to protect patients, when all of the weaknesses in these precautions align big errors can occur. So, **A** is correct. While **E, C, B** and **D** may well be true, they are not the overall conclusion of the statement.

**Question 38: B**

Though not the first to be cited, the original error is cited as being the incorrect copying of the sidedness of the kidney to be removed, hence **B** is the correct option. The other options represent errors that in the 'Swiss cheese model' would have not been allowed to occur if the original had not taken place.

**Question 39: D**

In this instance the 'tip of the iceberg' refers to the number of medical errors reported, implying there may be a significantly larger proportion that go unreported; hence the correct option is **D**, and not **B**.

**Question 40: A**

The description given about the consultant's performance versus emotional arousal is described as initially increasing then eventually decreasing over time, which is best represented by graph **A**.

**Question 41: B**

The consultant says that the 'public perception is that medical knowledge increases steadily over time' which is best represented by graph **B**. The consultant says the regarding the acquisition of medical knowledge, 'many doctors [reach] their peak in the middle of their careers', which is best described by the graph **D**.

**Question 42: B**

Obesity is not mentioned in the passage, so **E** is incorrect. There is no mention of exercise specifically as it relates to old age, so **A** and **D** are also wrong. The diseases associated with lack of exercise are not specifically stated to cause early death, only that they are associated with older people, so **C** is also incorrect. The passage does, however, argue that lack of exercise is associated with illness. It follows from this that exercise would be linked to a lack of illness, or good health, so **B** is correct.

**Question 43: E**

The preference of women to have their babies at hospital versus home is not commented upon so **B** is incorrect. **A** and **D** are possible inferences from the passage but not conclusions. **C** is never implied, only that normal home births are no riskier than those in hospital. The overall conclusion of the statement is that home births should be encouraged where possible as they do not carry more risk, and hospital births are an unsustainable cost for the NHS.

**Question 44: B**

While **A**, **C** and **D** would, if true, make the practicalities of increasing home births more difficult they would not weaken the argument as much as **B** would. Where the statement's whole argument rests on home births being as safe as hospital births, **B**, if true, would negate this.

**Question 45: D**

The statement says, 'With the increase in availability of health resources we now, too often, use services such as a full medical team for a process that women have been completing single-handedly for thousands of years.' Thus, implying **D**, 'excessive availability of health resources' is the cause of 'medicalisation of childbirth'.

**Question 46: E**

Statements **1** and **3** identify weaknesses in the argument. If campaigns help keep deaths by fire low, they can be seen as 'necessary', and their necessity may be proven by low rates of fire-related mortality. If there are more people with hernias than people injured in fires, it follows that more people could die from hernias, but this does not mean that fires are less dangerous to the individuals involved. Statement **2** is irrelevant, as the argument is about how dangerous fires are in their entirety, not in relation to their constituent parts. Therefore **E**, '1 and 3 only', is correct.

**Question 47: B**

Since the group of 'some footballers' that like maths are not necessarily the same 'some' who like history we can exclude **A** and **D**. Equally, while **C** may or may not be true, we are not given any information about rugby players' preference for history, so it is incorrect. We know that all basketball players like English and chemistry, and that none of them like history, but as we do not know about a third subject that they may like, **E** is incorrect. We know all of the rugby players like English and geography and some of them like chemistry, hence there must be a section of rugby players that like all three subjects, so **B** is correct.

**Question 48: D**

The passage discusses the problems surrounding controlling drugs and focuses on the rapid manufacture of new 'legal highs': it is therefore implied that this is the current major problem. The passage also suggests that as the authorities cannot keep up with drug manufacture, the legal category of drugs doesn't reflect their relative risks. **1** is incorrect as the passage says health professionals feel legality is less relevant now, but it doesn't say that it is not still important. **3** is incorrect as the last sentence says a potential problem of legal highs is that the risks are not as clear, which contradicts the statement that the public are not concerned about any risks.

**Question 49: B**

The passage argues that it is essential to ban those with the mentioned medical conditions from climbing for safety reasons. It does not claim that this is *sufficient* to ensure safety, but simply that it is *necessary* to do so. Thus, **C** is irrelevant, as the risks of other activities do not influence the risk posed by mountain climbing. **D** is also irrelevant, because the argument discusses how it is essential to ensure safety of people on WilderTravel holidays, so those using other companies are not considered in this argument. **A** is an irrelevant statement because the passage is discussing what should be done *to ensure safety*, not whether this is the morally correct course of action.

Thus, a discussion of whether people should choose to accept the risks is not relevant. However, **B** *is* a flaw, because the guidelines only mention those with *severe* allergies, so thinking those with less severe allergies are in danger is a false assumption that has been made by the directors.

**Question 50: D**

The hospital director's comments make it abundantly clear that the most important aspect of the new candidate is good surgical skills, because the hospital's surgical success record requires improvement. If we accept his reasoning as being true, then it is clear that the candidate who is most proficient at surgery should be hired, and patient interaction should not be the deciding factor. Thus, Candidate 3 should be hired, as suggested by statement **D**.

**Question 51: A**

Answers **B** and **D** are irrelevant to the conclusion, since the argument only talks about how medical complications could be avoided *if* winter tyres were fitted. Discussion of whether this is possible (as in **B**) or whether there are other options (as in **D**) is irrelevant to this conclusion. **C** is not an assumption because the passage explicitly states that delays cause many complications, which could be avoided with quicker treatment. However, the argument does not state that winter tyres would allow ambulances to reach patients more quickly, so **A** is an assumption.

**Question 52: B**

The passage discusses how anti-vaccine campaigns cause deaths by spreading misinformation and reducing vaccination rates. It claims that *in order to protect* people, we should block the campaigners from spreading such misinformation freely. Thus, it is made clear that this action should be taken *because the campaigners cause deaths*, not simply because they are spreading misinformation. Thus, **B** is the principle embodied by the passage, and **C** is incorrect. **A** actually demonstrates an opposite principle, whilst **D** is a somewhat irrelevant statement, as the passage makes no reference to whether we should promote successful public health programmes.

**Question 53: D**

The passage states that the tumour has established its own blood supply (it says this was shown during the testing), and that a blood supply is *necessary* for the tumour to grow beyond a few centimetres. Thus, **A** and **B** are not assumptions. **C** is not an assumption, as it actually disagrees with something the passage has implied. The passage has actually said that action *must* be taken, implying that something *can* be done to stop the tumour. However, at no point has it been said that a blood supply is *sufficient* for a tumour to grow larger than a few centimetres. If this is not true, then the argument's conclusion that we should expect the tumour to grow larger than a few centimetres, and that action must be taken, no longer readily follows on from its reasoning. It is possible the tumour will still fail to grow larger than a few centimetres. Thus, **D** is an assumption made by the passage, and also constitutes a flaw in its reasoning.

**Question 54: A**

**D** is incorrect, as the passage has stated the runners are people running to raise money for the GNAA. **B** and **C**, meanwhile, are incorrect as the passage is only talking about whether the GNAA *will be able to* get a new helicopter. Thus, references to whether it wishes to, or whether this is the best use of money, are irrelevant. **A**, however, is an assumption on the part of the writer. The passage says that the GNAA will be able to get a helicopter if £500,000 is raised, but this does *not* mean that it won't be able to if the £500,000 is not raised by the runners. It could well be that they secure funding from elsewhere, or that prices drop. The money being *sufficient* to get a new helicopter does not mean it is *necessary* to get one.

**Question 55: C**

**B** and **D** somewhat strengthen this argument, suggesting that more people going on courses leads to better growth, and that people who have gone on these courses are more attractive to employers. **A** does not really affect the strength of the argument, as the current rate of growth does not affect whether government subsidies would lead to increased growth. **C**, however, weakens the argument significantly by suggesting that people would not be more likely to attend the courses if the government were to subsidise them, as the cost has little effect on the numbers of people attending.

**Question 56: D**

**B** is simply a fact stated in the passage. It does not draw upon any other reasons given in the passage, so it is not a conclusion. **C** is not a conclusion because it does not follow on from the reasoning given in the passage. The passage discusses what should be done *if* Pluto is to be classified as a planet, it does not make any mention of whether this *should* happen. **A** and **D** are both valid conclusions from the passage. However, on closer examination we can see that if we accept **A** as being true, it gives us good reason to believe the statement in **D**. Thus, **D** is the *main* conclusion in the passage, whilst **A** is an *intermediate* conclusion, which goes on to support this main conclusion.

**Question 57: C**

**A**, **B** and **D** would all affect whether the calculation of the Glasgow train's arrival time is correct, but none are assumptions because all of these things have been stated in the passage. However, the passage has *not* stated that the trains will travel at the same speed, and if this is not true, then the conclusion that the Glasgow train will arrive at 8:30pm is no longer valid. Thus, **C** is an assumption.

**Question 58: A**

**C** can actually be seen to be probably untrue, as the passage mentions a need to escape immune responses, suggesting that the immune system *can* tackle these cells. **E** is true but not representative of the main argument made in the passage. **B** and **D** are not *definitely* true. The passage mentions several *essential* steps that *must* occur, but this does not mean that they are *sufficient* for carcinogenesis to occur, or guaranteed to occur. Equally, the passage makes no reference to multiple mechanisms by which carcinogenesis can occur. It could be there is only one pattern in which these steps can occur. **A**, however, can be reliably concluded, because the passage does mention several steps that are *essential* for carcinogenesis to occur.

**Question 59: D**

Answers **A** and **C** are stated in the passage (the passage states 'deservedly known'), so these can be reliably concluded. **B** can also be concluded, as it is stated that in over 50% of cancers, a loss of functional P53 is identified. **D** however, cannot be concluded, as the passage simply states that any cell that has a mutation in P53 *is at risk* of developing dangerous mutations. Thus, it cannot be concluded that a given cell *will* develop such a mutation.

**Question 60: D**

**D** is not an assumption because Sam's calculations are based on the *cost per 1000 miles*, not on a given amount of fuel being used up. Thus, he has *not* assumed anything about whether the fuel usage is the same for each car. All of the others are assumptions, which have not been considered. Each of these will affect the total saving he will make if they are not true. For example, if the diesel car costs £100 more than the petrol car, the total saving will be £1700, *not* £1800 as calculated.

**Question 61: D**

The passage discusses how alcohol is more dangerous than cannabis, and states that this highlights the gross inconsistencies in UK drugs policy. Thus, **D** is the main conclusion of the passage, while **A** is a reason given to support this conclusion. The passage simply highlights that the policy is grossly inconsistent, and does not mention whether it should be changed, or how (whether alcohol should be banned, or cannabis allowed). Thus, **B** and **C** are not valid conclusions from this passage. The fact alcohol is freely advertised is only mentioned briefly in the passage to add strength to the argument that alcohol is more accessible than cannabis, but no judgment is made on whether this should not be so, so **E** is also not a valid conclusion from this passage.

**Question 62: B**

The passage argues that if first aid supplies were available, many accidents could be avoided. **B** correctly points out that this is a flaw – first aid supplies may help treat accidents and reduce the prevalence of *injuries and deaths*, but there is no reason why first aid supplies should reduce the incidence of *accidents*. Answers **C** and **D** are irrelevant, since the argument is talking about how first aid supplies could reduce *accidents*, not *injuries* or deaths. Thus, discussing cases in which they could not treat the injuries, or whether they need other components to do so is irrelevant. Equally **A** is irrelevant, as the argument is simply talking about what could happen *if* first aid supplies were stocked in homes, and makes no reference to whether this is financially viable.

**Question 63: C**

Answers **A** and **D** are not flaws because the passage does not conclude the things mentioned in these. No mention is made to the safety of the drug, and the argument only states that it is thought the compound *may* be of use in combating cancer. No premature conclusions are drawn, only suggestions are made. **B** is not a flaw because we can see that the experiments *may* produce misleading results if the wrong solutions are used, suggesting that DNA replication is inhibited even if it is not. **C**, however, is a valid flaw because the argument erroneously concludes that the wrong solutions must have been used when it says the experiments *do not reflect what is actually happening*. This clearly indicates a conviction that the wrong solutions were used, which does not follow on from the experiments being old.

**Question 64: B**

The passage has not said anything about who scored the winning goal, so **A** is not an assumption. **C** is also incorrect because the passage states that South Shields won the game. **B** correctly identifies that while beating South Shields was *sufficient* to win the league, it was *not* necessary. If Rotherham wins their other 2 games, they will still win the league, so **B** demonstrates an assumption in the passage. **D** is not relevant, as it does not affect the erroneous nature of the claim that Rotherham *will not* win the league having lost the match to South Shields.

**Question 65: B**

**C** and **D** actually strengthen or reinforce the CEO's reasoning, with **C** suggesting as time progresses Middlesbrough will have more and more people compared to Warrington, whilst **D** suggests that the market share in Warrington may not be as high as suggested, adding further reasons to build in Middlesbrough. **A** somewhat weakens the CEO's argument, but it is not a flaw in the reasoning, because the CEO is simply talking about how Middlesbrough will bring them within the range of more people, so the market share comment is a counterargument, not a flaw in his reasoning. **B**, however, is a valid flaw in this argument. Just because Warrington's population is falling, and Middlesbrough's is rising, does not necessarily mean that Middlesbrough's will be higher.

**Question 66: D**

1 and 2 are assumptions. The information given does *not* necessarily lead on to the conclusion that these extinction events will continue without further conservation efforts. Equally, there is nothing in the passage that says conservation efforts cannot be stepped up without increased funding. However, 3 is not an assumption, because the passage *states* that global warming has caused changes in weather patterns, which have since caused destruction of many habitats, leading to many extinction events. Thus, the passage demonstrates that global warming has indirectly caused these extinctions, and so the answer is **D**.

**Question 67: E**

The argument is suggesting that in Austria, the high passenger numbers and approval ratings of the rail service are accounted for by the fact that road travel is difficult in much of Austria. The passage then concludes that the public subsidies have no effect. We can see that 1 instantly weakens this argument by providing evidence to the contrary, (in France, difficult road travel is not prevalent and so cannot account for the high passenger numbers/approval ratings the country possesses). Statement 3 also weakens this conclusion by suggesting multiple factors affect the situation. This makes the conclusion based on the evidence from Austria less strong. Thus, the answer is **E**. 2 actually strengthens the argument that the public subsidies do not cause high passenger numbers/approval ratings, as Italy has high subsidies but low passenger numbers/approval ratings.

**Question 68: C**

**A** is incorrect; in 2011 24% of men and 26% of women were obese (one should not confuse this with the rates of combined obese and overweight). **B** is also incorrect, as what it states is true for adults; however, the figures for children aged 2-15 have changed little over the past year. **D** is not stated or implied by the passage. **C** is implied in the last two sentences of the article, and so this is the correct answer.

**Question 69: E**

None of the given statements can be concluded from the information based on the passage.

**Question 70: D**

Be careful of using your own knowledge (outside of what is given in the passage) here! Whilst **A** and **B** may be true, they are not the main message of the passage. **C** may be true but is not discussed in the passage. **E** is speculative, as the passage does not say if the transplant would be a 'good alternative'. **D** is correct as it echoes the main message of the passage.

**Question 71: F**

Smoking and diabetes are risk factors for vascular disease (not a cause). Vascular disease does not always lead to infarction. The passage does not give sufficient detail about necrotic tissue to conclude **C** or **D**.

**Question 72: B**

**A** is not relevant to the conclusion of the passage. Meanwhile, **E** does nothing to alter the conclusion, as the fact that schools receive similar funds does not affect the fact that more funding could provide better resources, and thus improve educational attainment. **C** actually weakens the argument, by implying that banning the richer from using the state school system would not raise many funds, as most do not use it anyway. **D** does not strengthen the conclusion as stating that a gap exists does not do anything to suggest that more funding will help close it. **B** clearly supports the conclusion that more funding, and better resources, would help close the gap in educational attainment.

**Question 73: A**

**D** and **E** are irrelevant to the argument's conclusion. **C** is actually contradicting the argument. **B** is stated in the passage, so is not an assumption of the passage. **A** describes an assumption: the increase of DVDs does not, necessarily, cause the loss of cinema customers.

**Question 74: C**

The question refers to aeroplanes being the fastest form of transport, and states that this means that travelling by air will allow John to arrive as soon as possible. **C** correctly points out that the argument has neglected to take into account other delays induced by travelling by aeroplane. Cost and legality are irrelevant to the question, so **B** and **E** are incorrect. Meanwhile, **D** actually reinforces the argument, and **A** refers to future possible developments that will not affect John's current journey.

**Question 75: D**

The argument states that people should not seek to prevent spiders from entering their homes. It does not say anything about whether people should like spiders being in their home, so **A** is incorrect. The argument also makes no allusion to the notion of people preventing flies from entering their homes, so **B** is incorrect. The argument also does not mention or implies that any efforts should be made to encourage spiders to enter homes, or that they should be cultivated, so **C** and **E** are also incorrect.

**Question 76: A**

**A** correctly identifies an assumption in the argument. At no point is it stated that bacterial infections in hospitals are resulting in deaths. **B**, **C**, **D** and **E** are all valid points, but they do not affect the notion that pressure for more antibiotic research would save lives. Therefore, none of these statements affect the conclusion of the argument and as such they are not assumptions in this context.

**Question 77: B**

The passage does not state that John disregards arguments because of the gender of the speaker, so **D** is incorrect. **A** and **C** are also wrong, as John states he finds women with armpit hair necessarily unattractive, so a different face or the knowledge of concealed hair would not make him find the female in question more appealing to his aesthetic. John does not state Katherine wants other women to stop shaving, so **E** is incorrect.

**B** is the correct answer, as Katherine was simply speaking about societal norms, and at no point is it said she was trying to convince John to find her, with armpit hair, attractive.

**Question 78: D**

**A** is irrelevant to the argument, which says nothing about what will happen to medicine in the future. The argument is describing how Sunita is incorrect, and how better medicine is not responsible for a high death rate from infectious disease in third world countries, and how better medicine will actually decrease this rate. **C** is a direct contradiction to this conclusion, so is incorrect. **E** is a fact stated in the argument to explain some of its reasoning, and is not a conclusion, therefore **E** is incorrect.

Both **B** and **D** are valid conclusions from the argument. However, **B** is not the main conclusion, because the fact that 'Better medicine is not responsible for a high death rate from infectious disease in third world countries' actually supports the statement in **D**, 'Better medicine will lead to a decrease in the death rate from infectious disease in third world countries'. Therefore, **B** is an example of an intermediate conclusion in this argument, which contributes to supporting the main conclusion, which is that given in **D**.

**Question 79: A**

The statement in **A**, that housing prices will be higher if demand for housing is higher, is not stated in this argument. However, it is implied to be true, and if it is not true, then the argument's conclusion is not valid from the reasoning given. Therefore, **A** correctly identifies an assumption in the argument. The other statements do not affect how the reasons given in the argument lead to the conclusion of the argument and are therefore not assumptions made in the passage to support the argument.

**Question 80: B**

**A** and **E** are both contradictory to the argument, which concludes that because of the new research, Jellicoe motors should hire a candidate with good team-working skills. **C** refers to an irrelevant scenario, as the argument is referring to only one candidate being hired, and at no point does it state or imply that several should be hired. **B** correctly identifies the conclusion of the argument; that Jellicoe motors should hire a new candidate with good team-working skills in order to boost their productivity and profits. **D** meanwhile exaggerates the consequences of not following this course of action. The argument does not make any reference to the notion that Jellicoe motors will struggle to be profitable if they do not hire a candidate with good team-working skills.

**Question 81: E**

**D** is a direct contradiction of the argument, so is not the conclusion. Meanwhile, **B** is a reason stated in the argument to explain some of the situations described. It is not a conclusion, as it does not follow on from the reasons given in the argument.

**A** and **E** are both valid conclusions drawn from the argument presented in the passage. However, only **E** is the *main* conclusion. This is because both **A** goes on to support the statement in **E**. If bacterial resistance to current antibiotics could result in thousands of deaths, this supports the notion that the UK government must provide incentives for pharmaceutical firms to research new antibiotics if it does not wish to risk thousands of deaths.

Meanwhile, **C** appears to be another intermediate conclusion in the argument that also supports the main conclusion. However, on close inspection this is not the case. **C** refers to the UK government directly investing in new antibiotic research, whilst the argument refers to the government providing incentives for pharmaceutical firms to do so. Therefore, **C** is not a valid conclusion from the argument.

**Question 82: B**

**E** is completely irrelevant because the question is referring to an unsustainable solution, "*if*" the UN's development targets are met. The likelihood of the targets being met is irrelevant. **C** is irrelevant because they do not affect the fact that the situation would be unsustainable if everybody used the amount of water used by those in developed countries, as stated in the question. **A** is also irrelevant, as the passage does not mention price as a factor to be considered within the argument.

Meanwhile, **D** would actually strengthen the argument's conclusion.

Therefore, the answer is **B**. Statement **B** correctly identifies that if those in developed countries use less water, it may be possible for everyone to use the same amount as these people and still be in a sustainable situation.

**Question 83: C**
There is no mention of treatment, so **A** is incorrect. A need to travel abroad for the post is not stated either, so **B** is incorrect. The need for a cool head is stated explicitly, but not necessarily that this is required to be a leader, so **D** is also wrong. Other qualities are irrelevant to the argument, so **E** is also incorrect. **C** would only be relevant if there was indeed a link between 'a specific phobia' and 'a general tendency to panic'. Thus, **C** highlights the flaw: if a fear of flying does not indicate a general disposition of panic, the argument for not hiring this employee crumbles.

**Question 84: C**
The passage does not suggest there are no more university places, nor does it make a distinction between the qualities of different universities, so **A** is incorrect, and **D** is irrelevant. The argument does not deny the fact that people can be successful without a university education, so **B** is also wrong. **C** is correct, as the passage specifically states 'many more graduates', but not all, are equipped with better skills and better earning potential. This suggests not all degrees produce these skill-sets in their graduates, and so not all university places will create high-earning employees.

**Question 85: D**
**B** is unrelated to the argument, as other contributing factors would not negate the damaging potential of TV. Watching sport on television would not be akin to actually playing sport, so **A** is also incorrect. The possibility of eye damage is stated as caused by TV, so **C** is incorrect. However, if people watch television *and* partake in sport, which the passage seems to imply cannot happen, they may not suffer the negative effects of obesity and social exclusion. For example, they may play sport during the day and watch television in the evening, thus experiencing the benefits of exercise and also enjoying the sedentary activity. Therefore, various potential threats supposedly posed by watching excessive television are undermined, and **D** is correct.

**Question 86: C**
**D** directly counters the above argument, and so is incorrect. Though **A**, **B** and **D** are all suggested or stated by the passage, they each act as evidence to support the main conclusion, **C**, describing the 'multiple reasons to legalise cannabis'.

**Question 87: C**
**C** is not an assumption as it has been explicitly stated in the passage that the salary is fixed, and therefore it will not change. The rest of the statements are all assumptions that Mohan has made. At no point has it been stated that any of the other statements are true, but they are all required to be true for Mohan's reasoning to be correct. Therefore, they are all assumptions Mohan has made.

**Question 88: A**
The answer is not **B** because, although the Holocaust was a tragedy, this is not explicitly stated in the passage. It cannot be **C** or **E**, as these are also not directly stated above. **D** provides an intermediate conclusion that leads to the main conclusion of **A**: we should not let terrible things happen again, and through teaching we can achieve this, so therefore 'we should teach about the Holocaust in schools'.

**Question 89: C**

DVDs are irrelevant – though one could access disturbing material through a DVD, this does not mean the material available on TV is less disturbing. The argument also is not concerned with adults, and the suggestion is that violence in any quantity may have a detrimental effect, even if a show is not entirely made up of it. **A, B** and **D** are thus not the correct answers. **C** contradicts the argument, as it suggests there is no link between witnessing violence and re-enacting what one has witnessed.

**Question 90: C**

**A** is irrelevant, as the passage states it *could* teach children, not that it necessarily would. **B** and **C** are also irrelevant, as the entertainment quality of the show or the likeability of its protagonist would not undermine the logic of the argument. **C** is the correct answer, as it shows how the question uses one model of success and projects it onto all other models, which is illogical: just because Frank succeeds without morality, does not mean all others must reject morality to succeed.

**Question 91: A**

**B, C, D** and **E** are all irrelevant to Freddy's argument that he cannot say a sexist thing because he is a feminist. The woman's discomfort, Neil's feminist stance, the appropriateness of making comments about men, or lewd comments in general do not affect his claim. The presumed link between the two (inability to say something sexist, and feminist self-description) is the flaw in Freddy's argument: someone may believe in equal rights for the genders, and still make a sexist remark.

**Question 92: A**

At no point is it stated or implied that car companies should prioritise profits over the environment, so **C** is incorrect. Neither is it stated that the public do not care about helping the environment, so **E** is incorrect.
**B** is a reason given in the argument, whilst **D** is impossible if we accept the argument's reasons as true, so neither of these statements are conclusions.

**Question 93: D**

It is important not to add your own knowledge and only use what is written in front of you. The last sentence leaves us with a sense that something needs to be done, so we are looking for an answer describing a change of some sort. **A** is addressed in the paragraph, but it is not the main conclusion. **B** refers to parking, which is not discussed in the paragraph. **C** is also not mentioned. **E** seems to be a true statement but is not the main takeaway from the paragraph. **D** is the only answer which mentions reducing car usage.

**Question 94: D**

After reading the short paragraph, we can see that higher salaries are what we are looking for as the main conclusion is mentioned at both the start and at the end. Only **D** and **E** mention higher salaries, so we should look at these options. **E** states the firm will be big and successful, but the last sentence of the paragraph says, 'could help', and we see it is a prediction, not a certainty. **D** is also a prediction, but it is stated more definitively.

**Question 95: C**

We do not know from the passage if bushfires are a yearly occurrence, or if they will happen next year, so **A** is incorrect. **B** seems logical, but we also do not know that bushfires are the sole cause of furthering global warming. The control of bushfires is also not discussed. **C** is correct: the passage clearly states that a huge amount of carbon dioxide was released. **D** is incorrect, since current world targets are not discussed, and the fact that 'some scientific studies' suggest a number of 100 million tonnes does not mean that these are world targets. **E** is also incorrect. Although the figure given is a large one, we do not know the carbon emissions of other nations.

**Question 96: B**

**A** is not a flaw but a simple factual statement supported by the paragraph. **B** links the author's statements with their conclusion and addresses the flawed assumption behind it. **C** is not correct as the author does not suggest anywhere that we would find life like that on Earth. **D** is stated in the passage as a factual statement, but is not a flaw in the argument. **E** is incorrect, since the passage states that there might be life, not that there definitely is.

**Question 97: D**

**A** is not mentioned by the author, so we cannot comment on what the author thought about compensation. **B** is the opposite of the author's argument. **C** is one of the arguments used, but it is not the conclusion. **D** is correct, since it is in line with the author's conclusion. **E** is incorrect; the author explains why the criticism is unfair.

**Question 98: E**

**A**, if true, would not be a flaw in the argument. **B** is incorrect. While the statement may be true, it does not address what the passage is arguing. **C** is also irrelevant, and not referred to in the argument. **D** is the opposite of what the author is saying. **E** is correct since it identifies that the author's reasoning is backwards. The arts might thrive in freer, wealthier countries, rather than causing countries to become more successful.

**Question 99: D**

**A** does not address the news stories, which is what the author makes issue with. **B** might be a true statement, but it does not address the main conclusion about the news stories and how people react to them. **C** cannot be deduced from the paragraph alone. **D** is correct since it is relevant to this specific argument; it talks about the reaction the author wants us to have to the news stories, and not just the news stories themselves. **E** is not correct; the prediction is not outrageous.

**Question 100: B**

**A** is not correct, as 450 boys versus 300 girls as cyclists getting killed or seriously injured is not more than double. **B** is correct, as 1900 boys versus 900 girls is more than twice as likely. **C** cannot be correct since we are unable to comment on the supervision of girls or boys, as this is not referred to in the passage. **D** cannot be concluded as we have no information on the total number of boys or girls that ride bicycles or walk on the streets – only the accident data. **E** is similar. While the statement may be true, it is not a conclusion based on the information in the passage so cannot be correct in this case.

**Question 101: D**

There is no clear indication that the author wants the state to express a view on separate, urgent and non-urgent surgeries. **B** is not correct - whether the public can distinguish between urgent and non-urgent care is not mentioned in the passage. **C** is not stated in the passage. **D** is correct since it refers to the workload outside of office hours, and the public being a contributing factor, as stated in the first sentence. **E** is not included in the passage.

**Question 102: B**

**A** is a true statement but is not the main conclusion of the entire passage. **B** refers to government change, and the inaccessibility of justice as a result of policy changes. This refers to most of the passage, so is the best answer. **C** is an inference from the passage but is not the main conclusion of the whole passage. **D** is the opposite of the conclusion, as the fees hinder rather than aid people's ability. **E**, like **C**, may be inferred but is not the main conclusion.

## Question 103: E

**A** is not correct, because the author has added the conditional 'if' in the final sentence. **B** is not correct because education is not discussed in the passage at all. **C** is not correct because the author only states that intelligence 'tends to' result in more wealth, not that it always does. **D** is not the main assumption, although the author appears to assume they are representative. **E** is the best answer as it is the assumption that links to the conclusion, that there is a link between the professions and intelligence.

## Question 104: E

**A** refers to optimum quality of life, however the passage only talks about cognitive function, which may or may not be related to quality of life. **B** is mentioned briefly at the start of the passage, but is an inference made rather than a reliable conclusion. **C** is not mentioned, so is not a conclusion of the passage. **D** is incorrect. While true, there may be other factors involved so is not a full conclusion. **E** is a reasonable conclusion from the evidence given in the passage.

## Question 105: B

**B** is the answer because it follows the same logic as the passage; people who drive more will use roads more, so should pay more for that service in the form of a road tax. **A** is incorrect since wealth is not mentioned in the passage. **C** is focused on convenience rather than fairness. **D** is a different argument about money not being wasted. At face value, **E** appears to be a similar argument, but it is not a financial argument, so **B** is a better answer.

## Question 106: C

**A** is contrary to the passage. **B** is incorrect as the statement is too strong; the passage is only illustrating one specific instance. **C** is the best answer as the statement is less strong and uses the word 'sometimes', which is all we can conclude from the passage. **D** does not match the content of the passage as there is no comparison between citizens of other countries at all. **E** also does not match the argument in the passage, which argues for the less economically expedient option.

## Question 107: E

The columnist is saying that anyone should be able to express themselves however they see fit
**A** is incorrect since it argues for freedom of expression but states that it may be immoral to do so, which the columnist does not. **B** is incorrect since it argues for the limitation of something not the freedom to do something. **C** is incorrect since it argues expression in poor taste should be discouraged not rewarded. **D** is incorrect since it argues that artists should be able to create whatever they want as long as they do not offend people. **E** is correct: it argues for free speech and makes no moral judgements.

## Question 108: A

**A** is correct since the author is using direct evidence as refutation. **B** is incorrect because the author never extends the argument to all animals in the passage. **C** is incorrect because the author never attacks the link between the premise and the conclusion. **D** is incorrect because the author is not trying to establish their own claim but rather undermine someone else's claim. **E** is incorrect because it is the opposite of what the author is arguing.

**Question 109: A**

Analogy is being used to make a case for a specific scenario. **A** is correct since it matches the passage as it argues for specific circumstances. **B** is incorrect because there are no observed facts that the arguer is trying to explain. **C** is incorrect because there are no experimental results. **D** is incorrect because the argument is not about correcting an explanation. **E** is incorrect because the argument does not use empirical evidence to reach a conclusion about a particular case.

**Question 110: D**

**A, B, C and E** - All took actions to save face or for profit. Only **D** acted on a moral principle, making it the correct option.

**Question 111: A**

**A** is the most accurate summary of the author's strategy. In the last two sentences, the author said that not enough people voted to make this sample representative. **B** is incorrect since the author does not criticize the view. **C** is incorrect since the author is complaining about the size of the voter pool, not their motives. **D** is incorrect since the author does not argue that statistical data has been manipulated. **E** is incorrect since the author is not arguing about the premise, but the sample size.

**Question 112: C**

We can summarise the argument as follows: All of animal X have attribute Y, and all of animal Z have attribute Y. Therefore, X and Z are similar. (X = sharks, Y = fins, Z = dolphins). The argument closest to this is **C**, where X = bats, Y = wings, Z = eagles. **A** says they are similar but have differences. **B** does not tell us both share the same trait - the conclusion is based on the fact that they are similar, not that they both have teeth (if they both have teeth). **D** does not claim cats and dogs are similar as a result of both having eyes. **E** argues which category one species belongs to.

**Question 113: D**

In this argument, two things cannot be done simultaneously, and doing one means you cannot do the other. The conclusion is that you cannot be required to do both things. **A** is incorrect: it is not a trade-off and is incorrect. **B** is also incorrect: it appears similar, but it is a condition of certain people. **C** cannot be correct as it argues that of two options, both are equally risky. **D** is the correct answer; in order to do one thing, we must sometimes neglect the other. **E** is an argument about the probability that one of several things have happened, and therefore cannot be correct.

**Question 114: D**

**A** is wrong, because it is about market niches, which are not mentioned in the passage. **B** is wrong; the designer may still create appealing features. **C** is wrong as the passage does not contrast external with internal components. **D** is the only option stated in the passage so is correct. **E** is wrong because we do not know that phone companies always use extensive post-market surveys.

**Question 115: C**

**A** is wrong: the performer is not sacrificing something practical; he is convincing others to give him something expensive to impress the audience. B is wrong: it is altruistic. **C** is correct: the choice is impractical but more impressive. **D** is wrong: the choice of comfort and taste is in addition to safety. **D** is wrong: we can only guess at the motives of the man buying the car.

**Question 116: B**

This question demonstrates the importance of only using information given in the passage and not using outside knowledge & logic. **A** is incorrect; the passage never tells us that the driver's education programs that Chris donated to were successful. **B** is correct since Chris' business has benefited from his support of a good cause. C is wrong: we do not know that the young drivers benefited from the driving program. **D** is wrong; we do not know if it usually is, just that it was in this instance. E is wrong; we do not know that the action had broad community support just that some members of the community supported what Chris did.

**Question 117: C**

**A** is wrong; the commentator said that the universities should pick the kind of software that matches with their mission, not the most advanced. **B** is wrong because, although price is mentioned, it is not the determining factor. **C** is correct, as it re-states the conclusion that universities should choose the type of software technology that best matches the values embodied in the activities that are central to the mission of university. **D** is incorrect as efficiency is not mentioned as a determining factor. **E** is incorrect as we do not know from the passage if using the software would block the universities' goals.

**Question 118: D**

The conclusion to this argument is found in the middle of the paragraph: not all efforts to increase productivity are beneficial to the business as a whole. We know this is the conclusion because the rest of the arguments explain it. **A** and **B** are incorrect: they are pieces of evidence, not the conclusion. **C** is never argued in the passage; nothing is said about the employees being the owners, so this cannot be the conclusion. **D** is a slight rephrasing of the conclusion. **E** is never mentioned in the argument.

**Question 119: A**

**A** is correct since the rejection of evidence does not prove the opposite argument is true. **B** mentions an unrepresentative sample, but we don't know anything about the sample of products that the report used so it cannot be correct. **C** is wrong since Sainos' motivations are irrelevant to this argument. **D** is wrong as Tesoc are entirely separate from this argument. **E** assumes without providing justification that Tesoc's public relations department would not approve a draft report that was hostile to Tesoc's products. There was no report about Tesoc's products.

**Question 120: B**

**A** is wrong as we do not know what other conditions must be fulfilled to be an eligible board member. **B** is correct; if only people who are eligible to be on the board can be the executive administrator, Jim cannot be on the board, so, Jim can't be the executive administrator. **C** cannot be right as we do not know either way, and likewise with **D**. **E** is also wrong as we know nothing about the charges against Jim.

**Question 121: D**

The conclusion is that double-blind techniques should be used whenever possible in scientific experiments, because they help prevent misinterpretations. **A** is a piece of evidence, not the conclusion. **B** is accurate but does not refer to double blind techniques so cannot represent the conclusion. **C** is evidence for the conclusion, not the conclusion itself. **D** is a rephrasing of the conclusion, making it the correct answer. **E** is implied in the passage but is not the conclusion.

## Question 122: C

The conclusion is that Group B contains twice as many cans as Group A, and we need to prove this with a new piece of information. **A** is irrelevant: whatever happens to Group B is beyond the scope of the question. **B** is wrong since quality is not an issue in the argument, quantity is. **C** is correct, because if you do not lose any aluminium in the recycling process there are twice as many cans. **D** is wrong since it does not matter where else aluminium came from before we made Group A cans, as the passage focuses on the transition from Group A to B only. **E** is outside the scope of the argument, and so is irrelevant.

## Question 123: D

Every year it will be necessary for all high-risk individuals to receive a vaccine for a different strain of the virus. We need to prove this with a new piece of information. **A** is wrong as the number of people is not relevant to this argument. **B** is irrelevant. **C** does not provide proof we need a different vaccine every year. We already know the vaccine is only going to work against the strain most prevalent. **D** is correct; if a different virus is prevalent each year, then there will be a different vaccine every year. **E** is wrong since side effects are irrelevant to the argument.

## Question 124: B

The conclusion is the last sentence, and the evidence comes before it. The flaw is about the nature of the experts and their expertise. **A** is incorrect: the argument never mentions the causes of the problems. **B** is correct since the argument relies solely on the testimony of computer experts. **C** is wrong as the argument never mentions causes. **D** is wrong as the conclusion is just about a hospital, not about a group. **E** is another version of **D**. No claims about institutions are made.

## Question 125: A

Minivans are correlated with a low accident rate, but the argument relies on the assumption that the reason they do not get into accidents is because of the minivans, not the drivers. A reckless driver in a safe car is still reckless. **A** is therefore correct as we do not know what the cause of lower rate of accidents is. **B** is wrong: we do not know what sample the argument is based on. **C** is wrong: the driver never concludes a certain result, just a lower risk. **D** is wrong: the argument claims it is sufficient to get a minivan to bring the risk down, but it does not say it is necessary (necessary vs sufficient is a key point for many BMAT questions). **E** is wrong: we do not know enough about the source to comment.

## Question 126: C

**A** states only wrong actions hurt people. It is stated so is not an assumption. **B** is close to the answer. We know that neutral actions do not hurt people, so are not morally wrong. **C** states that any action that is not morally wrong is morally right. If something is not wrong, it is right. So, if it is neutral, it is right. This makes it a better answer than B. **D** is wrong since these actions exist, but this does not prove to us that they are right or wrong. **E** is irrelevant: the passage only covers reasonable expectations.

**Question 127: E**

The intended purpose of the posters is to boost employee motivation, but the evidence isn't about whether it's being boosted, just whether they are already motivated to work productively. Even if you are motivated, you can have your motivation boosted.

**A** is not relevant; what happens when companies do not use motivational posters is beyond the scope of the argument.

**B** is wrong; the argument is not about companies in general.

**C** is about other effects, but we are only looking for the intended effect.

**D** is irrelevant; whether motivation is affected by other things does not really matter.

**E** demonstrates the difference between being motivated already and the potential to be motivated further, making it the correct answer.

**Question 128: C**

**A** does not tell us about the particles or food, so does not lead us to the conclusion of the passage. **B** is wrong: weak evidence is not zero evidence, so it is still possible for the entomologist to be correct if the weak evidence is correct. **C** states if dump sites had no food, then the ants were not giving food to their neighbours. With this assumption, the conclusion now works. **D** is irrelevant: the argument is about the ants that the particles were brought to. **E** is unknown: the entomologist may have retracted their conclusion.

**Question 129: E**

Hopefully, you can tell that this is not a great survey. The conclusion is about Febrooze versus all available fabric softeners, but only Febrooze was used. Just because people prefer Febrooze to having no softener doesn't mean that they prefer Febrooze to every other fabric softener available. **A** is wrong; allergies are not relevant here. **B** is also irrelevant, as the product can be effective regardless of the environmental cost. **C** is wrong as expense is not related to how effective it is. **D** is also not about effectiveness. **E** is correct since Febrooze was not compared to other products.

**Question 130: C**

The principle is that those who use the healthcare system should pay for it out of their own pocket and those who are not using it should not have to pay for it. **A** does not address the argument that users pay for the services they use, so is extraneous. **B** is wrong as the principle established is not concerned with amount of usage, but who is using the service. **C** concerns the people who benefit from medical care, and their responsibility to pay, making it the correct answer. **D** is irrelevant; the argument was not concerned with incentives to seek care. **E** is irrelevant as the principle was about refusing services offered.

**Question 131: C**

The principle is that there are people who are able to apply fairly sophisticated rules without being able to specify those rules. **A** is wrong; it is a narrative description and poems are fairly distinct from each other. **B** makes a different argument, comparing those who apply and those who discover. **C** makes the same argument as the passage; people can recognise something but cannot articulate the defining characteristics. **D** is wrong; the argument is about recognition not describing. **E** is the reverse; people may understand rules but not apply them.

## Question 132: A

The moral principle applied here underlies the final decision to not press charges. **A** matches what is said in the passage about repenting, and then not pressing charges to punish the criminal. **B** applies to the wrong group, as the robber is not yet a convicted criminal. **C** does not apply since the robber did repent. **D** is not applicable since the criminal did cause permanent damage. **E** cannot be correct since we do not know if there are other reasons to show mercy from the above paragraph.

## Question 133: B

The principle is that even though each individual at an institution can be acting selfishly, the institution as a whole can accomplish good things for the public.

**A** is wrong; there isn't any such comparison between some social organisations and other social organisations. The passage instead compares the motivations of the individual staff members with the purpose of the institution.

**B** is correct as it states that an organisation (hospitals, universities, etc) can have a property (working for the public good) that not all of its members possess.

**C** is irrelevant; what people claim to be motivated by is not addressed in the paragraph.

**D** is also irrelevant; the passage never addresses those who founded the social institutions, nor does it address unintended consequences.

**E** is wrong since the institution discussed does fulfil its intended purpose not an unintended one.

## Question 134: B

In this situation, there is no strong opinion or argument. The key point is the discrepancy between what drivers think is happening and what is happening. **A** states that alcohol causes drivers to be poor judges, so they will not know if they are too drunk to drive. **B** is not a physical condition which prevents students from being able to do something. **C** provides a physical condition which causes the workers to be poor judges of whether they should keep working. **D** also presents a physical condition- being faint. **E** introduces the condition of schizophrenia.

## Question 135: C

**A** gives an argument is about what deserves criticism. **B** is similar to **A**. **C** is correct, as it justifies the author's reasoning. It connects the gap between accurate information and public interest and what constitutes good journalism. **D** is wrong since we do not know what the public desire or need. **E** does not strengthen the argument; it is accurate information and does satisfy curiosity.

## Question 136: D

The principle is that you should always have your own work checked by someone else. **A** focuses on who is better able to explain something, not who's better at detecting mistakes in someone's work. **B** emphasises making a special effort to explain one's views—it does not address the detection of mistakes. **C** is also wrong as the focus is on who is in a better position to detect 'good legal arguments', not who's in a better position to detect mistakes. **D** is correct. This choice illustrates the passage's principle that you should have your work (writing) checked (proofread) by someone else, because people are better at detecting mistakes in others' work (because that someone does not know in advance what is meant to be said) than in their own. **E** is wrong, it states the goal is to have a more enjoyable meal, whereas the goal in the passage is to spot mistakes more easily.

**Question 137: D**

We have two 'all' statements, then a mixture that is halfway between the two. A presents a scenario in which there are two things mixed together rather than one thing with a mixture of properties. **B** is wrong as Edward's family has two different properties; they live in two different places. **C** is irrelevant. It states Tom can do two different things. **D** is correct. It starts with two 'all' statements. It has parts that correspond to each of the parts in the original argument. It uses the same type of evidence and has the same type of conclusion. **E** does not have a second 'all' statement. We need 'all' and then another 'all'.

**Question 138: C**

Disproving a piece of evidence or an argument does not prove the opposite is true. **A** is wrong as the reasoning here isn't that there's a group who we should oppose and then do the opposite of what they say. It's just that we should do something, and there are some people who might not agree. **B** is in opposition to the argument. **C** takes the same line of argument as the one in the paragraph but in a different context. Beauticians argue something that is in their interest not in everybody else's. **D** is wrong because in this argument, the people are getting what they want. **E** is in opposition to something, unlike the main argument.

**Question 139: C**

The argument assumes that if all A are B, then all B must be A. A = dogs, B = barks. That is the central flaw of the argument, because it may be true that all dogs bark, but other animals may also bark. Similarly, although it may be true that all high interest debt should be avoided, there may be other debt that should be avoided as well.
A = high interest debt, B = avoid.
**A** is more accurate than the flawed argument given, singling out specific, rather than general, cases. **B** brings in another factor, which is low interest debt, a third part to the argument. The initial argument does not bring a third element. **C** follows the parallel reasoning, uses 'all', and only refers to high interest debt. **D** argues for 'some' cases rather than for all. **E** also argues using a 'some' statement.

**Question 140: B**

The first argument (Raiders winning title) is dismissed on the basis that the second argument presented (Jackie winning award) is false. **A** is not the same, as both arguments (health class and eating before exercise) are dismissed. **B** dismisses the belief that seagulls migrate using advanced spatial recognition patterns based on the second argument (highly developed frontal cortices). **C** dismisses both arguments together, like A. **D** dismisses both arguments without much reasoning. **E** has the same structure as **D**.
**B** is the answer.

**Question 141: C**

The original argument uses a structure of AB, BC, therefore -C, -A. A = winning, B = willingness to cooperate, C = motivation. **A** uses AB, BC, but then does not have two negatives, it just has one negative (no exercise). It follows AB, BC, therefore A, -B. **B** also has one negative (no mistakes). It follows AB, AC, therefore -B C. **C** has two negatives, and follows a similar structure using the ABC rule we outlined above. AB, BC, -C, -A. **D** follows the structure AB, BC, therefore -A, -C, so is similar but not quite parallel. **E** is the same as **D** in structure.

**Question 142: E**

If won, three questions were answered; Angela answered three questions, Angela won. A leads to B, and B leads to A. AB; BA. A - AB; AB The first statement matches, but the second doesn't. In fact, this argument makes sense, and the sentence confirms the condition. B - AB; not A - not B. This is a bad argument, but it denies the first condition. C - Is just a series of statements because no argument is being made. D - AB; BC; AC. This is a chain of events argument. E - AB; BA. This answer is longer than the stimulus, uses different language and tone, and even has a couple of extra arguments, but it is parallel in its reasoning to the example.

**Question 143: B**

The argument is a conditional statement, so A leads to B. It is likely, but not definite that B did not happen, so A is unlikely. **A** has a conditional statement with A leading to B and uses the word 'unlikely'. However, the second statement does not include the fact that 'B happened', we need to know the team did win the tournament. **B** has a conditional statement with A leading to B. The conclusion is that it is unlikely that A happened, matching the original statement. Order does not matter. **C** matches the structure of A, with one parallel statement, but the second statement does not match, because we do not know if Oliver actually won. **D** has similar wording, but the second half of the argument is different. **E** is close but does not tell us whether the first choice keeper is healthy or not at the end, so we cannot conclude this is parallel, as different reasoning is used.

**Question 144: D**

The passage concerns intelligence across different species. We are told that absolute brain size is not an indication of intelligence. The conclusion drawn is that relative brain size is a better indicator of intelligence than absolute brain size – **D**. **A**, **B** and **C** cannot be concluded from the passage. **E** is an argument but not a conclusion from the passage.

**Question 145: B**

**A** is not a necessary assumption of the argument; opposition to raising the driving age is not factored into the argument. **C** is not assumed by the argument. **D** is not assumed by the argument - it assumes that most of the individuals who do drive dangerously are young people. **E** is not assumed by the argument. The argument seeks to explain the root cause of road traffic accident deaths. It concludes that young drivers cause a large portion of traffic accidents. The underlying assumption is that most of the accidents involving young people were the fault of the young drivers – **B** is therefore the correct answer.

**Question 146: D**

The argument concludes that all public buildings should install ramps to enable accessibility for all disabled people.

**A** is irrelevant; the text does not make any arguments about non-public buildings.

**B** is also irrelevant; cost is not mentioned in the text.

**C** is beyond the scope of the discussion.

**D** is wrong since the conclusion is based on the assumption that older buildings are invariably inaccessible and fails to take into account the existence of older public buildings which are already accessible.

**E** is not a flaw in the argument.

## Question 147: E

This passage concerns the advantages of developing a 4-day work week. **A** is not supported by the passage, as pay is not mentioned. **B** cannot be drawn from the passage – although reduced stress is mentioned, they are not linked to health outcomes. **C** does not follow from the passage, as there is there is no mention of the macroeconomic impact of the proposed change. **D** cannot be drawn from the passage – there is nothing about who should implement the proposed change. **E** is correct since the passage argues for many benefits.

## Question 148: C

The argument seeks to explain the impact of wind farms on bird migration. It concludes that the plans to build electricity-generating wind farms on the hills surrounding the Straits of Gibraltar will negatively impact bird migration, making **C** the correct answer. **A**, **B**, **D** and **E** cannot be drawn from the passage – remember not to use any outside knowledge

## Question 149: E

**A** cannot be the case, as the passage does not mention research into microwave penetration. Nor can **B**, as text message popularity with various groups is not mentioned either. **C** might be a flaw in this argument, but it does not address the argument's central claim. **D** is an example of 'whataboutery', where a superficially similar issue is used as a counterargument. **E** is the answer, because it identifies the argument's key failing, which is that less call usage does not mean that the supposed danger is eliminated.

## Question 150: C

This passage compares fast food restaurants to factories. **C** correctly states the passage concludes that they are similar. **A** cannot be confidently concluded from this passage, as only two examples are given. **B** cannot be concluded by causation, as a relationship is not implied. **D** is an argument, not a summary of the conclusion. **E** cannot be correct as it is implied that they are similar, but it is an exaggeration to say that there is no difference.

## Question 151: D

The easiest thing to do is draw the relative positions. We know Harrington is north of Westside and Pilbury. We know that Twotown is between Pilbury and Westside. Crewville is south of Twotown, Westside and Harrington but we do not know but its location relative to Pilbury.

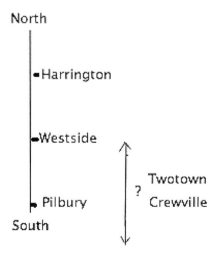

**Question 152: B**

By making a grid and filling in the relevant information the days Dr James works can be deduced:

|  | Sunday | Monday | Tuesday | Wednesday | Thursday | Friday | Saturday |
|---|---|---|---|---|---|---|---|
| Dr Evans | X | √ | X | X | √ | √ | √ |
| Dr James | X | √ | √ | √ | √ | X | √ |
| Dr Luca | X | X | √ | √ | X | √ | √ |

- No one works Sunday.
- All work Saturday.
- Dr Evans works Mondays and Fridays.
- Dr Luca cannot work Monday or Thursday.
- So, Dr James works Monday.
- And, Dr Evans and Dr James must work Thursday.
- Dr Evans cannot work 4 days consecutively so he cannot work Wednesday.
- Which means Dr James and Luca must work Wednesday.
- (Mentioned earlier in the question) Dr Evans only works 4 days, so cannot work Tuesday.
- Which means Dr James and Luca work Tuesday.
- Dr James cannot work 5 days consecutively so cannot work Friday.
- Which means Dr Luca must work Friday.

**Question 153: E**

Working algebraically, using the call out rate as C, and rate per mile as m.

So, C + 4m = 11

C + 5m = 13

Hence; (C + 5m) – (C + 4m) = £13 - £11

M = £2

Substituting this back into C + 4m = 11

C + (4 x 2) = 11

Hence, C = £3

Thus, a ride of 9 mile will cost £3 + (9 x £2) = £21.

**Question 154: E**

Use the information to create a Venn diagram.

We don't know the exact position of both Trolls and Elves, so **A** and **D** are true. Goblins are mythical but not magical, so **C** is true. Gnomes are neither so **B** is true. But **E** is not true.

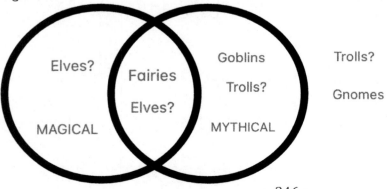

**Question 155: D**

The best method may be work backwards from 7pm. The packing (15 minutes) of all 100 tiles must have started by 6:45pm, hence the cooling (20 minutes) of the last 50 tiles started by 6:25pm, and the heating (45 minutes) by 5:40pm. The first 50 heating (45 minutes) must have started by 4:35pm, and cooling (20 minutes) by 5:20pm. The decoration (50 minutes) of the second 50 can occur anytime during 4:35pm- 5:40pm as this is when the first 50 are heating and cooling in the kiln, and so does not add time. The first 50 take 50 minutes to decorate and so must be started by 3:45pm.

**Question 156: E**

Speed = distance/time. Hence for the faster pain impulse the speed is 1m/ 0.001 seconds. Hence the speed of the pain impulse is 1000 metres per second. The normal touch impulse is half this speed and so is 500 metres per second.

**Question 157: E**

Using the months of the year, Melissa could be born in March or May, Jack in June or July and Alina in April or August. With the information that Melissa and Jack's birthdays are 3 months apart, the only possible combination is March and June. Hence Alina must be born in August, which means it is another 7 months until Melissa's birthday in March.

**Question 158: A**

PC Bryan cannot work with PC Adams because they have already worked together for 7 days in a row, so **C** is incorrect. **B** is incorrect because if PC Dirk worked with PC Bryan that would leave PC Adams with PC Carter, who does not want to work with him. PC Carter can work with PC Bryan.

**Question 159: C**

Paying for my next 5 appointments will cost £50 per appointment before accounting for the 10% reduction, hence the cost counting the deduction is £45 per appointment. So, the total for 4 appointments = 5 x £45 = £225 for the hair. Then add £15 for the first manicure and £10 x 2 for the subsequent manicures using the same bottle of polish giving an overall total of £260.

**Question 160: D**

Elena is married to Alex or David, but we are told that Bertha is married to David and so Alex must be married to Elena. Hence David, Bertha, Elena and Alex are the four adults. Bertha and David's child is Gemma. So, Charlie and Frankie must be Alex and Elena's two children. Leaving only options **A** or **D** as possibilities. Only Frankie and Gemma are girls so Charlie must be a boy.

**Question 161: C**

Using, x (minutes) as the unknown amount of time the second student took to examine, we can plot the time taken with the information provided thus:

|  | 1st student | | 2nd student | | 3rd student |
|---|---|---|---|---|---|
| 1st examination | $4x$ | 1 min | $2x$ | 1 min | $2x$ |
|  | 8 mins break | | | | |
| 2nd examination | $x$ | 1 min | $x$ | 1 min | $x$ |

Hence the total time taken, 45minutes (14:30-15:15)

Is represented by:   $4x + 2x + 2x + x + x + x + 1 + 1 + 8 + 1 + 1$

45 minutes = $11x$ (minutes) + 12 minutes

33 minutes = $11x$ (minutes)

Hence, $x = 3$ minutes, so the amount of time the second student took the first time, $2x$, is 6 minutes.

**Question 162: C & E**

Calculate the amount of change: £5 - (2 x £1.65), which = £3.30.

Logically we can then work out that the 3 coins in the change that are the same must be 1p as no other 3-coin combination can yield £1.70 when made up with 5 more coins. Thus, we know that 3 of the coins are 1p, 1p & 1p. We can then deduce that there must also have been 2p and 5p coins in the change as £1.70 is divisible by ten. The only way then to make up the remaining £1.60 in 3 different coins is to have £1, 50p and 10p, Hence the change in coins is 1p, 1p, 1p, 2p, 5p, 10p, 50p and £1. So, the two coins not given in change are £2 and 20p.

**Question 163: D**

If we express the speed of each train as W ms$^{-1}$, the relative speed of the two trains is 2W ms$^{-1}$.

Using Speed = distance / time: 2W = (140 + 140)/ 14.

2W = 20, and W = 10, so the speed of each train is 10 ms$^{-1}$.

To convert from metres to kilometres, divide by 1,000. To convert from seconds to hours, divide by 3,600. Therefore, the conversion factor is to divide by 1,000/3,600 = 10/36 = 5/18

To convert from ms$^{-1}$ to kmph, multiply by 18/5. Therefore, the final speed of the train is 18/5 x 10 = 36km/hr.

**Question 164: C**

Taking the day to be 24 hours long, this means the first tap fills 1/6 of the pool in an hour, the second 1/48, the third $\frac{1}{72}$ and the fourth $\frac{1}{96}$.

Taking 288 as the lowest common denominator, this gives: $\frac{48}{288} + \frac{6}{288} + \frac{4}{288} + \frac{3}{288}$ which = $\frac{61}{288}$ full in one hour.

Hence the pool will be $\frac{244}{288}$ full in 4 hours.

The pool fills by approximately $\frac{15}{288}$ every 15 minutes.

Thus, in 4 Hours 15: $\frac{244 + 15}{288} = \frac{249}{288}$

Thus, in 4 Hours 30: $\frac{244 + 30}{288} = \frac{274}{288}$

Thus, in 4 Hours 45: $\frac{244 + 45}{288} = \frac{289}{288}$

## Question 165: B

Each day until day 28, the ant gains a net distance of 1cm, so at the end of day 27 the ant is at 27cm height and therefore only 1cm below the top. On day 28, the 3cm the ant climbs in the day is enough to take it to the top of the ditch and so it is able to climb out.

## Question 166: A

To solve this question, three different sums are needed to use the information given to deduce the costs of the various items. With the information that 30 oranges cost £12, £12/30 = 40p per orange with the 20% discount, so oranges must cost 50p at full price. With the information that 5 sausages and 10 oranges cost £8.50, we know that the oranges at a 10% discount account for 10 x 45p = £4.50 so 5 undiscounted sausages cost £4 so each full price sausage is £4/5 = 80p. Finally, we know that 10 sausages and 10 apples cost £9, at 10% discount the sausages cost 72p each, thus accounting for 10 x 72p = £7.20 of the £9, hence the 10 apples at a 10% discount must cost £1.80, so each apple costs 18p at 10% discount. So, an apple is 20p full price. Now to add up the final total: 2 oranges + 13 sausages + 2 apples = (2 x 50p) + (13 x 72p) + (12 x 18p) = £12.52.

## Question 167: C

If we take the number of haircuts per year to be x, the information we have can be shown:

| Membership | Annual Fee | Cost per cut | Total Yearly cost |
|---|---|---|---|
| None | None | £60 | 60x |
| VIP | £125 | £50 | £125 + 50x |
| Executive VIP | £200 | £45 | £200 + 45x |

We know that changing to either membership option would cost the same for the year. We can express the cost for the year, y as;

VIP:     $y = £125 + 50x$

Executive VIP:   $y = £200 + 45x$

Therefore:   $£125 + 50x = £200 + 45x$

Simplified   $5x = £75$, therefore the number of haircuts a year, x is 15.

Substituting in x, we can therefore work out:

| Membership | Annual Fee | Cost per cut | Total Yearly cost |
|---|---|---|---|
| None | None | £60 | £900 |
| VIP | £125 | £50 | £875 |
| Executive VIP | £200 | £45 | £875 |

Hence the amount saved by buying membership is £25.

## Question 168: B

All thieves are criminals. So, the circle must be fully inside the square. We are told judges cannot be criminals so the star must be completely separate from the other two.

**Question 169: C**

We are told that March and May have the same last number, which must be either 3 or 13.

Taking the information from the question, that one of the factors is related to the letters of the month names, we can interpret that 13 represents the M which starts both March and May. Therefore, we know the rule is that the last number is the position of the starting letter.

Knowing that there is another factor about the letters of the month that controls the code, we can work out that one of the numbers may code for the number of letters. Which, in March, would be 5, which is the second letter, so we have the rule of the 2nd number.

Finally, through observation we may note that the first number codes for the months' relative position in the year. Hence, the code of April will be 4, (for its position), 5 (for the number of letters in the name) and 1 for the position of the starting letter 'A', and so 451 is the code.

**Question 170: D**

If $b$ is the number of years older than 5, and $a$ is the number of A*s, the money given to the children can be expressed:

£5 + £3b + £10a

Hence for Josie £5 + (£3 × 11) + (£10 × 9) = £128

We know that Carson receives £44 less yearly, and his b value is 13, so his amount can be expressed:

£5 + (£3 × 13) + (£10a) = £84

Simplified: £44 + £10a = £84

I.e. £10a = £40,

Carson's 'a' value, i.e. his number of A*s is 4, so the difference between Josie and Carson is 5.

**Question 171: B & C**

Using the information to make a diagram:

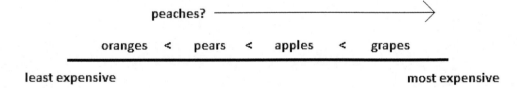

Hence **A** is incorrect. **D** and **E** may be true, but we do not have enough information to say for sure. **B** is correct, as we know peaches are more expensive than oranges, but not about their price relative to pears. Equally, we know **C** to be true, as grapes are more expensive than apples, so they must be more expensive than pears.

**Question 172: B**

It's easy to assume all the cuts should be in the vertical plane as a cake is usually sliced, however there is a way to achieve this with fewer cuts. Only three cutting motions are needed. **Start by cutting in the horizontal plane** through the centre of the cake to divide the top half from the bottom half. Then slice in the vertical plane into quarters to give 8 equally sized pieces with just three cuts.

## Question 173: B & D

After the changes have been made, at 12 PM (GMT +1):

- Russell thinks it is 11 AM
- Tom thinks it is 12 PM
- Mark thinks it is 1 PM

Thus, in current GMT+1 time zone, Mark will arrive an hour early at 11 AM, Russell an hour late at 1 PM and Tom on time at 12 PM. There is therefore a two-hour difference between the first and last arrival. For options E and F, be careful: the time zone listed is **NOT** GMT +1 that everyone else is working in. 1PM in GMT +3 = 11am GMT +1 (the time zone just entered) so that is Mark's actual arrival time; 12pm GMT +0 is the old time zone that Russell didn't change out of so that is Russell's correct arrival time.

## Question 174: D

Using Bella's statements, she must contradict herself with her two statements, as one of them must be true, we know that it was definitely either Charlotte or Edward. Looking to the other statements, e.g., Darcy's, we know that it was either Charlotte or Bella, as only one of the two statements saying it was both of them can have been a lie. Hence it must have been Charlotte.

## Question 175: E

The only way to measure 0.1 litres or 100ml, is to:

- Fill the 300ml beaker
- Pour into the half litre/ 500 ml beaker
- Fill the 300ml again and pour (200ml) into the 500ml
- This will make the 500ml full, leaving 100ml left in the 300ml beaker

The process requires 600ml of solution to fill the 300ml beaker twice.

## Question 176: D

If you know how many houses there are on the street it is possible to work out the average, which then you can round up and down and to find the sequence of numbers, e.g. if you know there are 6 houses in the street 870/6 = 145. Thus, we need to know the number of houses in the street (**statement 2 is correct**).

145 is not a house number because they are even so going up and down one even number consequentially one discovers that the numbers are 146, 144, 148, 150, 142 and 140.

But it is not possible to determine Francis' house number without knowing its relative position i.e. highest, 3rd highest, lowest etc. (**statement 1 is correct**).

**Statement 3 is incorrect**, as we can work out at least 3 of the house numbers without being given these house numbers!

## Question 177: D

Expressed through time:

| Event | People Present |
|---|---|
| There were 20 people exercising in the cardio room | 20 |
| Four people were about to leave | 20 |
| A doctor was on the machine beside him (one of the original 20) | 20 |
| Emerging from his office one of the personal trainers called an ambulance. | 21 |
| Half of the people who were leaving, left (-2) | 19 |
| Eight people came into the room to hear the man being pronounced dead. (+8) | 27 |
| The two paramedics arrived, (+2) | 29 |
| The man was pronounced dead (-1) | 28 |

## Question 178: B & D

Blood loss can be described as 0.2 L/min.

**For the man:**

8 litres – 40% (3.2 L) = 4.8 L when he collapses, taking 16 minutes (3.2 / 0.2 = 16)

**For the woman:**

7 litres – 40% (2.8L) = 4.2: when she collapses, taking 14 minutes (2.8 / 0.2 = 14)

Hence the woman collapses 2 minutes before the man, so **B** is correct, and **A** is incorrect. The total blood loss is 3.2L + 2.8L which = 6L so **C** is incorrect. The man's blood loss is 3.2L when he collapses so **E** is incorrect. The woman has a remaining blood volume of 4.2L when she collapses so **D** is correct.

## Question 179: B

Work out the times taken by each girl – (distance/pace) x 60 (converts to minutes) + lag time to start

Jenny: (13/8) x 60 = 97.5 minutes

Helen: (13/10) x 60 + 15 = 93 minutes

Rachel (13/11) x 60 + 25 = 95.9 minutes

## Question 180: C

Work through each statement and the true figures given in the question.

A.  Overlap of pain and flu-like symptoms must be at least 4% (56+48-100).  4% of 150: 0.04 x 150=6

B.  30% high blood pressure and 20% diabetes, so maximum percentage with both must be 20%.  20% of 150: 0.2*150 = 30

C.  Total number of patients – patients with flu-like symptoms – patients with high blood pressure.  Assume different populations to get minimum number without either.  150 – (0.56 x 150) – (0.3 x 150) = 21

D.  This is an obvious trap that you might fall into if you added up the percentages and noted that the total was >100%. However, this isn't a problem as patients can discuss two problems.

**Question 181: C**
This is easiest to work out if you give all products an original price. We used £100 as an example. You can then work out the higher price, and the subsequent sale price, and thus the discount from the original £100 price. As the price increases and decreases are in percentages, they will be the same for all items regardless of the price, so it does not matter what the initial figure you start with is.
Marked up price: 100 x 1.15 = £115
Sale price: 115 x 0.75 = £86.25
Percentage reduction from initial price is 100 – 86.25 = 13.75%

**Question 182: D**
The recipe states 2 eggs make 12 pancakes, therefore each egg makes 6 pancakes, so the number Steve must make should be a multiple of 6 to ensure he uses a whole egg.
Steve requires a minimum of 15 x 3 = 45 pancakes. To ensure use of whole eggs, this should be increased to 48 pancakes.
The original recipe is for 12 pancakes, therefore, to make 48 pancakes you use 4 times the original recipe.
Total quantities: 8 eggs, 400g plain flour and 1200 ml milk.

**Question 183: B**
Work through the question backwards.
In 6 litres of diluted bleach, there are 4.8 litres of water and 1.2 litres of partially diluted bleach.
In the 1.2 litres of partially diluted bleach, there are 9 parts water to one part original warehouse bleach.
Remember that a ratio of 1:9 means 1/10 bleach and 9/10 water. Therefore, working through the example, 120ml of warehouse bleach is needed.

**Question 184: C**
We know that Charles is born in 2002, therefore in 2010 he must be 8 years old. There are 3 years between Charles and Adam, and Charles is the middle grandchild. As Bertie is older than Adam, Adam must be younger than Charles. Therefore, Adam must be 5 in 2010. In 2010, if Adam is 5, Bertie must be 10 (the question states he is double the age of Adam).
The question asks for ages in 2015: Adam = 10, Bertie = 15, Charles = 13

**Question 185: B**
Make the statements into algebraic equations and then solve them as you would simultaneous equations. Let $a$ denote the flat fixed rate for hire, and $b$ the price per half hour.
Cost = $a + b$ (time in mins/30)
Peter: $a + 6b$ (6 half hours) = 14.50 (equation 1)
Kevin: $2a + 18b = 41$, or this can be simplified → cost per kayak, $a + 9b = 20.5$ (equation 2)
If you subtract equation 1 from equation 2:
$3b = 6$, therefore $b = 2$

Substitute $b$ into either equation to calculate a, using equation 1, $a + 12 = 14.50$.
Therefore, $a = 2.50$
Finally use these values to work out the cost for 2 hours:
2.50 (flat fee) + 4 × 2 (4half hours ×cost/half hour) = £10.50

**Question 186: E**

It is most helpful to write out all the numbers from 0 – 9 in digital format to most easily see which light elements are used for each number. You can then cross out any numbers which don't use all the lights from the digit 7.

Go through the digits methodically and you can cross out 1, 2, 4, 5, and 6 as they don't contain all three bars from the digit 7.

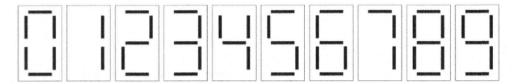

**Question 187: B**

In this question it is worth remembering it will take more people a shorter amount of time.
Work out how many man hours it takes to build the house (days x hours x builders)
12 x 7 x 4 = 336 hours
Work out how many hours it will take the 7man workforce: 336/7 = 48 hours
Convert to 8 hour days: 48/8 = 6 days

**Question 188: D**

By far the easiest way to do these types of questions is to draw a Venn diagram (use question marks if you are unsure about the exact position):

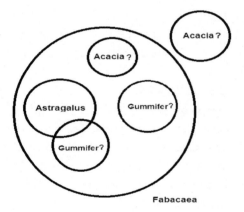

Now, it is a case of going through each statement:
A.  Incorrect - Acacia may be fabacaea. Acacia are not astragalus, but does not logically follow that they therefore can't be fabacaea.
B.  Incorrect – astragalus and gummifer are not necessarily separate within fabacaea.
C.  Incorrect – the statement is not reversible so the fact that all astragalus and gummifer are fabacaea does not mean all facacaea are gummifer and/or astragalus. E.g. Fabacaea could be acacia.
D.  Correct
E.  Incorrect – Whilst some acacia could be gummifer, there is no certainty that they are.

**Question 189: D**

Area of a trapezium = (a+b)/2 x h
Area of cushion = (50+30)/2 x 50 = 2000cm²
Since each width of fabric is 1m wide, both sides of one cushion can fit into one width. The required length is therefore 75cm x 4 = 3m with a cost of 3 x £10 = £30.
Cost of seamstress = £25 x 4 = £100
Total cost is £130

**Question 190: C**

There are 30 days in September, so Lisa will buy 30 coffees.

In Milk, every 10th coffee is free, so Lisa will pay for 27 coffees at 2.40 = £64.80

In Beans, Lisa gets 20 points each day and needs 220 points to get a free coffee, which is 11 days, with 5 points left over. Therefore, in 30 days she will get 2 free coffees. The cost for 28 coffees at 2.15 is £60.20

Beans is cheaper, and the difference is £64.80 - £60.20 = £4.60.

**Question 191: C**

For this question, it is best to work backwards and take note of how often each bus comes.

Paula must get off the 220 bus at 10.57 latest (she walks 3 minutes to her meeting).

Therefore, she could get the 10:40 bus, arriving at 10:54.

The latest that she can get on the 283 bus is 10:15, so as to make it to the 220 bus connection.

The 283 bus comes every 10mins (beware, the question doesn't state at what points past the hour it arrives/leaves), so Paula should be at the bus stop at 10.06 to ensure a bus arrives by 10.15 at the latest.

If the bus comes every 10mins, even if a bus comes at 10.05 which Paula will miss, the next bus will come at 10.15 and therefore she will still be on time. This gives the answer: Paula must leave at 10.01

**Question 192: B**

You are working out the time taken to reach the same distance (D). Make sure to take into account changing speeds of train A, and that train B leaves 20 minutes earlier.

$Speed = \frac{distance}{time}$

Make sure you keep the answers consistent in the time units you are using. The worked answer is all in minutes (hence the need to multiply by 60).

**Train A:** time for first 20 kilometres = $\frac{20}{100} \times 60 = 12$ minutes

So, the distance where it equals B is $12 + (\frac{D-20}{150}) \times 60$

You need to use D-20 to account for the fact you have already calculated the time at the slower speed for the first 20km

**Train B:** $(\frac{D}{90}) \times 60 - 20$

Make the equations equal each other as they describe the same time and distance, and then solve.

Simplifies to $32 + \frac{2D}{5} - 8 = \frac{2D}{3}$ so $D = 90$km

Train B will take 60 minutes to travel 90 km and train A will take 40 minutes (but as it leaves 20 minutes later, this will be point at which it passes).

**Question 193: C**

Work out the annual cost of local gym: 12 x 15 = £180

Upfront cost + class costs of university gym must therefore be >£180.

Subtract upfront cost to find number of classes: 180 – 35 = £145

Divide by cost per class (£3) to find number of classes: 145/3 = 48 1/3

48 1/3 classes would make the two gyms the same price, so for the local gym to be cheaper, you would need to attend 49 classes.

**Question 194: C**

**A** is definitely true, since the question states that all herbal drugs are not medicines. **B** is also definitely true as all antibiotics are medicines which are all drugs. **C** is definitely false, because all antibiotics are medicine, yet no herbal drugs are medicines. **D** is true as all antibiotics are medicines.

**Question 195: C**

Answer **A** cannot be reliably concluded, because from the information given a non-"Fast" train could stop at Newark, but not at Northallerton or Durham. We have no information on whether *all* trains stopping at Newark also stop at Northallerton.

Answer **B** is not correct because 8 is the *average* number of trains that stop at Northallerton. It is possible that on some days more than 16 trains run, and more than 8 will thus stop at Northallerton.

Answer **D** is incorrect because it is mentioned that *all* trains stopping at Northallerton also stop at Durham, giving a total 6 stops as a minimum for a train stopping at Northallerton (the others being the 4 stops which *all* trains stop at).

Answer **E** is incorrect for a similar reason to **A**. We have no information on whether all trains stopping at Newark also stop at Northallerton, so cannot determine that they must also stop at Durham.

Answer **C** is correct because "Fast" trains make less than 5 stops. Since all trains already stop at 4 stops (Peterborough, York, Darlington and Newcastle), they cannot then stop at Durham, as this would give 5 stops.

**Question 196: D**

From the information we are given, we can compose the following image of how these towns are located (not to scale, but shows the direction of each town with respect to the others):

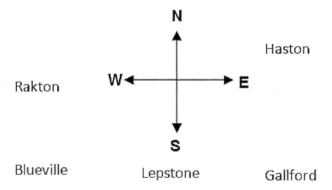

From this "map", we can see that all statements apart from **D** are true. Statement **D** is definitely *not true*: since Blueville is southwest of Haston, it cannot be east of Haston.

**Question 197: C**

We are told that in order to form a government, a party (or coalition) must have *over* 50% of the seats in parliament. Thus, they must have at least 50% of the total seats plus 1, which is 301 seats.

We are told that we are looking for the *minimum* number of seats the Greens can have in order to form a coalition with the Red and Orange parties. Thus, Red and Orange must have the *maximum* number of seats possible, under the criteria given.

Thus we can calculate as follows:

- No party has over 45% of seats, so the maximum that the Red party can have is 45%, which is 270 seats.

- No party except for Red and Blue has won more than 4% of seats. We are told that the Green party won the 4th highest number of seats, so it is possible that the Orange party won the 3rd highest.

- Thus, the maximum number of seats the Orange party can have won is 4% of the total, which is 24 seats.

- Thus, the maximum possible combined total of the Red and Orange party's seats won is 294.

Thus, in order to achieve a total of 301 seats in a Red-Orange-Green coalition, the Green party have to have won at least 7 seats. However, in addition to satisfy the criteria of the Green party coming 4th place they must have won the majority of the remaining 36 seats giving a final breakdown of votes as: Red 270, Blue 270, Orange 24, Green 13, Yellow 12, Purple 11.

**Question 198: E**

Expressing the amount each child receives:

| Youngest | $M$ |
|---|---|
| 2nd youngest | $M + D$ |
| 3rd youngest/ 3rd oldest | $M + 2D$ |
| 4th youngest/ 2nd oldest | $M + 3D$ |
| Oldest | $M + 4D$ |

**Question 199: D**

The total amount of money received:

£100 = M + M + D + M + 2D + M + 3D + M + 4D

Simplified, thus is:

£100 = 5M + 10D

**Question 200: C**

The two youngest are expressed as $M$ and $M + D$. This can be simplified as $2M + D$.

The three oldest are expressed as $M + 2D$, $M + 3D$ and $M + 4D$, which can be simplified as $3M + 9D$

Hence, 7 times the two youngest together can be expressed $7(2M + D)$, so altogether the answer is $7(2M + D)$ = $3M + 9D$.

## Question 201: A

To work this out, simplify the two equations:

- $7(2M + D) = 3M + 9D$
- $14M + 7D = 3M + 9D$
- $11M = 2D$
- $M = \frac{2D}{11}$

## Question 202: A

Substitute $M$ into the equation $£100 = 5M + 10D$

$$5\left(\frac{2D}{11}\right) + 10D = £100$$

$$\frac{10D}{11} + 10D = \frac{10D}{11} + \frac{110D}{11} = \frac{120D}{11}$$

## Question 203: C & E

The easiest way to work this out is using a table. With the information we know:

| | | |
|---|---|---|
| 1st | | Madeira |
| 2nd | | |
| 3rd | Jaya | |
| 4th | | |

Ellen made carrot cake, and it did not come last. It now cannot be in 1st or 3rd place, as these places are taken, so it must be second:

| | | |
|---|---|---|
| 1st | | Madeira |
| 2nd | Ellen | Carrot cake |
| 3rd | Jaya | |
| 4th | | |

Aleena's was better than the tiramisu, so she can't have come last. Therefore, Aleena must have placed first

| | | |
|---|---|---|
| 1st | Aleena | Madeira |
| 2nd | Ellen | Carrot cake |
| 3rd | Jaya | |
| 4th | | |

And the girl who made the Victoria sponge was better than Veronica:

| | | |
|---|---|---|
| 1st | Aleena | Madeira |
| 2nd | Ellen | Carrot cake |
| 3rd | Jaya | Victoria Sponge |
| 4th | Veronica | Tiramisu |

## Question 204: D

The information given can be expressed to show the results that the teams must have had to make their points total.

| Team | Points | Game Results | | | |
|---|---|---|---|---|---|
| Celtic Changers | 2 | L | L | D | D |
| Eire Lions | ? | ? | ? | ? | ? |
| Nordic Nesters | 8 | W | W | D | D |
| Sorten Swipers | 5 | W | D | D | L |
| Whistling Winners | 1 | D | L | L | L |

The results so far total 3 wins, 6 losses and 7 draws. Since, the number of draws must be even, there must have been another draw. So, we know one of the Eire Lions results is a draw.

The difference between wins (3) and losses (6) is 3. Thus, there must be another 3 wins to account for this difference. So, the Eire Lions results must be 3 wins and 1 draw. Thus, they scored 3 x 3 + 1 = 10.

## Question 205: D

Remember to consider the gender of each person. Then draw a quick diagram to show the given information you can see that only D is correct.

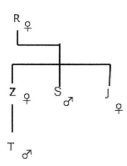

## Question 206: B

After the first round, he knocks off 8 bottles to leave 8 left on the shelf. He then puts back 4 bottles. There are therefore 12 left on the shelf. After the second round, he has hit 3 bottles and damages 6 bottles in total, and an additional 2 at the end. He then puts up 2 new bottles to leave 12 − 8 + 2 = 6 bottles left on the shelf. After the final round, John knocks off 3 bottles from the shelf to leave 3 bottles standing.

## Question 207: D

Based on the information we have we can plot the travel times below. Changeover times are in a smaller font.

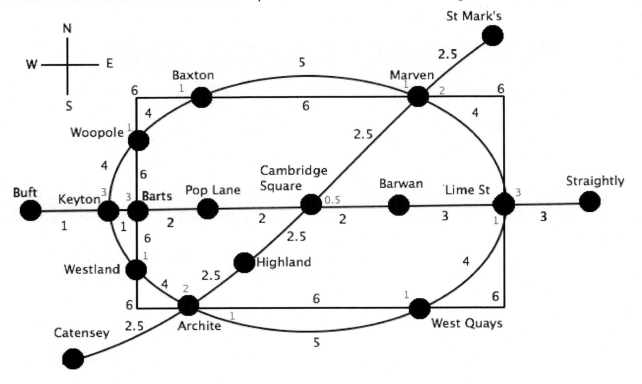

Hence on the St Mark's line, St Mark's to Archite takes 4 x 2.5 minutes = 10 minutes.

## Question 208: A

Going from stop to stop on the Straightly line end Buft to Straightly would take 14 minutes, but we are told earlier in the question that there is an express train that goes end to end which only takes 6 minutes.

## Question 209: B

The quickest route from Baxton to Pop Lane is via Marven and Cambridge Square, which takes 5 + 2 + 2.5 + 0.5 + 2 = 12 minutes. Baxton to Pop Lane via Barts would take 4 + 1 + 6 + 3 + 2 = 16 minutes, which is longer, so **E** is incorrect. Other options include times failing to take account of, or incorrectly adding changeover times, and so are incorrect.

## Question 210: C

From Cambridge Square:

- Catensey is (2.5 x 3 =) 7.5 minutes away.
- Woopole, is ( 4 + 3 + 1 +2 + 2 =) 12 minutes.
- Buft is (1 + 1 + 2 + 2 =) 6 minutes.
- Westland is (4 + 2 + 2.5 + 2.5 =) 11 minutes.

## Question 211: B

With the new delay information, we can plot the travel times as before, adjusted for the delays. Plus a 5 minute delay on the platforms when waiting on any platform for a train.

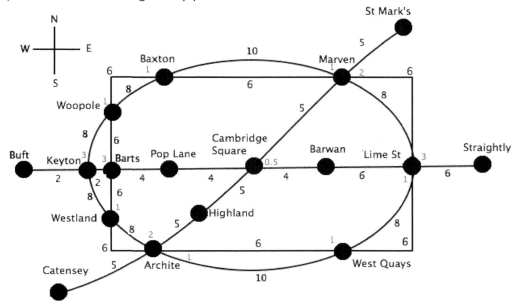

The quickest way from Westland to Marven now uses the non-delayed reliable rectangle line. Four stops on the rectangle line take 6 mins each so 24 minutes in total on the train. Add to this the additional 5 minutes platform waiting time to give a total journey time of 29 minutes.

## Question 212: C

- Baxton to Archite via Barts using only the Rectangle line takes (5 + 6 +6+ 6 +6) 29 minutes.
- Baxton to Woopole on the Rectangle line, then Oval to Archite via Keyton takes (5 + 6 + 1 + 5 + 8 + 8 + 8) 41 minutes
- Baxton to Archite on the Oval line only takes (5 + (8 x 4)) 37 minutes
- Baxton to Woopole on the Oval line, then Rectangle to Archite via Barts takes (5 + 8 + 1 + 5 + 6 + 6 + 6) 37 minutes
- As the bus takes 27-31 minutes, it is not possible to tell from between the options which will be slower/quicker, so option **C** is the right answer.

## Question 213: D

Remember the 5-minute platform wait. We are not told that the St Mark's express train from end to end is no longer running so we must assume that it is, which takes 5 minutes (plus the wait at St Mark's to go to Catensey).

Then, there is a 5-minute wait at Catensey to Archite, and a 2 + 5 minute changeover at Archite onto the Rectangle line, which then takes 6 minutes to West Quays. 5 + 5 + 5 + 5 + 2 + 5 + 6 = 33 minutes. Via Lime St the journey takes 5 + 5 + 5+ 2 + 5 + 6+ 6 = 29 minutes.

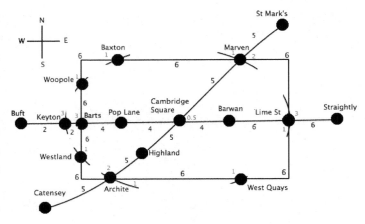

## Question 214: D

From the information:

- "Simon's horse wore number 1."
- "...the horse that wore 3, which was wearing red..."
- "the horse wearing blue wore number 4."

We can plot the information below:

| Place | Owner | Number | Colours |
|---|---|---|---|
| | Simon | 1 | |
| | | 2 | |
| | | 3 | Red |
| | | 4 | Blue |

In addition: "The horse wearing green; Celia's, came second"

This means Celia's horse must have worn number two because it cannot have worn number 1 because that is Simon's horse. Also, it cannot have worn number three or four because they wore red and blue respectively. So, we can plot this further deduction:

| Place | Owner | Number | Colours |
|---|---|---|---|
| | Simon | 1 | |
| 2nd | Celia | 2 | Green |
| | | 3 | Red |
| | | 4 | Blue |

We also know that

- "Arthur's horse beat Simon's horse"
- "Celia's horse beat the horse that wore number 1." i.e. Simon's

We know Celia's horse came second, and that both Celia's and Arthur's horses beat Simon's. This means that Simon's horse must have come last. So;

| Place | Owner | Number | Colours |
|-------|-------|--------|---------|
| 4th | Simon | 1 | |
| 2nd | Celia | 2 | Green |
| | | 3 | Red |
| | | 4 | Blue |

And knowing that:

- "Only one horse wore the same number as the position it finished in."

The horses wearing numbers 3 and 4 must have placed 1st and 3rd respectively. Hence:

| Place | Owner | Number | Colours |
|-------|-------|--------|---------|
| 4th | Simon | 1 | |
| 2nd | Celia | 2 | Green |
| 1st | | 3 | Red |
| 3rd | | 4 | Blue |

"Lila's horse wasn't painted yellow nor blue"

So, Lila's must have been red, and Simon's yellow. Leaving the only option for Arthur's to be blue. So we now know:

| Place | Owner | Number | Colours |
|-------|-------|--------|---------|
| 4th | Simon | 1 | Yellow |
| 2nd | Celia | 2 | Green |
| 1st | Lila | 3 | Red |
| 3rd | Arthur | 4 | Blue |

**Question 215: C**

Year 1 – 40 x 1.2 = 48

Year 2 – 48 x 1.2 = 57.6

Year 3 – 57.6 x 1.1 = 63.36

Year 4 – 63.36 x 1.1 = 69.696.

**Question 216: C**

To minimise the total cost to the company, they want the wage bills for each site to be less than £200,000. Working this out involves some trial and error; you can speed this up by splitting employees who earn similar amounts between the sites e.g. Nicola and John as they are the top two earners. Trial-and-error gives the following:

Nicola + Daniel + Luke = £ 198,500 and John + Emma + Victoria = £ 199,150

**Question 217: C**

Remember that pick up and drop off stops may be the same stop, therefore the minimum number of stops the bus had to make was 7. This would take 7 x 1.5 = 10.5 minutes.

Therefore, the total journey time = 24 + 10.5 = 34.5 minutes.

**Question 218: A**

The best method here is to work backwards. We know the potatoes have to be served immediately, so they should be finished roasting at 4pm, so they should start roasting 50 minutes prior to that, at 3:10. We also know they have to be roasted immediately after boiling, so they should be prepared by 3:05, in order to boil in time. She should therefore start preparing them no later than 2:47, though she could prepare them earlier.

The chicken needs to be cooked by 3:55 to give it time to stand, so it should begin roasting at 2:40, and Sally should begin to prepare it no later than 2:25.

You can construct a rough timeline:

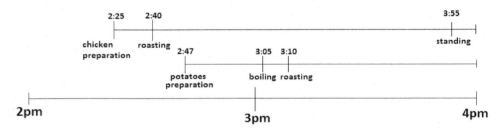

We can see from this timeline that from 2:40 onwards, there will be no long enough period of time in which there is a free space in the cooker for the vegetables to be boiled. They therefore must be finished cooking at 3:05. The latest time prior to this that Sally has time to prepare them (5 minutes) is at 2:40, between preparing the chicken and the potatoes. She should therefore begin preparing the vegetables at 2:42, then begin boiling at 2:47, so they can be finished cooking by 2:55, in time for the potatoes to boil at 3:05.

Chicken: 2:25

Potatoes: 2:47

Vegetables: 2:42

**Question 219: C**

The quickest way to do this is via looking at the options given and seeing which fits! However, for the sake of completion: let each child's age be denoted by the letter of their name, and form an equation for their total age:

$P + J + A + R = 80$

The age of each child can be written in terms of Paul's age.

$P = 2J$, therefore $J = \frac{P}{2}$

$A = \frac{P+J}{2}$

Now substitute in $J = \frac{P}{2}$ to get in terms of P only: $A = \frac{P+\frac{P}{2}}{2} = \frac{P}{2} + \frac{P}{4} = \frac{3P}{4}$

$R = P + 2$

Thus: $P + \frac{P}{2} + \frac{3P}{4} + P(+2) = 80$

Simplify to give: $\frac{13P}{4} = 78$

$13P = 312$. Thus, $P = 24$

Substitute P = 24 into the equations for the other children to get: J = 12, A = 18, R = 26

**Question 220: A**

The total number of buttons is 71 + 86 + 83 = 240. The total number of suitable buttons is 22 + 8 = 30. Thus, she will have to remove a maximum of 210 buttons in order to guarantee picking a suitable button on the next attempt.

**Question 221: E**

This question requires you to calculate the adjusted score for Ben for each segment. If Ben has a 50% chance of hitting the segment he is aiming for, we can assume he hits each adjacent segment 25% of the time. Thus:

$Adjusted\ Score = \frac{Segment\ aimed\ at}{2} + \frac{First\ Adjacent\ Segment}{4} + \frac{Second\ Adjacent\ Segment}{4}$

$Adjusted\ Score = \frac{Segment\ aimed\ at}{2} + \frac{Sum\ of\ Adjacent\ Segments}{4}$

E.g. if he aims at segment 1: He will score $\frac{1}{2} + \frac{18+20}{4} = 10$

Now it is a simple case of trying the given options to see which segment gives the highest score. In this case, it is segment 19: $\frac{19}{2} + \frac{7+3}{4} = 12$

**Question 222: C**

The total cost is £8.65, and Victoria uses a £5.00 note, leaving a total cost of £3.65 to be paid using change.

Up to 20p can be paid using 1p and 2p pieces, so she could use 20 1p coins to make up this amount.

Up to 50p can be paid using 5p and 10p pieces, so she could use 10 5p pieces to make up this amount. This gives a total of 30 coins, and a total payment of £0.70.

Up to £1.00 can be paid using 20p pieces and 50p pieces. Thus, she could use up to 5 20p pieces, giving a total of 35 coins used, and a total payment of £1.70.

The smallest denomination of coin that can now be used is a £1.00 coin. Hence Victoria must use 2 £1.00 coins, giving a total of 37 coins, and a total payment of £3.70. However, we know that the total cost to pay in change was £3.65, and that Victoria paid the exact amount, receiving no change. Thus, we must take away coins to the value of 5p, removing the smallest number of coins possible. This is achieved by taking away 1 5p piece, giving a grand total of 36 coins.

**Question 223: B**

The time could be 21:25, if the first 2 digits were reversed by the glass of water (21 would be reversed to give 15). **A** cannot be the answer, because this would involve altering the last 2 digits, and we can see that 25 on a digital clock, when reversed simply gives 25 (the 2 on the left becomes a 5 on the right, and the 5 on the right becomes a 2 on the left). **C** cannot be the answer, as this involves reversing the middle 2 digits. As with the right two digits, the middle 2 digits of 2:5 would simply reverse to give itself, 2:5. **D** could be the time if the 2nd and 4th digits were reversed, as they would both become 2's. However, the question says that 2 *adjacent* digits are reversed, meaning that the 2nd and 4th digits cannot be reversed as required here. **E** is not possible as it would require all four numbers to be reversed.

Thus, the answer is **B**.

**Question 224: B**

We can see from the question that Lorkdon is a democracy and therefore cannot have been invaded by a democracy because of the treaty (we are assuming this treaty is upheld, as said in the question). Thus, Nordic (which has invaded Lorkdon) *must* be a dictatorship. Now, we can see that Worsid has been invaded by a dictatorship, *and* has invaded a dictatorship. The question states that no dictatorship has undergone both of these events. Thus, we know that Worsid cannot be a dictatorship. We also know from the question that each of these countries is *either* a dictatorship or a democracy. Thus, Worsid must be a democracy.

**Question 225: C**

The total price of the items is: $(3.25 + 0.75 + (0.75 \times 0.6) + \left(9 \times \frac{2}{3}\right) = £10.45$

$50 - 10.45 = £39.55$ in change.

**Question 226: B**

To answer this, we simply calculate how much of the total room in the pan will be taken up by the food for each guest:

- 2 rashers of bacon, giving a total of 14% of the available space.
- 4 sausages, taking up a total of 12% of the available space.
- 1 egg takes up 12% of the available space.

Adding these figures together, we see that each guest's food takes up a total of 38% of the available space.

Thus, Ryan can only cook for 2 guests at once, since 38% multiplied by 3 is 114%, and we cannot use up more than 100% of the available space in the pan.

**Question 227: C**

To calculate this, let the total number of employees be termed "Y".

We can see that £60 is the total cost for providing cakes for 40% of "Y".

We know that £2 is required for each cake. Thus, we can work out that 30 must be 40% of Y.

$0.4Y = 60/2$
$0.4Y = 30$
$Y = 75$

Thus, we can calculate that the total number of employees must be 75.

**Question 228: E**

The normal waiting time for treatment is 3 weeks. However, the higher demand in Bob's local district means that this waiting time is extended by 50%, giving a total of 4.5 weeks.

Then, we must consider the delay induced because Bob is a lower risk case, which extends the waiting time by another 20%. 20% of 4.5 is 0.9, so there is a delay of another 0.9 weeks for treatment.

Thus, Bob can expect to wait 5.4 weeks for specialist treatment on his tumour.

**Question 229: D**

In the class of 30, 40% drink alcohol at least once a month, which is 12 students. Of these, 75% drink alcohol once a week, which is 9. Of these, 1 in 3 smoke marijuana, which is 3 students.

In the class of 30, 60% drink alcohol less than once a month, which is 18. Of these, 1 in 3 smoke marijuana, which is 6.

Therefore, the total number of students who smoke marijuana is 3+6, which is 9.

**Question 230: C**

The sequence can either be thought of as doubling the previous number then adding 2, or adding 1 then doubling. Double 46 is 92, plus 2 is 94.

**Question 231: B**

If the mode of 5 numbers is 3, it must feature at least two threes. If the median is 8, we know that the 3rd largest number is an 8. Hence, we know that the 3 smallest numbers are 3, 3, and 8. Because the mean is 7, we know that the 5 numbers must add up to 35. The three smallest numbers add up to 14. Hence the two largest must add up to 21.

**Question 232: E**

The biggest difference in the weight of potatoes will be if the bag with only 5 potatoes in weighs the maximum, 1100g, and the bag with 10 potatoes weighs the minimum, 900g. If there are 5 equally heavy potatoes in a bag weighing 1100g, each potato weighs 220g. If there are 10 equally heavy potatoes in a 900g bag, each potato weighs 90g. The difference between these is 130g.

**Question 233: D**

There are 60 teams, and 4 teams in each group, so there are 15 groups. In each group, if each team plays each other once, there will be 6 matches in each group, making a total of 90 matches in the group stage. There are then 16 teams in the knockout stages, so 8 matches in the first-round knockout, then 4, then 2, then 1 final match when only two teams are left. Hence there are 105 matches altogether (90 + 8 + 4 + 2 + 1 = 105).

**Question 234: A**

We know the husband's PIN number must be divisible by 8 because it has been multiplied by 2 a total of 3 times and had a multiple of 8 added to it. The largest 4-digit number which is divisible by 8 is 9992. Minus 200 is 9792. Dividing by 2 gives us 4896. Hence the largest the husband's last 4 card digits can be is 4896. Minus 200 gives 4696. Dividing by 2 gives us 2348. Hence the largest my last 4 card digits can be is 2348. Minus 200 is 2148. Dividing by 2 gives us 1074. Hence the largest my PIN number can be is 1074.

**Question 235: C**
If the first invitation is sent as early as possible, it will be sent on the 50th birthday. It will be accepted after 2 reminders and hence conducted at 50 years 11 months. The time between each screening will be 3 years 11 months. Hence, the second screening will be at 54 years 10 months. The third screening will be at 58 years 9 months. Hence, the fourth screening will be at 62 years 8 months.

**Question 236: A**
Ellie has worked for the company for more than five, but less than six whole years. At the end of each whole year, she receives a pay rise in thousands equal to the number of years of her tenure. Therefore, at the end of the first year the raise is £1,000, then at the end of the second year it is £2,000, and so on to year 5. Thus, the total amount of her pay comprised of the pay rises is £15,000. Using this, we can calculate the basic pay before accounting for these rises was £40,000 - £15,000 = £25,000.

**Question 237: B**
The trains come into the station together every 40 minutes, as the lowest common multiple of 2, 5 and 8 is 40. Hence, if the last time trains came together was 15 minutes ago, the next time will be in 25 minutes.

**Question 238: C**
If you smoke, your risk of getting Disease X is 1 in 24. If you drink alcohol, your risk of getting Disease X is 1 in 6. Each tablet of the drug halves your risk. Therefore, a drinker taking 1 tablet means their risk is 1 in 12, and taking 2 tablets means their risk is 1 in 24, the same as someone who smokes.

**Question 239: A**
There are 10 red and 8 green balls. Clearly the most likely combination involves these colours only. Since there are more red balls than green, the probability of red-red is greater than green-green. However, there are **two** possible ways to draw a combination, either red first followed by green or green first followed by red. The probability of red-red = $\left(\frac{10}{20} \times \frac{9}{19}\right) = \frac{9}{38}$.
The probability of red and green = $\left(\frac{8}{20} \times \frac{10}{19}\right) + \left(\frac{10}{20} \times \frac{8}{19}\right) = \frac{8}{38} + \frac{8}{38} = \frac{16}{38}$.
Therefore, the combination of red and green is more likely.

**Question 240: B**
The least likely combination of balls to draw is blue and yellow. You are much more likely to draw a green ball than either a blue or yellow one because there are many more green balls in the bag. Since the balls are drawn and not replaced, yellow and yellow is an impossible combination because there is only one yellow ball.

**Question 241: E**
Since there is only 1 blue and 1 yellow ball, it is possible to take 18 balls which are red or green. You would need to take 19 of the 20 balls to be certain of getting either the blue ball or the yellow ball.

**Question 242: C**

The smallest number of parties required would theoretically be 3 – namely Labour, the Liberal Democrats and UKIP, giving a total of 355 seats. However, the Liberal Democrats will not form a coalition with UKIP, so this will not be possible. Thus, there are 2 options:

- Labour can form a coalition with the Greens and UKIP, which is not contradictory to anything mentioned in the question. This would give a total of 325 seats, and would thus need the next 2 largest parties (The Scottish National Party and Plaid Cymru) in order to get more than 350 seats, meaning 5 parties would need to be involved.

- Alternatively, Labour can form a coalition with the Liberal Democrats and the Green Party. This would give a total of 340 seats. Only one more party (e.g. the SNP) would be required to exceed 350 seats, giving a grand total of 4 parties.

Thus, the smallest number of parties needed to form a coalition would be 4.

**Question 243: E**

360 appointments are attended and only 90% of those booked are attended

From this, we can calculate there were originally 400 appointments booked in, and 40 have been missed.

1 in 2 of the booked appointments were for male patients, so 200 appointments were for male patients. Male patients are three times as likely to miss booked appointments; this means that of the 40 that were missed, 30 were missed by men. Given that of 200 booked appointments, 30 were missed, this means 170 were attended.

**Question 244: B**

If every one of 60 students studies 3 subjects, this is 180 subject choices altogether. 60 of these are maths, because everyone takes maths. 60% of 60 is 36, so 36 are biology. 50% of 60 is 30, so 30 are economics and 30 are chemistry. 60+36+30+30=156, so there are 24 subject choices left which must be physics.

**Question 245: B**

If 100,000 people are diagnosed with chlamydia and for each case, an average of 0.6 partners are informed, this equates to 60,000 people, of which 80% (so 48,000) have tests. 12,000 of the partners who are informed, as well as 240,000 who are not (300,000 – 60,000) do not have tests. This makes 252,000 who are not tested. We can assume that half of these people would have tested positive for chlamydia, which is 126,000 people. So, the answer is 126,000.

**Question 246: C**

Tiles can be added at either end of the 3 lines of 2 tiles horizontally or at either end of the 2 lines of 2 tiles vertically. This is a total of 10, but in two cases these positions are the same (at the bottom of the left-hand vertical line and the top of the right-hand vertical line). So, the answer is 10 – 2 = 8.

**Question 247: C**

Harry needs a total of 4000ml + 1200ml = 5200ml of squash. He has 1040ml of concentrated squash, which is a fifth of the total dilute squash he needs. So, he will need 4 parts water to every 1 part concentrated squash, therefore the resulting liquid is 1/5 squash and 4/5 water.

**Question 248: C**

There are 24 different possible arrangements (4 x 3 x 2 x 1), which means that there are 23 further possible arrangements other than the current arrangement of Alex, Beth, Cathy, Daniel.

**Question 249: E**

**A** is incorrect because the distance travelled is only 10 miles. **B** is incorrect because the distance travelled is 19 miles. **C** is incorrect because no town is visited twice. **D** is incorrect because Hondale and Baleford are both visited twice. Therefore, **E** is the correct answer.

**Question 250: C**

Georgia is shorter than her mum and dad, and each of her siblings is at least as tall as mum. We know mum is shorter than dad because Ellie is between the two, so we know Georgia is the shortest.

We know that Ellie, Tom, and dad are taller than mum, so mum is second shortest. Ellie is shorter than dad and Tom is taller than dad, so we can work out that Ellie must be third shortest.

**Question 251: A**

Danielle must be sat next to Caitlin. Bella must be sat next to the teaching assistant. Hence these two pairs must sit in different rows. One pair must be sat at the front with Ashley, and the other must be sat at the back with Emily. Since the teaching assistant has to sit on the left, this must mean that Bella is sat in the middle seat and either Ashley or Emily (depending on which row they are in) is sat in the right-hand seat. However, Bella cannot sit next to Emily, so this means Bella and the teaching assistant must be in the front row. So, Ashley must be sat in the front right seat.

**Question 252: C**

The dishwasher is run $2 + p$ times a week, where $p$ is the number of people in the house. Let the number of people in the house when the son is not home be $s$, and when the son is home, it is $s + 1$. In 30 weeks when the son is home, she would buy 6 packs of dishwasher tablets.

In 30 weeks when the son is not home, she would buy 5 packs of dishwasher tablets.

So, when he is home, she buys $1.2(normal\ number\ of\ packs\ of\ dishwasher\ tablets)$.

So, $2 + s + 1 = 1.2 \times (2 + s)$.

i.e. $2.4 + 1.2s = 2 + s + 1$

Therefore $0.2s = 0.6$

$s = 3$

When her son is home, there are $s + 1 = 4$ people in the house.

**Question 253: A**

No remaining days in the year obey the rule. The next date that does is 01/01/2015 (integers are 0, 1, 2, 5). This is 6 days later than the specified date.

**Question 254: B**

If each town is due north, south, east or west of at least two other towns and we know that one is east and one is north of a third, then they must be arranged in a rectangle. So Yellowtown is 4 miles east of Bluetown to make a rectangle, which means it must be 5 miles north of Redtown. So Redtown is 5 miles south of Yellowtown.

**Question 255: B**

Jenna pours 4/5 of 250 ml into each glass, which is 200 ml. Since she has 1500 ml of wine, she pours 100 ml into the last glass, which is 2/5 of the 250 ml full capacity.

**Question 256: E**

The maximum number of girls in Miss Ellis's class with brown eyes and brown hair is 10, because the two thirds of the girls with brown eyes could also all have brown hair. The minimum number is 0 because it could be that all the boys, and the third of the girls without brown eyes, all had brown hair, which would be 2/3 of the class.

**Question 257: E**

A negative "score" results from any combination of throws which includes a 1 but from no other combination. Given that a negative score has a 0.75 probability, a positive or zero score has a 0.25 probability. Therefore, throwing two numbers that are not 1 twice in a row has a probability of 0.25. Hence, the probability of throwing a non-1 number on each throw is √0.25 = 0.5. So the probability of throwing a 1 on an individual throw is 1 − 0.5 = 0.5.

**Question 258: C**

We can work out from the information given the adult flat rate and the charge per stop. Let the charge per stop be s and the flat rate be f. Therefore: 15s + f = 1.70
8s + f = 1.14
We can hence work out that: 7s = 0.56, so s = 0.08. Hence, f = 0.50
Megan is an adult, so she pays this rate. For 30 stops, the rate will be 0.08 x 30 + 0.50 = 2.90.

**Question 259:  B**

We found in the previous question that the flat rate for adults is £0.50 and the rate per stop is £0.08. We know that the child rate is half the flat rate and a quarter of the "per stop" rate, so the child flat rate is £0.25 and the rate per stop is 2p. So, for 25 stops, Alice pays:
0.02 x 25 + 0.25 = 0.75

**Question 260: C**

We should first work out how many stops James can travel. For £2, he can afford to travel as many stops as £1.50 will take him once the flat rate is taken into account. The per stop rate is 8p per stop, so he can travel 18 stops. This means he will need to go to the 18th stop from town. So he will need to walk past 7 stops to get to the stop he can afford to travel from.

**Question 261: D**

The picture will need a 12-inch by 16-inch mount, which will cost £8. It will need a 13 inch by 17-inch frame, which will cost £26. So, the cost of mounting and framing the picture will be £8 + £26 = £34.

**Question 262: C**

Mounting and framing an 8 by 8-inch painting will cost £5 for the mount and £22 for the frame, which is £27. Mounting and framing a 10 by 10-inch painting will cost £6 for the mount and £26 for the frame, which is £32. The difference is £32 - £27 = £5.

**Question 263: B**

We found in the last question that mounting and framing a 10 by 10-inch painting will cost £6 for the mount and £26 for the frame, which is £32 total. We can calculate that each additional inch of mount and frame for a square painting will cost £2.50; £2 for the frame and £0.50 for the mount. So, an 11-inch painting will cost £34.50 to frame and mount, a 12 inch £37, a 13 inch £39.50, a 14 inch £42. The biggest painting that can be mounted and framed for £40 is a 13-inch painting.

## Question 264: D

Recognise that the pattern is *"consonants move forward by two consonants; vowels stay the same"*. This allows coding of the word MAGICAL to PAJIFAN to RALIHAQ.

| Forward two | | | Forward two |
|---|---|---|---|
| M | $\Rightarrow$ | O (skips to) P | $\Rightarrow$ R |
| A | $\Rightarrow$ | Stays the same | $\Rightarrow$ A |
| G | $\Rightarrow$ | I (skips to) J | $\Rightarrow$ L |
| I | $\Rightarrow$ | Stays the same | $\Rightarrow$ I |
| C | $\Rightarrow$ | E (skips to) F | $\Rightarrow$ H |
| A | $\Rightarrow$ | Stays the same | $\Rightarrow$ A |
| L | $\Rightarrow$ | N | $\Rightarrow$ Q |

## Question 265: C

If $f$ denotes the flat rate, and $k$ denotes the rate per km, we can form simultaneous equations:

f + 5k = £6 AND f + 3k = £4.20

Subtract equation two from equation one:

(f + 5k) - (f + 3k) = £6 - £4.20

Thus, 2k = £1.80 and k = £0.90

Therefore, f + (5 x 0.90) = £6

So, f + £4.50 = £6. Thus, f = £1.50

7k will be £1.50 + 7 x £0.90 = £7.80

## Question 266: C

The increase from 2001/2 to 2011/12 was 1,019 to 11,736, which equals a linear increase of 10,717 admissions. So, in 20 years, we would expect to see an increase by 10,717 x 2 = 21,434. Add this to the number in 2011 to give 33,170 admissions.

## Question 267: A

As the question uses percentages, it does not matter what figure you use.

To make calculations easier, use an initial price of £100. When on sale, the dress is 20% off, so using a normal price of £100, the dress would be £80. When the dresses are 20% off, the shop is making a 25% profit. Therefore: £80 = 1.25 x purchase price.

Therefore, the purchase price is: $\frac{80}{1.25}$ = £64. Thus, the normal profit is £100 - £64 = £36. i.e. when a dress sells for £100, the shop makes £36 or 36% profit.

**Question 268: C**

1.  Incorrect. There must be 6 general committee clinical students, plus the treasurer, and 2 sabbatical roles, none of whom can be preclinical, so there must be a maximum of 11 preclinical students.
2.  Correct. There must be two general committee members for each year plus welfare and social officers, totalling 6 students.
3.  Incorrect. The committee is made up of 20 students, 2 roles are sabbatical, so there are 18 studying students, and therefore there can be 3 from each year.
4.  Correct. There are 18 studying students on the committee, and there must be 6 general committee members from pre-clinical, plus welfare and social, therefore there must be a minimum of 8 pre-clinical students, so there must be 10 clinical students.
5.  Incorrect. You need to count up the number of specific roles on the committee, which is 5, and there must be 2 students from each year, which is 12. This leaves 3 more positions, which the question doesn't state can't be first years. Therefore, there could be up to 5 first years.
6.  Incorrect. There must be at least 2 general committee members from each year. However, the worked answer to 5 shows there are 15 general committee members which are split across the 6 years, and so there must be an uneven distribution.

**Question 269: B**

Remember 2012 was a leap year. Work through each month, adding the correct number of days, to work out what day each 13th would be on. If a month was 28 days, the 13th would be the same day each month, therefore, to work this out quickly, you only need to count on the number of days over 28. For example, in a month with 31 days, the 13th will be 3 weekdays (31-28) later. Thus, if 13th January is a Friday, 13th February is a Monday, (February has 29 days in 2012), 13th March is a Tuesday and 13th April is a Friday.

**Question 270: E**

There are 18 sheep in total. The question states there are 8 male sheep, which means there are 10 female sheep before some die. 5 female sheep die, so there are 5 female sheep alive to give birth to lambs. Each female delivers 2 lambs, giving 10 lambs in total. There are 4 male sheep and 5 mothers, so the total is 10 + 4 + 5 = 19 sheep.

**Question 271: D**

We can see from the fact that all the possible answers end "AME" that the letters "AME" must be translated to the last 3 letters of the coded word, "JVN", under the code. J is the 10th letter of the alphabet, so it is 9 letters on from A (V is the 21st letter of the alphabet and M is the 13th, and N is the 14th letter of the alphabet and E is the 5th, therefore these pairs are also 9 letters apart). Therefore, P is the code for the letter 9 letters before it in the alphabet. P is the 16th letter of the alphabet, therefore it is the code for the 7th letter of the alphabet, G. Therefore, from these solutions the only possibility for the original word is GAME.

**Question 272: C**

Let x be the number of people who get on the bus at the station.

It is easiest to work backwards. After the 4th stop, there are 5 people on the bus. At the 4th stop, half the people who were on the bus got off (and therefore half stayed on) and 2 people got on. Therefore, 5 is equal to 2 plus half the number of people who were on the bus after the 3rd stop. So half the number of people who were on the bus after the 3rd stop must be 3. Therefore, after the 3rd stop, there must have been 6 people on the bus. We can then say that 6 is equal to 2 plus half the number of people who were on the bus after the 2nd stop. Therefore, there were 8 people on the bus after the 2nd stop.

We can then say that 8 is equal to 2 plus half the number of people who were on the bus after the 1st stop. Therefore, there were 12 people on the bus after the 1st stop.

We can then say that 12 is equal to 2 plus half the number of people who got on the bus at the station. Therefore, the number of people who got on the bus at the station is 20.

**Question 273: B**

We know from the question that I have purchased small cans of blue and white paint, and that blue paint accounted for 50% of the total cost. Since a can of blue paint is 4 x the price of a can of white paint, we know I must have purchased 4 cans of white paint for each can of blue paint. Each can of small paint covers a total of $10m^2$, and I have painted a total of $100m^2$, in doing so using up all the paint. Therefore, I must have purchased 10 cans of paint. Therefore, I must have purchased 2 cans of blue paint and 8 cans of white paint. So, I must have painted $20m^2$ of wall space blue.

**Question 274: E**

The cost for x cakes under this offer can be expressed as: $x(42-x^2)$

Following this formula, we can see that 2 cakes would cost 76p, 3 cakes would cost 99p, and 4 cakes would cost 104p. As the number of cakes increases beyond 4, we see that the overall price actually drops, as 5 cakes would cost 85p and 6 cakes would cost 36p. This confirms Isobel's prediction that the offer is a bad deal for the baker, as it ends up cheaper for the customer to purchase more cakes. It is clear that 6 cakes is the smallest number for which the price will be under 40p, and the price will continue to drop as more cakes are purchased.

**Question 275: C**

Adding up the percentages of students in University A who do science subjects gives:

23.50 + 6.25 + 30.25 = 60%.

60% of 800 students is 480, so 480 students in University A do science subjects.

Adding up the percentages of students in University B who do science subjects gives:

13.25 + 14.75 + 7.00 = 35%. 35% of 1200 students is 420, so 420 students in University B do science subjects.

Therefore:

480 – 420 = 60

60 more students in University A than University B take a science subject.

## Question 276: C

Let the number of miles Sonia is travelling be $x$. Because she is crossing 1 international border, travelling by Traveleasy Coaches will cost Sonia: £$(5 + 0.5x)$

Travelling by Europremier coaches will cost Sonia: £$(15 + 0.1x)$.

Because we know the cost is the same for both companies, the number of miles she is travelling can be found by setting these two expressions equal to each other: $5 + 0.5x = 15 + 0.1x$.

This equation can be rearranged to give: $0.4x = 10$   Therefore: $x = 10/0.4 = 25$

## Question 277: E

To find out whether many of these statements are true it is necessary to work out the departure and arrival times, and journey time for each girl.

Lauren departs at 2:30pm and arrives at 4pm, therefore her journey takes 1.5 hours

Chloe departs at 1:30pm and her journey takes 1 hour longer than 1.5 hours (Lauren's journey), therefore her journey takes 2.5 hours, and she arrives at 4pm

Amy arrives at 4:15pm and her journey takes 2 times 1.5 hours (Lauren's journey), therefore her journey takes 3 hours, and she departs at 1:15pm.

Looking at each statement, the only one which is definitely true is **E**: Amy departs at 1:15pm and Chloe departs at 1:30pm therefore Amy departed before Chloe.

**D** *may* be true, but nothing in the question shows it is *definitely* true, so it can be safely ignored.

## Question 278: B

First consider how many items of clothing she can take by weight. The weight allowance is 20kg. Take off 2kg for the weight of the empty suitcase, then take off another 3kg (3 X 1000g) for the books she wishes to take. Therefore, she can fit 15kg of clothes in her suitcase. To find out how many items of clothing this is, we can divide 15kg=15000g by 400g: $15000/400 = 150/4 = 37.5$

So, she can pack up to 37 items of clothing by weight.

Now consider the volume of clothes she can fit in. The total volume of the suitcase is:

50cm x 50cm x 20cm = 50000cm³

The volume of each book is: 0.2m x 0.1m x 0.05m = 1000cm³

So, the volume of space available for clothes is: 50000 − (3 x 1000) = 47000cm³

To find out how many items of clothing she can fit in this space, we can divide 47000 by 1500: $47000/1500 = 470/15 = 31\ 1/3$

So, she can pack up to 31 items of clothing by volume.

Although she can fit 37 items by weight, they will not fit in the volume of the suitcase, so the maximum number of items of clothing she can pack is 31.

**Question 279: D**

We can work out the answer by considering each option:

Bed Shop A: £120 + £70 = £190

Bed Shop B: £90 + £90 = £180

Bed Shop C: £140 + (1/2 x £60) = £170

Bed Shop D: (2/3) x (£140+£100) = (2/3) x (£240) = £160

Bed Shop E: £175

Therefore, the cheapest is Bed Shop **D**.

**Question 280: C**

The numbers of socks of each colour is irrelevant, so long as there is more than one of each (which there is). There are only 4 colours of socks, so if Joseph takes 5 socks, it is guaranteed that at least 2 of them will be the same colour.

**Question 281: D**

Paper comes in packs of 500, and with each pack 20 magazines can be printed. Each pack costs £3.

Card comes in packs of 60, and with each pack 60 magazines can be printed. Each pack costs £3 x 2 = £6.

Each ink cartridge prints 130 sheets, which is 130/26 = 5 magazines. Each cartridge costs £5.

The lowest common multiple of 20, 60 and 5 is 60, so it is possible to work out the total cost for printing 60 magazines. Printing 60 magazines will require 3 packs of paper at £3, 1 pack of card at £6 and 12 ink cartridges at £5. So, the total cost of printing 60 magazines is: (3 x 3) + 6 + (12 x 5) = £75.

The total budget is £300.

£300/£75 = 4

So, we can print 4x60 magazines in this budget, which is 240 magazines.

**Question 282: E**

We can express the information we have as: $\frac{1}{4} - \frac{1}{5} = \frac{1}{20}$

So, the six additional lengths make up 1/20 of Rebecca's intended distance. So, the number of lengths she intended to complete was: 20 x 6 = 120.

**Question 283: B**

Sammy has a choice of 3 flavours for the first sweet that he eats. Each of the other sweets he eats cannot be the same flavour as the sweet he has just eaten. So, he has a choice of 2 flavours for each of these four sweets. So, the total number of ways that he can make his choices is:

3 x 2 x 2 x 2 x 2 = 48

**Question 284: C**

Suppose that today Gill is $x$ years old. It follows that Granny is $15\,x$ years old. In 4 years' time, Gill will be $(x +4)$ years old and Granny will be $15x + 4$ years old. We know that in 4 years' time, Granny's age is equal to Gill's age squared, so: $15x + 4 = (x + 4)^2$

Expanding and rearranging, we get: $x^2 - 7x + 12 = 0$

We can factorise this to get: $(x - 3)(x - 4)$

So, $x$ is either 3 or 4. Gill's age today is either 3 or 4 so Granny is either 45 or 60. We know Granny's age is an even number, so she must be 60 and hence Gill must be 4. So, the difference in their ages is 56 years.

**Question 285: C**

If Pierre is telling the truth, everyone else is not telling the truth. But, also in this case, what Qadr said is not true, and hence Ratna is telling the truth. So, we have a contradiction. So, we deduce that Pierre is not telling the truth. Therefore, Qadr is telling the truth, and so Ratna is not telling the truth. So, Sven is also telling the truth, and hence Tanya is not telling the truth. So Qadr and Sven are telling the truth and the other three are not telling the truth.

**Question 286: D**

Angus walks for 20 minutes at 3 mph and runs for 20 minutes at 6 mph. 20 minutes is one-third of an hour. So, the number of miles that Angus covers is: $3 \times \frac{1}{3} + 6 \times \frac{1}{3} = 6$

Bruce covers the same distance. So, Bruce walks $\frac{1}{2} \times 3$ miles at 3 mph which takes him 30 minutes and runs the same distance at 6 mph which takes him 15 minutes. So altogether it takes Bruce 45 minutes to finish the course.

**Question 287: B**

Although you could do this quickly by forming simultaneous equations, it is even quicker to note that $72 \times 4 = 288$. Since Species 24601 each have 4 legs; it leaves a single member of species 8472 to account for the other 2 legs.

**Question 288: E**

None of the options can be concluded for certain. We are not told whether any chicken dishes are spicy, only that they are all creamy. Whilst all vegetable dishes are spicy, some non-vegetable dishes could also be spicy. There is no information on whether dishes can be both creamy and spicy, nor on which, if any, dishes contain tomatoes. Remember, if you're really stuck, draw a Venn diagram for these types of questions.

**Question 289: C**

At 10mph, we can express the time it takes Lucy to get home as: $60 \times 8/10 = 48$

Since Simon sets off 20 minutes later, his time taken to get home, in order to arrive at the same time, must be: $48 - 20 = 28$

Therefore, his cycling speed must be: $48/28 \times 10 = 17$mph

**Question 290: A**

The total profit from the first transaction can be expressed as: 2000 x 8 = 16,000p
The total profit from the second transaction is: 1000 x 6 = 6,000p

Therefore, the total profit is 22,000p or £220 before charges. There are four transactions at a cost of £20 each, therefore the overall profit is: £220 – (20 x 4) = £140

**Question 291: C**

For the total score to be odd, there must be either three odd or one odd and two even scores obtained. Since the solitary odd score could be either the first, second or third throw there are four possible outcomes that result in an odd total score. Additionally, there are the same number of possibilities giving an even score (either all three even or two odd and one even scores obtained), and the chance of throwing odd or even with any given dart is equal. Therefore, there is an equal probability of three darts totalling to an odd score as to an even score, and so the chance of an odd score is ½.

**Question 292: C**

This is a compound interest question. £5,000 must be increased by 5%, and then the answer needs to be increased by 5% for four more iterations. After one year: £5,000 x 1.05 = £5,250
Increasing sequentially gives 5512, 5788, 6077 and 6381 after five years. Therefore, the answer is £6,381.

**Question 293:  D**

If in 5 years' time the sum of their ages is 62, the sum of their ages today will be: 62 – (5 x 2) = 52
Therefore, if they were the same age, they would both be 26, but with a 12 year age gap they are 20 and 32 today. Michael is the older brother, so 2 years ago he would have been aged 30.

**Question 294: A**

Tearing out every page which is a multiple of 3 removes 166 pages. All multiples of 6 are multiples of 3, so no more pages are torn out with that instruction. Finally, half of the remaining pages are removed, which equates to an additional 167 pages. Therefore 333 pages are removed in total. The total surface area of these pages is 15 x 30 x 333 = 149,850 cm$^2$ = 14.9m$^2$. At 110 gm$^2$, 14.9 m$^2$ weighs 14.9 x 110 = 1,650g (1,648g unrounded).

**Question 295: D**

The cost of fertiliser is 80p/kg = 8p/100g. At 200g the incremental increase in yield is 65 pence/m. At each additional 100g it will be reduced by 30%, therefore at 300g/m it is 45.5p, at 400g/m it is 31.8p, at 500g/m it is 22.3p, at 600g/m it is 15.6p, at 700g/m it is 10.9p, and at 800g it is 7.6p. So at 800g the gain in yield is less than the cost of the fertiliser to produce the gain, and so it is no longer cost effective to fertilise more.

**Question 296: D**

Statements **A**, **C** and **E** are all definitely true. Meanwhile, statement **B** may be not true but is not definitely untrue, as this depends on the number of cats and rabbit owned.
Only statement **D** is definitely untrue. The type of animal requiring the most food is a dog, and as can be seen from the tables, Furry Friends actually sells the most expensive dog food, not the cheapest.

**Question 297: C**

The largest decrease in bank balance occurs between January 1st and February 1st, totalling £171, reflecting the amount spent during the month of January, £1171. However, because there is a pay rise beginning on March 10th, we need to consider that from April onwards, the bank balance will have increased by £1100, not £1000. This means that the same decrease in bank balance reflects £100 more spending if it occurs after March. This means that 2 months now have seen more spending than February. Between March 1st and April 1st, the bank balance has decreased by £139. With the salary increase, the salary is now £1100, so the total spending for the month of March is £1239. This is greater than the total spending during the month of January.

Similarly, the month of April has also seen more spending than January once the pay rise is considered, a total of £1225 of spending. However, this is still less than the month of March.

**Question 298: C**

If Amy gets a taxi, she can set off 100 minutes before 1700, which is 1520.

If Amy gets a train, she must get the 1500 train as the later train arrives after 1700, so she must set off at 1500. Since Northtown airport is 30 minutes from Northtown station, there is no way Amy can get the flight and still arrive at Northtown station by 1700. Therefore, Amy should get a taxi and should leave at 1520.

**Question 299: C**

We can decompose the elements of the multiplication grid into their prime factors, thus:

|   | C | D |
|---|---|---|
| **A** | $2 \times 2 \times 2 \times 3 \times 7$ | $2 \times 2 \times 2 \times 2 \times 3 \times 3 \times 5$ |
| **B** | $7 \times 17$ | $2 \times 3 \times 5 \times 17$ |

$B \times C = 7 \times 17$, so one of b and c must be 7 and the other must be 17. b must be 17 because bd is a multiple of 17 and not of 7, and c must be 7 because ac is a multiple of 7 and not of 17. ac is 168, so a must be 168 divided by 7, which is 24. ad is 720 so d must be 720 divided by 24, which is 30. Hence the answer is 30.

Alternatively approach the question by eliminating all answers which are not factors of both 720 and 510.

**Question 300: E**

48% of the students are girls, which is 720 students. Hence 80 is 1/9 of the girls, so 1/9 of boys are mixed race. The remaining 780 students are boys, so 87 boys are mixed race to the nearest person. There is a shortcut to this question. Notice that 80 girls are mixed race, and the proportion is the same for boys. As there are more boys than girls, we know the answer is greater than 80. Option **E** 90 is the only option for which this holds true.

**Question 301: A**

DNA consists of 4 bases: adenine, guanine, thymine, and cytosine. The sugar backbone consists of deoxyribose, hence the name DNA. DNA is found in the cytoplasm of prokaryotes (bacteria are prokaryotic!).

**Question 302: D**

**1 – correct** – Mitochondria are responsible for energy production by ATP synthesis.

**2 – incorrect** – Animal cells do not have a cell wall, only a cell membrane.

**3 – correct** – chloroplasts are only found in animal cells, they are the site of photosynthesis

**Question 303: B**

If you aren't studying A-level biology, this question may stretch you. However, it is possible to reach an answer by process of elimination.

**A, D, E – incorrect** – Mitochondria are the 'powerhouse' of the cell in aerobic respiration, responsible for cell energy production rather than DNA replication or protein synthesis.

**C – incorrect -** As energy producers they are required in muscle cells in large numbers.

**B – correct** – Hence, we can conclude that they are enveloped by a double membrane, possibly because they started out as independent prokaryotes engulfed by eukaryotic cells.

**Question 304: A**

The majority of bacteria are commensal, thus don't lead to disease. Each of the other statements are true.

**Question 305: C**

Bacteria carry genetic information on plasmids and not in nuclei like animal cells. They don't need meiosis for replication, as they do not require gametes. Bacterial genomes consist of DNA, just like animal cells.

**Question 306: C**

Active transport requires a transport protein and ATP, as work is being done against an electrochemical gradient. Unlike diffusion, the relative concentrations of the materials being transported aren't important.

**Question 307:  D**

Meiosis produces haploid gametes. This allows for fusion of 2 gametes to reach a full diploid set of chromosomes again in the zygote.

**Question 308: B**

Mendelian inheritance separates traits into dominant or recessive. It applies to all sexually reproducing organisms. Don't get confused by statement C – the offspring of 2 heterozygotes has a 25% chance of expressing a recessive trait, but it will be homozygous recessive.

**Question 309: A**

Hormones are released into the bloodstream and act on receptors in different organs in order to cause relatively slow changes to the body's physiology. Hormones frequently interact with the nervous system, e.g. adrenaline and insulin, however, they don't directly cause muscles to contract. Almost all hormones are synthesised.

**Question 310: D**

Neuronal signalling can happen via direct electrical stimulation of nerves or via chemical stimulation of synapses which produce a current that travels along the nerves. Electrical synapses are very rare in mammals; the majority of mammalian synapses are chemical.

**Question 311: D**

Remember that pH changes cause changes in electrical charge on proteins (= polypeptides) that could interfere with protein – protein interactions. Whilst the other statements are all correct to a certain extent, they are the downstream effects of what would happen if enzymes (which are also proteins) didn't work.

**Question 312: A**

The bacterial cell wall is made up of murein and protects the bacterium from the external environment, in particular from osmotic stresses, and is important in most bacteria.

**Question 313: C**

Sexual reproduction relies on formation of gametes during **meiosis**. Mitosis doesn't produce genetically distinct cells. Mitosis is, however, the basis for tissue growth.

**Question 314: A**

A mutation is a permanent change in the nucleotide sequence of DNA. Whilst mutations may lead to changes in organelles and chromosomes, or even be harmful, they are strictly defined as permanent changes to the DNA or RNA sequence.

**Question 315: E**

Mutations are fairly common, but in the vast majority of cases do not have any impact on phenotype due to the redundancy of the genome. Sometimes they can confer selective advantages and allow organisms to survive better (i.e. evolve by natural selection), or they can lead to cancers as cells start dividing uncontrollably.

**Question 316: D**

Antibodies represent a pivotal molecule of the immune system. They provide very pointed and selective targeting of pathogens and toxins without causing damage to the body's own cells.

**Question 317: A**

Kidneys are not involved in digestion, but do filter the blood of waste products. Glucose is found in high concentrations in the urine of diabetics. The lack of insulin production and/or tissue response to insulin means diabetics cannot absorb glucose and thus it must be excreted as a waste product.

**Question 318: D**

Hormones are slower acting than nervous signals and act for a longer time. Hormones also act in a more general way. Adrenaline is also a hormone released into the body causing the fight-or-flight response. Although it is quick acting, it still lasts for a longer time than a nervous response, as you can still feel its effects for a time after the response, e.g., shaking hands.

**Question 319: D**

Homeostasis is about minimising changes to the internal environment by modulating both input and output.

**Question 320: B**

There is less energy and biomass each time you move up a trophic level. Only 10% of consumed energy is transferred to the next trophic level, so only one tenth of the previous biomass can be sustained in the next trophic level up.

**Question 321: A**

In asexual reproduction, there is no fusion of gametes as the single parent cell divides. There is therefore no mixing of chromosomes and, as a result, no genetic variation.

## Question 322: E

The image is first formed on the retina which conveys it to the brain via a sensory nerve. The brain then sends an impulse to the muscle via a motor neuron.

## Question 323: D

1 – **correct** – the right-hand side of the heart contains deoxygenated blood, while the left-hand side contains oxygenated blood.

2 – **incorrect** – the aorta receives oxygenated blood from the left <u>ventricle</u>.

3 – **incorrect** – the heart pumps deoxygenated blood into the pulmonary <u>artery</u>.

4 – **incorrect** – valves prevent flow of blood backwards from ventricle to atrium, while walls are present to prevent flow from ventricle to ventricle (and atrium to atrium).

## Question 324: E

Clones are genetically identical by definition, and a large number of them could conceivably reduce the gene pool of a population. In adult cell cloning, the genetic material of an egg is replaced with the genetic material of an adult cell. Cloning is possible for all DNA based life forms, including plants and other types of animals.

## Question 325: E

Genetic variation gives rise to a variety of intraspecies phenotypes, e.g. different eye colours. If mutations confer a selective advantage, those individuals with the mutation will survive to reproduce and grow in numbers. Genetic variation is caused by a combination of parental genetic mixing and mutations. Species with similar characteristics often do have similar genes.

## Question 326: E

Alleles are different versions of the same gene. If you are a homozygous for a trait, you have two identical alleles for that particular gene, and if you are heterozygous, you have two different alleles for that gene. Recessive traits only appear in the phenotype when there are no dominant alleles for that trait, i.e. two recessive alleles are carried.

## Question 327: D

Remember that red blood cells don't have a nucleus and therefore have minimal DNA. In meiosis, a diploid cell divides in such a way so as to produce four haploid cells. Any type of cell division will require energy.

## Question 328: C

The hypothalamus detects too little water in the blood, so the pituitary gland releases ADH. The kidneys maintain the blood water level and allow less water to be lost in the urine until the blood water level returns to normal.

## Question 329: E

Venous blood has a higher level of carbon dioxide and lower level of oxygen. Carbon dioxide forms carbonic acid in aqueous solution, thus making the pH of venous blood slightly more acidic than arterial blood. This leaves only **D** and **E** as possibilities, but recall that under normal physiological conditions, pH is maintained under strict control, giving an answer of pH 7.4 as the most likely. Remember, the pH scale is logarithmic, so a pH of 8.0 would be a big difference in the number of H+ ions in the blood!

**Question 330: E**

1 – **correct** – the cytoplasm is 80% water.
2 – **incorrect** – the cytoplasm doesn't contain everything, e.g. DNA is found in the nucleus.
3 – **correct** – the cytoplasm contains, among other things, electrolytes and proteins.

**Question 331: D**
ATP is produced in mitochondria in aerobic respiration and in the cytoplasm during anaerobic respiration only.
1 – correct – ATP is produced in the cytoplasm during anaerobic respiration only.
2 – incorrect – plasmids are not a site of ATP production.
3 – correct – ATP is produced in the mitochondria during aerobic respiration only.
4 – incorrect – the nucleus is not a site of ATP production.

**Question 332: C**
The cell membrane allows both active transport (via specialised transport proteins) and passive transport (via diffusion) of certain ions and molecules and is found in eukaryotes and prokaryotes like bacteria. It is a phospholipid bilayer.

**Question 333: A**
1 and 2 only: 223 PAIRS = 446 chromosomes; meiosis produces 4 daughter cells with half of the original number of chromosomes each, while mitosis produces two daughter cells with the original number of chromosomes each.

**Question 334: E**
If Bob is homozygous dominant (RR) the probability of having a child with red hair is 0%. However, if Bob is heterozygous (Rr), there is a 50% chance of having a child with red hair, since Mary must be homozygous recessive (rr) to have red hair. As we do not know Bob's genotype, both possibilities must be considered.

**Question 335: A**
If an offspring is born with red hair, it confirms Bob is heterozygous (Rr). He cannot have a red-haired child if he is homozygous dominant (RR), and would himself have red hair were he homozygous recessive (rr).

**Question 336: A**
Monohybrid cross rr and Rr results in 50% Rr and 50% rr offspring. 50% of offspring will have black hair, but they will be heterozygous for the hair allele (Rr).

**Question 337: C**
When the chest walls expand, the intra-thoracic pressure decreases. This causes the atmospheric pressure outside the chest to be greater than pressure inside the chest, resulting in a flow of air into the chest.

**Question 338: A**
Producers are found at the bottom of food chains and always have the largest biomass of all the trophic levels.

**Question 339: E**

All the statements are true; the carbon and nitrogen cycles are examinable in Section 2, so make sure you understand them! The atmosphere is 79% inert $N_2$ gas, which must be 'fixed' to useable forms by high-energy lightning strikes or by bacterial mediation. Humans also manually fix nitrogen for fertilisers with the Haber process.

**Question 340: E**

None of the above statements are correct.

**1 – incorrect –** mutations can be silent, for example if the new triplet codes for the same amino acid as the original. Or, a mutation may cause a change in the amino acid, but if the amino acid is not in the active site or has similar properties to the original amino acid, this may not affect the function of the protein. Mutations can either be silent, cause loss of function, or even gain of function!

**2 – incorrect –** as outlined above, mutations can be silent – i.e. a substitution of one triplet codon for another that codes for the same amino acid. Or, if the mutation is in an exon (part of the protein that is cut out to make the protein functional), the structure of the end product protein won't be affected.

**3 – incorrect –** whilst cancer arises as a result of a series of mutations (the two-hit hypothesis), only a small percentage of mutations actually lead to cancer.

**Question 341: C**

Remember that heart rate is controlled via the autonomic nervous system, which isn't a part of the central nervous system.

**Question 342: E**

None of the above are correct. There is no voluntary input to the heart in the form of a neuronal connection. Parasympathetic neurones slow the heart and sympathetic nervous input accelerates heart rate.

**Question 343: B**

If lipase is not working, fat from the diet will not be broken down, and will be instead excreted in the stool. Lactase, for instance, is responsible for breaking down lactose, and its malfunctioning is the reason for lactose intolerance.

**Question 344: E**

None of the statements A-D are correct.

**A – incorrect –** oxygenated blood from the lungs flows to the heart via the pulmonary vein.

**B – incorrect –** the pulmonary artery is the exception to this rule! It carries deoxygenated blood from the heart to the lungs.

**C – incorrect –** some animals, such as fish, have single circulatory systems.

**D – incorrect –** the SVC contains deoxygenated blood, returning to the heart from the body.

**Question 345: E**

Enzymatic digestion takes place throughout the GI tract, including in the mouth (e.g. amylase), stomach (e.g. pepsin), and small intestine (e.g. trypsin). The large intestine is primarily responsible for water absorption, whilst the rectum acts as a temporary store for faecal matter (i.e. digestion has finished prior to the rectum).

**Question 346: B**

This is an example of the monosynaptic stretch reflex; these reflexes occur at the level of the spinal cord and therefore don't involve the brain. These reflexes are truly involuntary as they involve no higher processing. **Thermo-receptors** are involved in the reaction – they detect the heat and send the information to a **sensory nerve**. The sensory nerve takes the information to the **spinal cord**, where the information is relayed to a **motor nerve**. The motor nerve then relays the information to a **muscle** and causes muscular contraction to remove the hand from the hot stimulus.

**Question 347: A**

Statement 2 describes diffusion as $CO_2$ is moving along the concentration gradient. Statement 3 describes active transport, as amino acids are moving against the concentration gradient.

**Question 348: C**

3 is the correct equation for animals, and 4 is correct for plants.

**Question 349: C**

The mitochondria are only the site for aerobic respiration, as anaerobic respiration occurs in the cytoplasm. Aerobic respiration produces more ATP per substrate than anaerobic respiration, and therefore is also more efficient. The chemical equation for glucose being respired aerobically is: $C_6H_{12}O_6 + 6O_2 \rightarrow 6CO_2 + 6H_2O$. Thus, the molar ratio is 1:6 (i.e. 1 mole glucose produces 6 moles of $CO_2$).

**Question 350: B**

The nucleus contains the DNA and chromosomes of the cell. The cytoplasm contains enzymes, salts, and amino acids in addition to water. The plasma membrane is a bilayer. Lastly, the cell wall is indeed responsible for protecting the cell against increased osmotic pressures.

**Question 351: D**

When a solution is hypotonic/less concentrated relative to the cell cytoplasm, the cell will gain water through osmosis. When the solution is isotonic, there will be no net movement of water across the cell membrane. Lastly, when the solution is hypertonic/more concentrated relative to the cell cytoplasm, the cell will lose water by osmosis.

**Question 352: A**

Stem cells have the ability to differentiate and so produce other kinds of cells. However, they also have the ability to generate cells of their own kind and stem cells are able to maintain their undifferentiated state. This is totipotency. The two types of stem cells are embryonic stem cells and adult stem cells. The adult stem cells are present in both children and adults.

**Question 353: B**

All of the following statements are examples of natural selection, except for the breeding of horses. Breeding and animal husbandry are notable methods of artificial selection, which are brought about by humans.

**Question 354: C**

Enzymes create a stable environment to stabilise the transition state. Enzymes do not distort substrates. Enzymes generally have little effect on temperature directly. Lastly, they are able to provide alternative pathways for reactions to occur.

**Question 355: C**

A negative feedback system seeks to minimise changes in a system by modulating the response in accordance with the error that's generated. Salivating before a meal is an example of a feed-forward system (i.e. salivating is an anticipatory response). Throwing a dart does not involve any feedback (during the action). pH and blood pressure are both important homeostatic variables that are controlled via powerful negative feedback mechanisms, e.g. massive haemorrhage leads to compensatory tachycardia.

**Question 356: A**

1 – **correct** – one of the major functions of white blood cells is to defend the body against infectious agents, including bacterial and fungal infections (viral infections too!).
2 – **incorrect** – WBCs, not RBCs, are involved in phagocytosis.
3 – **correct** – WBCs, specifically plasma cells, produce antibodies. These stick to recognition sites on pathogens and help the immune system to target these pathogens.
4 – **incorrect** – antibodies are produced by white blood cells (specifically, plasma cells, a type of B cell).

**Question 357: B**

**A – correct** – the CVS does transport nutrients, such as glucose and oxygen, to all cells in the body.
**B – incorrect** – the <u>respiratory</u> system is responsible for oxygenating blood.
**C – correct** – the CVS transports hormones to target organs.
**D – correct** – via vasoconstriction in response to cold, and vasodilation in response to heat, the cardiovascular system contributes to thermoregulation.
**E – correct** – heart rate increases in response to exercise.

**Question 358: C**

Adrenaline always increases heart rate and is almost always released during sympathetic responses. It travels primarily in the blood and affects multiple organ systems. It is also a potent vasoconstrictor.

**Question 359: B**

Protein synthesis occurs in the cytoplasm. Proteins are usually coded for by several amino acids. Red blood cells lack a nucleus and, therefore, do not contain sufficient DNA to create new proteins. Protein synthesis is a key part of mitosis, as it allows the parent cell to grow prior to division.

**Question 360: C**

Remember that most enzymes work better in neutral environments (amylase works even better at slightly alkaline pH). Thus, adding sodium bicarbonate will increase the pH and hence increase the rate of activity, so **statement 1 is correct**.
Adding carbohydrate will have no effect, as the enzyme is already saturated, so **statement 2 is incorrect.**
Adding amylase will increase the amount of carbohydrate that can be converted per unit time, thus increasing the rate, so **statement 3 is correct**.
Increasing the temperature to 100° C will denature the enzyme and reduce the rate, so **statement 4 is incorrect.**

## Question 361: E

Taking the healthy allele to be C and the disease conferring allele to be c, this Punnet square models the potential offspring:

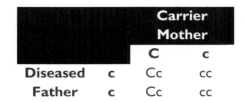

| | | Carrier Mother | |
|---|---|---|---|
| | | C | c |
| Diseased | c | Cc | cc |
| Father | c | Cc | cc |

The gender of the children is irrelevant as the inheritance is autosomal recessive, but we see that all children produced would inherit at least one disease-conferring allele (c).

## Question 362: F

All of the organs listed have endocrine functions.
The thyroid produces thyroid hormone.
The ovary produces oestrogen.
The pancreas secretes glucagon and insulin.
The testes produce testosterone.

## Question 363: A

Insulin works to decrease blood glucose levels. Glucagon causes blood glucose levels to increase; glycogen is a carbohydrate. Adrenaline works to increase heart rate.

## Question 364: A

The left side of the heart contains oxygenated blood from the lungs which will be pumped to the body. The right side of the heart contains deoxygenated blood from the body to be pumped to the lungs.

## Question 365: A

Since Individual 1 is homozygous and healthy, and individual 5 is heterozygous and affected, the disease must be dominant. Since males only have one X-chromosome, they cannot be carriers for X-linked conditions. If Nafram syndrome was X-linked, then parents 5 and 6 would produce sons who always have no disease and daughters that always do. As this is not the case shown in individuals 7-10, the disease must be **autosomal dominant.**

## Question 366: C

We know that the inheritance of Nafram syndrome is autosomal dominant, so using N to mean a disease conferring allele and n to mean a healthy allele, 5, 7 and 8 must be Nn because they have an unaffected parent. 2 is also Nn, as if it was NN all its progeny would be Nn and so affected by the disease, which is not the case, as 3 and 4 are unaffected.

## Question 367: A

Since 6 is disease free, his genotype must be nn. Thus, neither of 6's parents could be NN, as otherwise 6 would have at least one diseased allele.

**Question 368: A**
Urine passes from the kidney into the ureter and is then stored in the bladder. It is finally released through the urethra.

**Question 369: E**
**Deoxygenated** blood from the body flows through the **inferior vena cava** to the **right atrium**. From the RA, it flows to the **right ventricle** to be pumped via the **pulmonary artery** to the **lungs,** where it is **oxygenated**.

**Oxygenated** blood then returns to the heart via the **pulmonary vein** into the **left atrium,** then into the **left ventricle**, where it is pumped to the body via the **aorta.**

Correct passage of blood: Left Atrium → Left Ventricle → Aorta → Inferior Vena Cava → Right Atrium → Right Ventricle → Pulmonary Artery → Lungs → Pulmonary Vein → Left Atrium…

**Question 370: E**
During inspiration, the pressure in the lungs decreases as the diaphragm contracts, increasing the volume of the lungs. The intercostal muscles contract in inspiration, lifting the rib cage up and out to increase intrathoracic volume.

**Question 371: D**
Whilst **A**, **B**, **C** and **E** are true of the DNA code, they do not represent the property described, which is that more than one combination of codons can encode the same amino acid, e.g. Serine is coded by the sequences: TCT, TCC, TCA, TCG.

**Question 372: B**
The degenerate nature of the code can help to reduce the deleterious effects of point mutations. The several 3-nucleotide combinations (triplets) that code for each amino acid are usually similar such that a point mutation, i.e. a substitution of one nucleotide for another, can still result in the same amino acid as the one coded for by the original sequence. The degenerate nature of the code does little to protect against deletions/insertions/duplications, which will cause the bases to be read in incorrect triplets, i.e. result in a frame shift.

**Question 373: D**
The hypothalamus is the site of central thermoreceptors.
A decrease in environmental temperature decreases sweat secretion and causes vasoconstriction of the blood vessels near the skin, to minimise heat loss from the blood.

**Question 374: A**
The movement of carbon dioxide in the lungs and neurotransmitters in a synapse are both examples of diffusion. Glucose reabsorption is an active process, as it requires work to be done against a concentration gradient.

**Question 375: E**

Some enzymes contain other molecules besides protein, e.g. metal ions. Enzymes can increase rates of reaction that may result in heat gain/loss, depending on if the reaction is exothermic or endothermic. They are highly sensitive to variations in pH and their chemical structure is extremely specific to their individual substrate.

**Question 376: D**

Different isotopes are differentiated by the number of neutrons in the core. This gives them different molecular weights and different chemical properties with regards to stability. The number of protons defines each element, and the number of electrons determine its overall charge.

**Question 377: E**

A displacement reaction occurs when a more reactive element displaces a less reactive element in its compound. All 4 reactions are examples of displacement reactions as a less reactive element is being replaced by a more reactive one.

**Question 378: A**

There needs to be 3Ca, 12H, 14O and 2P on each side. Only option **A** satisfies this.

**Question 379: A**

To balance the equation there needs to be 9Ag, 9N, $9O_3$, 9K, 3P on each side. Only option **A** satisfies this.

**Question 380: D**

A more reactive halogen can displace a less reactive halogen. Thus, chlorine can displace bromine and iodine from an aqueous solution of its salts, and fluorine can replace chlorine. The trend is the opposite for alkali metals, where reactivity increases down the group as electrons are further from the core and easier to lose.

**Question 381: C**

$2Mg + O_2 = 2MgO$. So, $2 \times 24 = 48$ and $2 \times (24 + 16) = 80$. So, 48 g of magnesium produces 80g of magnesium oxide. So 1g of magnesium produces 1g $\times$ 80g/48g = 1.666g oxide. So 75g $\times$ 1.666 = 125g

**Question 382: B**

$H_2 + 2OH^- \rightarrow 2H_2O + e^-$
Thus, the hydrogen loses electrons i.e. is oxidised.

**Question 383: E**

1 – correct – this is the formula of ammonia.
2 – correct – ammonia is 1 nitrogen and 3 hydrogen atoms bonded covalently. N = 14g and H = 1g per mole, so percentage of N in $NH_3$ = 14g/17g = 82%.
3 – correct – it can be broken down to nitrogen and hydrogen, through decomposition.
4 – correct – the bonds between N and H are covalent.
5 – correct – ammonia is an important ingredient in fertilisers.
All of the statements are correct, thus the answer is **E.**

## Question 384: A

Whole milk has a roughly neutral pH (~7.0) and contains **fat**. This is broken down by **lipase** to form **fatty acids** - turning the solution slightly more acidic.

## Question 385: C

Glucose loses four hydrogen atoms; one definition of an oxidation reaction is a reaction in which there is loss of hydrogen.

## Question 386: C

Isotopes have the same number of protons and electrons, but a different number of neutrons. The number of neutrons has no impact on the rate of reactions or on the overall charge of the isotope.

## Question 387: E

$Mg + H_2SO_4 \rightarrow MgSO_4 + H_2$

Number of moles of $Mg = \frac{6}{24} = 0.25$ moles.

1 mole of Mg reacts with 1 mole $H_2SO_4$ to produce 1 mole of magnesium sulphate. Therefore, 0.25 moles $H_2SO_4$ will react to produce 0.25 moles of $MgSO_4$.

$M_r$ of $H_2SO_4 = 2 + 32 + 64 = 98g$ per mole

The mass of $H_2SO_4$ used = 0.25 moles x 98g per mole = 24.5g.

Since 30g of $H_2SO_4$ is present, $H_2SO_4$ is in excess and the magnesium is the limiting reagent.

$M_r$ of $MgSO_4 = 24 + 32 + 64 = 120g$ per mole

The mass of $MgSO_4$ produced = 0.25 moles x 120g per mole = 30g which is the same mass as that of sulphuric acid in the original reaction.

## Question 388: E

Reactivity series of metals:

Cu is more reactive than Ag and will displace it.

Ca is more reactive than H and will displace it.

2 and 4 are incorrect because Fe is higher in the reactivity series than Cu and Fe is lower in the reactivity series than Ca, so no displacement will occur.

## Question 389: E

1 – **incorrect** – moving left to right is the equivalent of moving down the metal reactivity series (i.e. Na is most reactive and Zn is least reactive). Therefore, moving from left to right, the reactivity of the metals **decreases**.

2 – **incorrect** – moving L to R, the reactivity decreases so the likelihood of corrosion of the metals decreases, rather than **increases**.

3 – **incorrect** – moving L to R, the reactivity decreases, so **less** energy is required to separate metals from their ores.

4 – **incorrect** – moving L to R, the reactivity decreases, so metals lose electrons **less** readily to form positive ions.

None of the statements given are correct, thus the answer is **E**.

## Question 390: E

Halogens become less reactive as you progress down group 17. Thus, in order of increasing reactivity from left to right: I→ Br→ Cl. Therefore, I will not displace Br, Cl will displace Br and Br will displace I.

## Question 391: A

Wires are made out of copper because it is a good conductor of electricity. Copper is also used in coins (not aluminium). Aluminium is resistant to corrosion but because of a layer of aluminium oxide (not hydroxide).

## Question 392: C

$2Li + 2H_2O \rightarrow 2LiOH + H_2$

Therefore, 2 moles of Li react to produce 1 mole of $H_2$ gas (24 dm³).

The number of moles of Li $= \frac{21}{7} = 3$ moles.

Thus, 1.5 moles of $H_2$ gas are produced = 36 dm³.

## Question 393: B

$MgCl_2$ contains stronger bonds than NaCl because Mg ions have a 2+ charge, thus having a stronger electrostatic pull for negative chloride ions. The smaller atomic radius also means that the nucleus has less distance between it and incoming electrons. Transition metals are able to form multiple stable ions e.g. $Fe^{2+}$ and $Fe^{3+}$. Covalently bonded structures do tend to have lower melting points than ionically bonded, but the giant covalent structures (diamond and graphite for example) have very high melting points. Graphite is an example of a covalently bonded structure which conducts electricity.

## Question 394: D

Energy is released from reaction **A**, as shown by a negative enthalpy. The reaction is therefore exothermic. Since energy is released, the product $CO_2$ has less energy than the reactants did. Therefore, $CO_2$ is more stable. Reaction **B** has a positive enthalpy, which means energy must be put into the reaction for it to occur i.e. it's an endothermic reaction. That means that the products (CaO and $CO_2$) have more energy and are less stable than the reactants ($CaCO_3$).

## Question 395: B

Solid oxides are unable to conduct electricity because the ions are immobile. Metals are extracted from their molten ores by electrolysis. Fractional distillation is used to separate miscible liquids with similar boiling points. $Mg^{2+}$ ions have a greater positive charge and a smaller ionic radius than $Na^+$ ions, and therefore have stronger bonds.

## Question 396: E

$Li^+$ (2) and $Na^+$ (2, 8)

$Mg^{2+}$ (2, 8) and Ne (2, 8)

$Na^{2+}$ (2, 7) and Ne (2, 8)

$O^{2+}$ (2, 4) and a Carbon atom (2, 4)

**Question 397: B**

Reactivity of both group 1 and 2 increases as you go down the groups because the valence electrons that react are further away from the positively charged nucleus (which means the electrostatic attraction between them is weaker). Group 1 metals are usually more reactive because they only need to donate one electron, whilst group 2 metals must donate two electrons.

**Question 398: D**

This is a straightforward question that tests basic understanding of kinetics. Catalysts help overcome energy barriers by reducing the activation energy necessary for a reaction.

**Question 399: D**

$H^1$ contains 1 proton and no neutrons. Isotopes have the same numbers of protons, but different numbers of neutrons. Thus, $H^3$ contains two more neutrons than $H^1$.

**Question 400: D**

Oxidation is the loss of electrons and reduction is the gain of electrons (therefore increasing electron density). Halogens tend to act as electron recipients in reactions and are therefore good oxidising agents.

**Question 401: D**

These statements all come from the Kinetic Theory of Gases, an idealised model of gases that allows for the derivation of the ideal gas law. The angle at which gas molecules move is not related to temperature; movement is random. Gas molecules lose no energy when they collide with each other. Collisions are assumed to be elastic. The average kinetic energy of gas molecules is the same for all gases at the same temperature as they are assumed to be point masses. Momentum = mass x velocity. Therefore, the momentum of gas molecules increases with pressure as a greater force is exerted on each molecule.

**Question 402: E**

An exothermic reaction is defined as a chemical reaction that releases energy. Thus, aerobic respiration, the burning of magnesium, and the reacting of acids/bases are almost always exothermic processes. Similarly, the combustion of most things (including hydrogen) is exothermic. Evaporation of water is a physical process in which no chemical reaction is taking place.

**Question 403:  E**

$2 C_3H_6 + 9 O_2 \rightarrow 6 H_2O + 6 CO_2$

Assign the oxidation numbers for each element:

For $C_3H_6$: C = -2; H = +1

For $O_2$: O = 0

For $H_2O$: H = +1; O = -2

For $CO_2$: C = +4; O = -2

Look for the changes in the oxidation numbers:

H remained at +1

C changed from -2 to +4. Thus, it was oxidized

O changed from 0 to -2. Thus, it was reduced.

**Question 404: B**

The equation for the reaction is: $Zn + CuSO_4 \rightarrow ZnSO_4 + Cu$

Assign oxidation numbers for each element:

For Zn: $Zn = 0$

For $CuSO_4$: $Cu = +2$; $S = +6$; $O = -2$

For $ZnSO_4$: $Zn = +2$; $S = +6$; $O = -2$

For Cu: $Cu = 0$

With these oxidation numbers, we can see that Zn was oxidized and Cu in $CuSO_4$ was reduced. Thus, Zn acted as the reducing agent and Cu in $CuSO_4$ is the oxidizing agent.

**Question 405: B**

Acids are proton donors which only exist in aqueous solution - a liquid state. Strong acids are fully ionised in solution and the reaction between an acid and a base $\rightarrow$ salt + water.

The pH of weak acids is usually between 4 and 6.

**Question 406: D**

Let x be the relative abundance of $Z^6$ and y the relative abundance of $Z^8$.

The average atomic mass takes the abundances of all 3 isotopes into account.

Thus, (Abundance of $Z^5$)(Mass $Z^5$) + (Abundance of $Z^6$)(Mass $Z^6$) + (Abundance of $Z^8$)(Mass $Z^8$) = 7

Therefore: $(5 \times 0.2) + 6x + 8y = 7$

So: $6x + 8y = 6$

Divide by two to give: $3x + 4y = 3$

The abundances of all isotopes = 100% = 1

This gives: $0.2 + x + y = 1$

Solve the two equations simultaneously:

$y = 0.8 - x \rightarrow 3x + 4(0.8 - x) = 3 \rightarrow 3x + 3.2 - 4x = 3$

Therefore, $x = 0.2$

$y = 0.8 - 0.2 = 0.6$

Thus, the overall abundances are $Z^5 = 20\%$, $Z^6 = 20\%$ and $Z^8 = 60\%$. Therefore, all the statements are correct.

**Question 407: A**

If a metal is more reactive than hydrogen, a displacement reaction will occur resulting in the formation of a salt made up of the metal cation and hydrogen.

**Question 408: B**

$6 FeSO_4 + K_2Cr_2O_7 + 7 H_2SO_4 \rightarrow 3 (Fe)_2(SO_4)_3 + Cr_2(SO_4)_3 + K_2SO_4 + 7 H_2O$

In order to save time, you have to quickly eliminate options (rather than try every combination out). The quickest way is to do this is algebraically:

**For Potassium:**

$2b = 2e = 2f$

Therefore, $b = f$.

Option **F** does not fulfil $b = e = f$.

**For Iron:**

$a = 2d$

Options **C, D** and **E** don't fulfil $a = 2d$.

**For Hydrogen:**

$2c = 2g$

Therefore, $c = g$. Option **A** does not fulfil $c = g$. This leaves option **B** as the answer.

**Question 409: E**

Atoms are electrically neutral. Ions have different numbers of electrons when compared to atoms of the same element. Protons provide just under 50% of an atom's mass; the other 50% is provided by neutrons, with a minimal contribution from the electrons. Isotopes don't exhibit significantly different kinetics. Protons do indeed repel each other in the nucleus (which is one reason why neutrons are needed: to reduce the electrical charge density).

**Question 410: B**

The noble gases are extremely useful, e.g. helium in blimps, neon signs, argon in bulbs. They are colourless and odourless and have no valence electrons. As with the rest of the periodic table, boiling point increases as you progress down the group. Helium is the most abundant noble gas (and indeed the 2nd most abundant element in the universe).

**Question 411: D**

**1 – correct** – all alkenes contain at least one double bond.

**2 – correct** – they can be reduced to alkanes.

**3 – incorrect** – it is an example of a hydrogenation or reduction reaction, not a hydration reaction.

Thus, the answer is **D.**

**Question 412: A**

The average atomic mass takes the relative abundance of both isotopes into account:

(Abundance of $Cl^{35}$)(Mass $Cl^{35}$) + (Abundance of $Cl^{37}$)(Mass $Cl^{37}$) = 35.453

34.969(Abundance of $Cl^{35}$) + 36.966(Abundance of $Cl^{37}$) = 35.453

The abundances of both isotopes = 100% = 1

I.e. abundance of $Cl^{35}$ + abundance of $Cl^{37}$ = 1

Therefore: $x + y = 1$ which can be rearranged to give: $y = 1-x$

Therefore: $x + (1 - x) = 1$.

$34.969x + 36.966(1-x) = 35.453$

$x = 0.758$

$1 - x = 0.242$

Therefore, $Cl^{35}$ is 3 times more abundant than $Cl^{37}$.

Note you could approximate the values here to arrive at the solution quicker, e.g. 34.969 → 35, 36.966 → 37 and 35.453 → 35.5

**Question 413: A**

A – correct - transition metals form multiple stable ions, which may have many different colours (e.g. green $Fe^{2+}$ and brown $Fe^{3+}$).

B – incorrect – transition metals usually for ionic bonds, not covalent.

C – incorrect – transition metals are commonly used as catalysts, e.g. iron in the Haber process.

D – incorrect – transition metals are excellent conductors of electricity.

E – incorrect – transition metals are known as the d-block elements of the periodic table, the alkali earth metals are found in group 2.

**Question 414: B**

$2Na + 2H_2O \rightarrow 2NaOH + H_2$

$8000 \text{ cm}^3 = 8 \text{ dm}^3 = \frac{1}{3}$ moles of $H_2$

2 moles of Na react completely to form 1 mole of $H_2$.

Therefore, $\frac{2}{3}$ moles of Na must have reacted to produce $\frac{1}{3}$ moles of hydrogen. $\frac{2}{3}$ x 23g per mole = 15.3g.

% Purity of sample $= \frac{15.3}{20}$ x 100 = 76.5%

**Question 415: C**

Assume total mass of molecule is 100g. Therefore, it contains 70.6g carbon, 5.9g hydrogen and 23.5g oxygen.

Now, calculate the number of moles of each element using $Moles = \frac{Mass}{Molar\ Mass}$

$Moles\ of\ Carbon = \frac{70.6}{12} \approx 6$  $Moles\ of\ Hydrogen = \frac{5.9}{1} \approx 6$  $Moles\ of\ Oxygen = \frac{23.5}{16} \approx 1.5$

Therefore, the molar ratios give an empirical formula of $C_6H_6O_{1.5} = C_4H_4O$.

Molar mass of the empirical formula = (4 x 12) + (4 x 1) + 16 = 68.

Molar mass of chemical formula = 136. Therefore, the chemical formula = $C_8H_8O_2$.

**Question 416: B**

$S + 6 HNO_3 \rightarrow H_2SO_4 + 6 NO_2 + 2 H_2O$

In order to save time, you have to quickly eliminate options (rather than try every combination out).

The quickest way to do this is algebraically:

For Hydrogen:

$b = 2c + 2e$

Options **A, C, D, E** and **F** don't fulfil $b = 2c + 2e$.

This leaves option **B** as the only possible answer.

Note how quickly we were able to get the correct answer here by choosing an element that appears in 3 molecules (as opposed to Sulphur or Nitrogen which only appear in 2).

**Question 417: A**

Alkenes undergo addition reactions, such as that with hydrogen, when catalysed by nickel, whilst alkanes do not as they are already fully saturated. The C=C bond is stronger than the C-C bond, but it is not exactly twice as strong, so will not require twice the energy to break it. Both molecules are organic and will dissolve in organic solvents.

**Question 418: E**

Diamond is unable to conduct electricity because all the electrons are involved in covalent bonds. Graphite is insoluble in water and organic solvents. Graphite is also able to conduct electricity because it has free electrons that are not involved in covalent bonds. Methane and ammonia both have low melting points. Methane is not a polar molecule, so cannot conduct electricity or dissolve in water. Ammonia is polar and will dissolve in water. It can conduct electricity in aqueous form, but not as a gas.

**Question 419: A**

Catalysts increase the rate of reaction by providing an alternative route for reaction with a lower activation energy, which means that less energy is required and as a result, costs are reduced. The point of equilibrium, the nature of the products, and the overall energy change are unaffected by catalysts.

**Question 420: E**

The 5 carbon atoms in this hydrocarbon make it a "pent" stem. The C=C bond makes it an alkene, and the location of this bond is the 2nd position, making the molecule pent-2-ene.

**Question 421: D**

Group 1 elements form positively charged ions in most reactions since they lose electrons. Thus, the oxidation number must increase. Their reactivity increases as the valence electrons are further away from the positively charged nucleus down group. All group one elements react spontaneously with oxygen – the less reactive ones form an oxide coating and the more reactive ones spontaneously burn.

**Question 422: E**

The cathode attracts positively charged ions. The cathode reduces ions and the anode oxidises ions. Electrolysis can be used to separate compounds but not mixtures (i.e. substances that are not chemically joined).

**Question 423: B**

Pentane, $C_5H_{12}$, has a total of 3 isomers. **A, C** and **D** are correctly configured. However, the 4th Carbon atom in option **B** has more than 4 bonds which wouldn't be possible. If you're stuck on this – draw them out!

**Question 424: E**

$3\ Cu + 8\ HNO_3 \rightarrow 3\ Cu(NO_3)_2 + 2\ NO + 4\ H_2O$

In order to save time, you have to quickly eliminate options (rather than try every combination out). The quickest way to do this is algebraically, by first assigning coefficients to the equation:

$aCu + bHNO_3 \rightarrow cCu(NO_3)_2 + dNO + eH_2O$. For Nitrogen: $b = 2c + d$. In this case, only option **E** satisfies $b = 2c + d$.

Note that using copper wouldn't be as useful, as all the options satisfy $a = c$.

**Question 425: D**

Alkenes are an organic series and have twice as many hydrogen atoms as carbon atoms. Bromine water is decolourised in their presence, and they take part in addition reactions. Alkenes are more reactive than alkanes because they contain a C=C bond.

**Question 426: A**

A – correct – group 17 elements are missing one valence electron, so form negative ions.

B – incorrect – reactivity decreases as you progress down group 17, so fluorine reacts **more** vigorously than iodine.

C – incorrect – all group 17 elements are found bound to each other e.g. $F_2$ and $Cl_2$.

**Question 427: D**

CO poisoning and spontaneous combustion do not occur in the electrolysis of brine. The products of cathode and anode in the electrolysis of brine are $Cl_2$ and $H_2$. If these two gases react with each other they can form HCl, which is extremely corrosive.

**Question 428: D**

The hydrogen produced is positively charged and therefore needs to be reduced by the addition of an electron before being released. This happens at the cathode. The chlorine produced is negatively charged and therefore needs to lose electrons. This happens at the anode. NaOH is formed in this process.

**Question 429: C**

Alkanes are made of chains of singly bonded carbon and hydrogen atoms. C-H bonds are very strong and confer alkanes a great deal of stability. An alkane with 14 hydrogen atoms is called hexane, as it has 6 carbon atoms. Alkanes burn in excess oxygen to produce carbon dioxide and water. Bromine water is decolourised in the presence of alkenes.

**Question 430: E**

Alcohols by definition contain an R-OH functional group and because of this polar group are highly soluble in water. Ethanol is a common biofuel.

**Question 431: E**

Alkanes are saturated (and therefore non-reducible), have the general formula $C_nH_{2n+2}$ and have no effect on Bromine solution. Alkenes are unsaturated (and therefore reducible), have the general formula $C_nH_{2n}$ and turn bromine water colourless because they can undergo an addition reaction with bromine.

**Question 432: D**

The balanced equation for the reaction between magnesium oxide and hydrochloric acid is:

$MgO + 2HCl \rightarrow MgCl_2 + H_2$

The relative molecular mass of MgO is $24 + 16 = 40g$ per mole.

Therefore, 10g of MgO represents $10/40 = 0.25$ moles.

As the ratio of MgO to $MgCl_2$ is 1:1, we know that the amount of $MgCl_2$ produced will also be 0.25 moles. One mole of $MgCl_2$ has a molecular mass of $24 + (2 \times 35.5) = 95g$ per mole.

Therefore, the reaction will produce $0.25 \times 95 = 23.75g$ of $MgCl_2$.

**Question 433: D**

Moving up the alkane series, as the size and mass of the molecule increases, the boiling point and viscosity increase, and the flammability and volatility decrease. Pentadecane will be more viscous than pentane.

**Question 434: E**

All of the factors mentioned will affect the rate of a reaction.

The temperature affects the movement rate of particles, which if moving faster in higher temperatures will collide more often, thus increasing the rate of reaction.

Collision rate is also increased with a higher **concentration** of reactants, and with a higher concentration of a **catalyst** or one with larger **surface area**, which will provide more active sites, thus increasing the rate of reaction.

**Question 435: C**

The total atomic mass of the end product is $C[12 + (2 \times 16)] + D[(2 \times 1) + 16] = 44C + 18D$

We know that $176 = 44C$. Therefore $C = 4$, and that $108 = 18D$ so $D = 6$.

Thus, the equation becomes: $C_aH_b + O_2 \rightarrow 4CO_2 + 6H_2O$.

This gives a ratio of 4C to 12H, which is a ratio of 1:3 carbon to hydrogen. This means the unknown hydrocarbon must be a multiple of this ratio. By balancing the equation, we can see that the unknown hydrocarbon must be ethane, $C_2H_6$: $2C_2H_6 + 7O_2 \rightarrow 4CO_2 + 6H_2O$.

**Question 436: A**

$C_2H_5OH \rightarrow C_2H_4O$. Thus, ethanol has lost two hydrogen atoms, i.e. it has been oxidised. Note that although another substrate may be reduced (therefore making it a redox reaction), ethanol itself has only been oxidised.

**Question 437: B**

This is fairly straightforward, but you can save time by doing it algebraically:

For barium: $3a = b$. For nitrogen: $2a = c$. Let $a = 1$, thus, $b = 3$ and $c = 2$

**Question 438: E**
There are 14 oxygen atoms on the left side. Thus: $3b + 2c = 14$.
Note also that for sulfur: $a = c$, and for Iron: $a = 2b$.
This sets up an easy trio of simultaneous equations:
Substitute $a$ into the first equation to give: $1.5a + 2a = 14$. Thus: $a = 14/3.5 = 4$.
Therefore, $a = c = 4$ and $b = 2$

**Question 439: C**
The average atomic mass takes the relative abundance of all isotopes found in nature into account:
Mass = (Abundance of $Mg^{23}$)(Mass $Mg^{23}$) + (Abundance of $Mg^{25}$)(Mass $Mg^{25}$) + (Abundance of $Mg^{26}$)(Mass $Mg^{26}$)
$Mass = 23 \times 0.80 + 25 \times 0.10 + 26 \times 0.10$
$= 18.4 + 2.5 + 2.6 = 23.5$

**Question 440: D**
$Cl_2$ and $Fe_2O_3$ are reduced in their reactions and are therefore oxidising agents. Similarly, CO and $Cu^{2+}$ are oxidised in their reactions and are therefore reducing agents. Cl is a stronger oxidising agent than Br as it is higher up in the reactivity series and will displace negative Br ions from its compounds to form the oxidised $Br_2$. Mg is a stronger reducing agent than Cu, as it is higher up in the reactivity series. Thus, Mg would displace a positive copper ion from its compound to form copper atoms. Therefore, Mg reduces Cu.

**Question 441: C**
NaCl is an ionic compound and therefore has a high melting point. It is highly soluble in water but only conducts electricity in solution/as a liquid.

**Question 442: C**
The equation for the reaction is: $2NaOH + Zn(NO_3)_2 \rightarrow 2NaNO_3 + Zn(OH)_2$
Therefore, the molar ratio between NaOH and $Zn(OH)_2$ is 2:1.
Molecular Mass of NaOH = $23 + 16 + 1 = 40$
Molecular Mass of $Zn(OH)_2$ = $65 + 17 \times 2 = 99$
Thus, the number of moles of NaOH that react = $80/40 = 2$ moles.
Therefore, 1 mole of $Zn(OH)_2$ is produced. Mass = 99g per mole x 1 mole = 99g

**Question 443: E**
Metal + Water $\rightarrow$ Hydroxide + Hydrogen gas; the reaction is always exothermic. Reactivity increases down the group, so potassium reacts more vigorously with water than sodium. Therefore, all four statements are correct.

**Question 444: C**
Electrolysis separates NaCl into sodium and chloride ions but not $CO_2$ (which is a covalently bound gas). Sieves cannot separate ionically bound compounds like NaCl. Dyes are miscible liquids and can be separated by chromatography. Oil and water are immiscible liquids, so a separating funnel is necessary to separate the mixtures. Methane and diesel are separated from each other during fractional distillation, as they have different boiling points.

**Question 445: B**

The reaction between water and caesium can cause spontaneous combustion, so it doesn't make the reaction safer. The reaction between caesium and fluoride is highly exothermic and does not require a catalyst. The reaction produces CsF, which is a salt.

**Question 446: B**

The nuclei of larger elements contain more neutrons than protons which reduces the charge density, e.g. $Br^{80}$ contains 35 protons but 45 neutrons. Stable isotopes very rarely undergo radioactive decay.

**Question 447: B**

The vast majority of salts contain ionic bonds that require a significant amount of thermal energy to break.

**Question 448: E**

306ml of water is 306g, which is the equivalent of 306g/18g per mole of $H_2O$ = 17 moles. 17 times Avogadro's constant gives the number of molecules present, which is $1.02 \times 10^{25}$. There are 10 protons and 10 electrons in each water molecule. Hence there are $1.02 \times 10^{26}$ protons.

**Question 449: D**

The number of moles of each element = Mass/Molar Mass. Let the % represent the mass in grams: Hydrogen: 3.45g/1g per mole = 3.45 moles. Oxygen: 55.2g/16g per mole = 3.45 moles
Carbon: 41.4g/12g per mole = 3.45 moles
Thus, the molar ratio is 1:1:1. The only option that satisfies this is option **D**.

**Question 450:  C**

Group 17 elements are non-metals, whilst group 2 elements are metals. Thus, the Group 17 element must gain electrons when it reacts with the Group 2 element, i.e. B is reduced.  The easy way to calculate the formula is to swap the valences of both elements: A is +2 and B is -1. Thus, the compound is $AB_2$.

**Question 451: E**

The amplitude of a wave does not determine the mass of the wave. Waves are not objects and thus do not have mass.

A – correct – microwaves are an example of using electromagnetic waves to heat things up!
B – correct – these waves have high energy and thus can knock electrons out of their orbits.
C – correct.
D – correct – this is a 'green' method of producing electricity.

**Question 452: A**

We know that displacement s = 30 m, initial speed u = 0 ms$^{-1}$, acceleration a = 5.4 ms$^{-2}$, final speed v = ?, time t = ?

And that $v^2 = u^2 + 2as$

$v^2 = 0 + 2 \times 5.4 \times 30$

$v^2 = 324$   so v = 18 ms$^{-1}$

and $s = ut + 1/2\ at^2$   so $30 = 1/2 \times 5.4 \times t^2$

To find 30/2.7 without a calculator, find a rough estimate by substituting 2.7 for 3, to give 30/3 = 10.

We now know that $t^2$ will be a shade over 10, as the actual number we should be dividing by (2.7) was smaller than the number we used in the estimate.

If $t^2$ is just over 10, we can exclude t = 3.1 as an option, as $3.1^2$ is 9.61 i.e. under 10, rather than over.

The only option that remains that gives $v = 18 ms^{-1}$ is option A, which gives 3.3 as an answer for t.

We can quickly calculate that $3.3^2$ would give us 10.89 for t, which is a shade over 10 – i.e. exactly what we are looking for!

**Question 453: D**

Consider the following equations:

- Velocity = λf
- Frequency = 1/T
- These 2 equations can be combined and rearranged to give λ = vT

The period T of one wave = $\frac{49s}{7}$ = 7s, so λ = 5 ms$^{-1}$ × 7 s = 35 m.

**Question 454:  E**

This is a straightforward question as you only have to put the numbers into the equation (made harder by the numbers being hard to work with).

$Power = \frac{Force \times Distance}{Time}$

$Force = mass \times acceleration = 37.5 \times 10$

$\frac{375\ N \times 1.3\ m}{5\ s}$

We can simplify 375/5 to 75, thus making the calculation easier.

$= 75 \times 1.3 = 97.5\ W$

**Question 455: E**

v = u + at

v = 0 + 5.6 × 8 = 44.8 ms$^{-1}$

And $s = ut + \frac{at^2}{2} = 0 + 5.6 \times \frac{8^2}{2} = 179.2$

**Question 456: C**

The skydiver leaves the plane and will accelerate until the air resistance equals their weight – this is their terminal velocity. The skydiver will accelerate under the force of gravity. If the air resistance force exceeded the force of gravity the skydiver would accelerate away from the ground, and if it was less than the force of gravity they would continue to accelerate toward the ground.

## Question 457: D

$s = 20$ m, $u = 0$ ms$^{-1}$, $a = 10$ ms$^{-2}$

and $v^2 = u^2 + 2as$

$v^2 = 0 + 2 \times 10 \times 20$

$v^2 = 400$; $v = 20$ ms$^{-1}$

Momentum = Mass x velocity = $20 \times 0.1 = 2$ kgms$^{-1}$

## Question 458: E

Electromagnetic waves have varying wavelengths and frequencies and their energy is proportional to their frequency – hence options 3 and 4 are incorrect.

Unlike sound waves, EM waves can all travel through a vacuum and can be reflected – hence options 1 and 2 are correct.

## Question 459: D

The total resistance in a series circuit can be found by adding the individual resistances – this is a 'series' circuit as the battery (resistance 0.8) and the drill (resistance 1) are in series.

Total resistance = $R + r = 0.8 + 1 = 1.8 \, \Omega$

and $I = \frac{e.m.f}{total\ resistance} = \frac{36}{1.8} = 20 \, A$

## Question 460: D

Use Newton's second law $\rightarrow F = ma$

Remember to work in SI units!

So $Force = mass \times accelaration = mass \times \frac{\Delta velocity}{time}$

$= 20 \times 10^{-3} \times \frac{100 - 0}{10 \times 10^{-3}}$

$= 200 \, N$

## Question 461: E

In this case, the work being done is moving the bag 0.7 m

i.e. $Work\ Done = Bag's\ Weight \times Distance = 50 \times 10 \times 0.7 = 350 \, N$

$Power = \frac{Work}{Time} = \frac{350}{3} = 116.7$ W

$= 117$ W to 3 significant figures

## Question 462: B

Firstly, use P = Fv to calculate the power [Ignore the frictional force as we are not concerned with the resultant force here].

So P = $300 \times 30 = 9000$ W

Then, use P = IV to calculate the current.

I = P/V = 9000/200 = 45 A

## Question 463: C

Work is defined as W = F x s. Work can also be defined as work = force x distance moved in the direction of force. Work is measured in joules and 1 Joule = 1 Newton x 1 Metre, and 1 Newton = 1 Kg x ms$^{-2}$ [F = ma]. Thus, 1 Joule = Kgm$^2$s$^{-2}$

**Question 464: E**

Joules are the unit of energy (and also Work = Force x Distance). Thus, 1 Joule = 1 N x 1 m.

Pa is the unit of Pressure (= Force/Area). Thus, Pa = N x m$^{-2}$. So J = Nm$^{-2}$ x m$^3$ = Pa x m$^3$. Newton's third law describes that every action produces an equal and opposite reaction. For this reason, the energy required to decelerate a body is equal to the amount of energy it possesses during movement, i.e. its kinetic energy, which is defined as in statement 1.

**Question 465: D**

Alpha radiation is of the lowest energy, as it represents the movement of a fairly large particle consisting of 2 neutrons and 2 protons. Beta radiation consists of high-energy, high-speed electrons or positrons.

**Question 466: E**

The half-life does depend on atom type and isotope, as these parameters significantly impact on the physical properties of the atom in general, so statement 1 is false. Statement 2 is the correct definition of half-life. Statement 3 is also correct: half-life in exponential decay will always have the same duration, independent of the quantity of the matter in question; in non-exponential decay, half-life is dependent on the quantity of matter in question.

**Question 467: C**

192 / 24 = 8 half-lives have elapsed. So, we can calculate: $56 \times 2^8 = 14,336$ = the original count rate.

**Question 468: A**

1 – correct – the rate of decay decreases exponentially as the material decays.

2 – incorrect – remember, not all nuclei of the same element are the same, as the number of neutrons can be different. Nuclei with different numbers of neutrons will have different half-lives. However, all nuclei of the same *isotope* of an element will have the same half-life.

3 – incorrect – radioactive decay is a highly unpredictable process.

**Question 469: E**

The total resistance of the circuit would be twice the resistance of one resistor and proportional to the voltage, as given by Ohm's Law. Since it is a series circuit, the same current flows through each resistor and since they are identical the potential difference across each resistor will be the same.

**Question 470: E**

The distance between Earth and Sun = Time x Speed = 60 x 8 seconds x 3 x 10$^8$ ms$^{-1}$ = 480 x 3 x 10$^8$ m

Approximately = 1500 x 10$^8$ = 1.5 x 10$^{11}$ m.

The circumference of Earth's orbit around the sun is given by 2πr = 2 x 3 x 1.5 x 10$^{11}$

= 9 x 10$^{11}$ = 10$^{12}$ m

**Question 471: E**

Speed is a scalar quantity whilst velocity is a vector describing both magnitude and direction. Speed describes the distance a moving object covers over time (i.e. speed = distance/time), whereas velocity describes the rate of change of the displacement of an object (i.e. velocity = displacement/time). The international standardised unit for speed is meters per second (ms$^{-1}$), while ms$^{-2}$ is the unit of acceleration.

**Question 472: E**

Ohm's Law only applies to conductors and can be mathematically expressed as $V \alpha I$. The easiest way to do this is to write down the equations for statements c, d and e. **C**: $I \alpha \frac{1}{V}$ ; **D**: $I \alpha V^2$ ; **E**: $I \alpha V$. Thus, statement **E** is correct.

**Question 473: E**

Any object at rest is not accelerating and therefore has no resultant force. Strictly speaking, Newton's second law is actually: Force = rate of change of momentum, which can be mathematically manipulated to give statement 2:

$$Force = \frac{momentum}{time} = \frac{mass \text{ x } velocity}{time} = mass \text{ x } accelaration$$

Thus, all of the statements are correct.

**Question 474: D**

Statement 3 is incorrect, as $Charge = Current \text{ } x \text{ } time$. Statement 1 substitutes $I = \frac{V}{R}$ and statement 2 substitutes $I = \frac{P}{V}$.

**Question 475: E**

Applying Newton's second law of motion gives:
Weight of elevator + people = mg = 10 x (1600 + 200) = 18,000 N
Thus, the resultant force is given by:
$F_M$ = Motor Force − [Frictional Force + Weight]
$F_M$ = M − 4,000 − 18,000
Use Newton's second law to give: $F_M$ = M − 22,000 N = ma
Thus, M − 22,000 N = 1,800a
Since the lift must accelerate at 1ms$^{-2}$: M = 1,800 kg x 1 ms$^{-2}$ + 22,000 N
M = 23,800 N

**Question 476: D**

Total Distance = Distance during acceleration phase + Distance during braking phase
Distance during the <u>acceleration phase</u> is given by:
$$s = ut + \frac{at^2}{2} = 0 + \frac{5 \text{ x } 10^2}{2} = 250 \text{ } m$$
$$v = u + at = 0 + 5 \text{ } x \text{ } 10 = 50 \text{ } ms^{-1}$$
And use $a = \frac{v-u}{t}$ to calculate the deceleration: $a = \frac{0-50}{20} = -2.5 \text{ ms}^{-2}$
Distance during the <u>deceleration phase</u> is given by:
$$s = ut + \frac{at^2}{2} = 50 \text{ } x \text{ } 20 + \frac{-2.5 \text{ x } 20^2}{2} = 1000 - \frac{2.5 \text{ x } 400}{2}$$
$$s = 1000 - 500 = 500 \text{ } m$$
Thus, $Total \text{ } Distance = 250 + 500 = 750 \text{ } m$

**Question 477: E**

It is not possible to calculate the power of the heater as we don't know the current that flows through it or its internal resistance. The 8 ohms refers to the external copper wire and not the heater. Whilst it's important that you know how to use equations like P = IV, it's just as important that you know when you **can't** use them!

**Question 478: E**

This question has a lot of numbers but not any information on time, which is necessary to calculate power. You cannot calculate power by using P= IV as you don't know how many electrons are accelerated through the potential difference per unit time. Thus, more information is required to calculate the power.

**Question 479: B**

When an object is in equilibrium with its surroundings, it radiates and absorbs energy at the same rate and so its temperature remains constant i.e. there is no *net* energy transfer. Radiation is slower than conduction and convection.

**Question 480: A**

The work done by the force is given by: $Work\ Done = Force \times Distance = 12\,N \times 3\,m = 36\,J$
Since the surface is frictionless, $Work\ Done = Kinetic\ Energy$.
$E_k = \frac{mv^2}{2} = \frac{6v^2}{2}$
Thus, $36 = 3v^2$
$v = \sqrt{12} = \sqrt{4}\sqrt{3} = 2\sqrt{3}\ ms^{-1}$

**Question 481: C**

$Total\ energy\ supplied\ to\ water = Change\ in\ temperature \times Mass\ of\ water \times 4{,}000\,J$
$= 40 \times 1.5 \times 4{,}000 = 240{,}000\,J$
$Power\ of\ the\ heater = \frac{Work\ Done}{time} = \frac{240{,}000}{50 \times 60} = \frac{240{,}000}{3{,}000} = 80\,W.$    Using $P = IV = \frac{V^2}{R}$:
$R = \frac{V^2}{P} = \frac{100^2}{80} = \frac{10{,}000}{80} = 125\ ohms$

**Question 482: C**

**1 – incorrect** – the half life of a radioactive substance is defined as the time taken for the radioactivity of a specific isotope to fall to half its original value.
**2 – correct** – a beta particle is essentially a high energy election, that is emitted from the nucleus. Beta emission occurs when a neutron is converted to a proton and an electron, and it occurs in elements which have too many neutrons relative to the number of protons. The element gains a proton in the process of beta emission, so it is converted to a new element.
**3 – incorrect** – this is true of beta emission, not alpha. An alpha particle is made up of 2 protons and 2 neutrons, the equivalent of a helium nucleus.

**Question 483: D**

Gravitational potential energy is just an extension of the equation work done = force x distance (force is the weight of the object, *mg*, and distance is the height, *h*). The reservoir in statement 3 would have a potential energy of $10^{10}$ Joules i.e. 10 Giga Joules ($E_p = 10^6$ kg x 10 N x $10^3$ m).

**Question 484: D**

Statement 1 is the common formulation of Newton's third law.

Statement 2 presents a consequence of the application of Newton's third law.

Statement 3 is false: the force of the rifle recoiling will be the same as the force of the bullet going forward, but the acceleration will be different as the masses of each are different (F = ma).

**Question 485: E**

Positively charged objects have lost electrons.

$$Charge \ = \ Current \ x \ Time \ = \ \frac{Voltage}{Resistance} \ x \ Time.$$

Objects can become charged by friction as electrons are transferred from one object to the other.

**Question 486: B**

Each body of mass exerts a gravitational force on another body with mass. This is true for all planets as well. Gravitational force is dependent on the mass of both objects. Satellites stay in orbit due to centripetal force that acts tangentially to gravity (not because of the thrust from their engines). Two objects will only land at the same time if they also have the same shape or they are in a vaccum (as otherwise air resistance would result in different terminal velocities).

**Question 487: A**

Metals conduct electrical charge easily and provide little resistance to the flow of electrons. Charge can also flow in several directions. However, all conductors have an internal resistance and therefore provide *some* resistance to electrical charge.

**Question 488: E**

First, calculate the rate of petrol consumption:

$$\frac{Speed}{Consumption} \ = \ \frac{60 \ miles/hour}{30 \ miles/gallon} = 2 \ gallons/hour$$

Therefore, the total power is:

$2 \ gallons \ = \ 2 \ x \ 9 \ x \ 10^8 = 18 \ x \ 10^8 J$

$1 \ hour \ = \ 60 \ x \ 60 \ = \ 3600 \ s$

Power $= \frac{Energy}{Time} = \frac{18 \ x 10^8}{3600} = \frac{18}{36} \ x \ 10^6 = 5 \ x \ 10^5 \ W$

Since efficiency is 20%, the power delivered to the wheels $= 5 \ x \ 10^5 \ x \ 0.2 = 10^5 \ W \ = \ 100 \ kW$

**Question 489: D**

Beta radiation is stopped by a few millimetres of aluminium, but not by paper. In β- radiation, a neutron becomes a proton plus an emitted electron. This means the atomic mass number remains unchanged.

**Question 490: E**

Firstly, calculate the mass of the car $= \frac{Weight}{g} = \frac{15,000}{10} \ = \ 1,500 \ kg$

Then using $v = u + at$ where v = 0 ms⁻¹ and u = 15 ms⁻¹ and t = 10 x 10⁻³ s

$a = \frac{0-15}{0.01} \ = \ 1500ms^{-2}$

$F \ = \ ma = 1500 \ x \ 1500 = 2 \ 250 \ 000 \ N$

**Question 491: E**

Electrical insulators offer high resistance to the flow of charge. Insulators are usually non-metals; metals conduct charge very easily. Since charge does not flow easily to even out, they can be charged with friction.

**Question 492: A**

The car accelerates for the first 10 seconds at a constant rate and then decelerates after t=30 seconds. It does not reverse, as the velocity is not negative.

**Question 493: B**

The distance travelled by the car is represented by the area under the curve (integral of velocity) which is given by the area of two triangles and a rectangle:

$$Area = \left(\frac{1}{2} \; x \; 10 \; x \; 10\right) + (20 \; x \; 10) + \left(\frac{1}{2} \; x \; 10 \; x \; 10\right)$$

$Area = 50 + 200 + 50 = 300 \; m$

Alternatively, you can use the area for a trapezium to get the same result:

$$area = \frac{1}{2}(a+b) \times height$$

**Question 494: C**

Using the equation force = mass x acceleration, where the unknown acceleration = change in velocity over change in time.

Hence: $\frac{F}{m} = \frac{change \; in \; velocity}{change \; in \; time}$

We know that F = 10,000 N, mass = 1,000 kg and change in time is 5 seconds.

So, $\frac{10,000}{1,000} = \frac{change \; in \; velocity}{5}$

So change in velocity $= 10 \; x \; 5 = 50 \; m/s$

**Question 495: D**

This question tests both your ability to convert unusual units into SI units and to select the relevant values from the information given in the question (e.g. the crane's mass is not important here).

0.01 tonnes = 10 kg; 100 cm = 1 m; 5,000 ms = 5 s

$$Power = \frac{Work \; Done}{Time} = \frac{Force \; x \; Distance}{Time}$$

In this case the force is the weight of the wardrobe $= 10 \; x \; g = 10 \; x \; 10 = 100N$. Thus, $Power = \frac{100 \; x \; 1}{5} = 20 \; W$

**Question 496: E**

Remember that the resistance of a parallel circuit ($R_T$) is given by: $\frac{1}{R_T} = \frac{1}{R_1} + \frac{1}{R_2} + \; ...$

Thus, $\frac{1}{R_T} = \frac{1}{1} + \frac{1}{2} = \frac{3}{2}$ and therefore $R = \frac{2}{3} \; \Omega$

Using Ohm's Law: I $= \frac{20 \; V}{\frac{2}{3} \Omega} = 20 \; x \; \frac{3}{2} = 30$ A

**Question 497: E**

Water is denser than air. Therefore, the speed of light decreases when it enters water and increases when it leaves water. The direction of light also changes when light enters or leaves water in comparison to air. This phenomenon is known as refraction and is governed by Snell's Law.

**Question 498: C**
The voltage in a parallel circuit is the same across each branch, i.e. branch A Voltage = branch B Voltage.
The resistance of Branch A = 6 x 5 = 30 Ω; the resistance of Branch B = 10 x 2 = 20 Ω.
Using Ohm's Law: I= V/R. Thus, $I_A = \frac{60}{30} = 2\ A$; $I_B = \frac{60}{20} = 3\ A$

**Question 499: C**
This is a very straightforward question, but it is made harder by the awkward units you have to work with. Ensure you are able to work comfortably with prefixes of $10^9$ and $10^{-9}$ and convert to decimals without difficulty.
50,000,000,000 nano Watts = 50 W and 0.000000004 Giga Amperes = 4 A.
Using $P = IV$: $V = \frac{P}{I} = \frac{50}{4} = 12.5\ V = 0.0125\ kV$

**Question 500: B**
Radioactive decay is highly random and unpredictable. Only gamma decay releases gamma rays and few types of decay release X-rays. The total electrical charge of an atom's nucleus decreases after alpha decay as two protons are lost.

**Question 501: D**
Using $P = IV$: $I = \frac{P}{V} = \frac{60}{15} = 4\ A$
Now using Ohm's Law: $R = \frac{V}{I} = \frac{15}{4} = 3.75\ \Omega$
So, each resistor has a resistance of $\frac{3.75}{3} = 1.25\ \Omega$. If two more resistors are added, the overall resistance = $1.25 \times 5 = 6.25\ \Omega$

**Question 502: E**
There is not enough information to answer this question. We would be required to know the resistive forces acting against the tractor and if there is any change in height in order to calculate the useful work done and hence the efficiency.

**Question 503: E**
Electromagnetic induction is defined by statements 1 and 2. An electrical current is generated when a coil moves in a magnetic field.
Thus, all 3 statements are correct.

**Question 504: D**
An ammeter will always give the same reading in a series circuit, but it will not in a parallel circuit where the current splits at each branch in accordance with Ohm's Law.

**Question 505: D**
1 – **correct** – note, this is not true in parallel circuits!
2 – **correct** – the current is directed from the positive terminal towards the negative terminal.
3 – **incorrect** – electrons move in the opposite direction to current, i.e. they move from negative to positive.

## Question 506: A

For a fixed resistor, the current is directly proportional to the potential difference. **This is shown in graph A.** For a filament lamp, as current increases, the metal filament becomes hotter. This causes the metal atoms to vibrate and move more, resulting in more collisions with the flow of electrons. This makes it harder for the electrons to move through the lamp and results in increased resistance. Therefore, the graph's gradient decreases as current increases. **This is shown in graph B.**

## Question 507: D

**A – correct** – vectors can be added to one another, although you must take into account the direction of each vector quantity in the sum!
**B – correct** – all vectors are comprised of both direction and magnitude.
**C – correct** – see explanation for B.

All of the statements are correct, thus the correct answer to the question is **D.**

## Question 508: C

The gravity on the moon is 6 times less than 10 ms$^{-2}$. Thus, $g_{moon} = \frac{10}{6} = \frac{5}{3}$ ms$^{-2}$.

Since weight = mass x gravity, the mass of the rock $= \frac{250}{\frac{5}{3}} = \frac{750}{5} = 150\ kg$

Therefore, the density $= \frac{mass}{volume} = \frac{150}{250} = 0.6\ kg/cm^3$

## Question 509: D

An alpha particle consists of a helium nucleus. Thus, alpha decay causes the mass number to decrease by 4 and the atomic number to decrease by 2. Five iterations of this would decrease the mass number by 20 and the atomic number by 10.

## Question 510: C

Using Ohm's Law: The potential difference entering the transformer ($V_1$) = 10 x 20 = 200 V
Now use $\frac{N1}{N2} = \frac{V1}{V2}$ to give: $\frac{5}{10} = \frac{200}{V2}$
Thus, $V_2 = \frac{2,000}{5} = 400$ V

## Question 511: D

For objects in free fall that have reached terminal velocity, acceleration = 0.
Thus, the sphere's weight = resistive forces.
Using Work Done = Force x Distance: Force = 10,000 J/100 m = 100 N.
Therefore, the sphere's weight = 100 N and since g = 10ms$^{-2}$, the sphere's mass = 10 kg

## Question 512: E

**A – incorrect** – the wavelength of ultraviolet waves is longer than that of x-rays.
**B – incorrect** – wavelength is inversely proportional to frequency.
**C – incorrect** – waves in the EM spectrum travel at the speed of light.
**D – incorrect** – humans are only able to visualise a very small part of the spectrum.
**E – correct** – none, of the above statements were correct, so E is the correct answer.

**Question 513: B**

If an object moves towards the sensor, the wavelength will appear to decrease and the frequency increase. The faster this happens, the faster the increase in frequency and decrease in wavelength.

**Question 514: A**

$Acceleration = \frac{Change\ in\ Velocity}{Time} = \frac{1,000}{0.1} = 10,000\ ms^{-2}$

Using Newton's second law: the braking force = Mass x Acceleration.

Thus, braking force = $10,000 \times 0.005 = 50\ N$

**Question 515: C**

Polonium has undergone alpha decay. Thus, Y is a helium nucleus and contains 2 protons and 2 neutrons.

Therefore, 10 moles of Y contain $2 \times 10 \times 6 \times 10^{23}$ protons = $120 \times 10^{23} = 1.2 \times 10^{25}$ protons.

**Question 516: C**

The rod's activity is less than 1,000 Bq after 300 days. In order to calculate the longest possible half-life, we must assume that the activity is just below 1,000 Bq after 300 days. Thus, the half-life has decreased activity from 16,000 Bq to 1,000 Bq in 300 days.

After one half-life: Activity = 8,000 Bq

After two half-lives: Activity = 4,000 Bq

After three half-lives: Activity = 2,000 Bq

After four half-lives: Activity = 1,000 Bq

Thus, the rod has halved its activity a minimum of 4 times in 300 days. 300/4 = 75 days

**Question 517: E**

There is no change in the atomic mass or proton numbers in gamma radiation. In β decay, a neutron is transformed into a proton (and an electron is released). This results in an increase in proton number by 1 but no overall change in atomic mass. Thus, after 5 rounds of beta decay, the proton number will be 89 + 5 = 94 and the mass number will remain at 200. Therefore, there are 94 protons and 200-94 = 106 neutrons.

NB: You are not expected to know about β⁺ decay.

**Question 518: C**

Calculate the speed of the sound $= \frac{distance}{time} = \frac{500}{1.5} = 333\ ms^{-1}$

Thus, the $Wavelength = \frac{Speed}{Frequency} = \frac{333}{440}$

Approximate 333 to 330 to give: $\frac{330}{440} = \frac{3}{4} = 0.75\ m$

## Question 519: B

Firstly, note the all the answer options are a magnitude of 10 apart. Thus, you don't have to worry about getting the correct numbers as long as you get the correct power of 10. So, you can make your life easier by rounding, e.g. approximate $\pi$ to 3, etc.

The area of the shell $= \pi r^2$.
$= \pi \times (50 \times 10^{-3})^2 = \pi \times (5 \times 10^{-2})^2$
$= \pi \times 25 \times 10^{-4} = 7.5 \times 10^{-3} \, m^2$

The deceleration of the shell $= \frac{u-v}{t} = \frac{200}{500 \times 10^{-6}} = 0.4 \times 10^6 \, ms^{-2}$

Then, using Newton's Second Law: $Braking \, force = mass \times acceleration = 1 \times 0.4 \times 10^6 = 4 \times 10^5 N$

Finally: $Pressure = \frac{Force}{Area} = \frac{4 \times 10^5}{7.5 \times 10^{-3}} = \frac{8}{15} \times 10^8 \, Pa \approx 5 \times 10^7 Pa$

## Question 520: B

The fountain transfers 10% of 1,000 J of energy per second into 120 litres of water per minute. Thus, it transfers 100 J into 2 litres of water per second.

Therefore, the total gravitational potential energy, $E_p = mg\Delta h$

Thus, $100 J = 2 \times 10 \times h$

Hence, $h = \frac{100}{20} = 5 \, m$

## Question 521: E

In step down transformers, the number of turns of the primary coil is larger than that of the secondary coil to decrease the voltage. If a transformer is 100% efficient, the electrical power input = electrical power output (P=IV).

## Question 522: C

The percentage of $C^{14}$ in the bone halves every 5,730 years. Since it has decreased from 100% to 6.25%, it has undergone 4 half-lives. Thus, the bone is 4 x 5,730 years old = 22,920 years

## Question 523: E

This is a straightforward question in principle, as it just requires you to plug the values into the equation: $Velocity = Wavelength \times Frequency$ – Just ensure you work in SI units to get the correct answer.

$Frequency = \frac{2 \, m/s}{2.5 \, m} = 0.8 \, Hz = 0.8 \times 10^{-6} MHz = 8 \times 10^{-7} \, MHz$

## Question 524: E

If an element has a half-life of 25 days, its count rate will be halved every 25 days.
A total of 350/25 = 14 half-lives have elapsed. Thus, the count rate has halved 14 times. Therefore, to calculate the original rate, the final count rate must be doubled 14 times = 50 x $2^{14}$.
$2^{14} = 2^5 \times 2^5 \times 2^4 = 32 \times 32 \times 16 = 16,384$.
Therefore, the original count rate = 16,384 x 50 = 819,200

**Question 525: D**

Remember that $V = IR = \frac{P}{I}$ and $Power = \frac{Work\ Done}{Time} = \frac{Force\ x\ Distance}{Time} = Force\ x\ Velocity$;

Thus, A is derived from: $V = IR$,

B is derived from: $= \frac{P}{I}$,

C is derived from: $Voltage = \frac{Power}{Current} = \frac{Force\ x\ Velocity}{Current}$,

Since $Charge = Current\ x\ Time$, E and F are derived from:

$Voltage = \frac{Power}{Current} = \frac{Force\ x\ Distance}{Time\ x\ Current} = \frac{J}{As} = \frac{J}{C}$,

D is incorrect as Nm = J. Thus, the correct variant would be NmC$^{-1}$

**Question 526: B**

Each three-block combination is mutually exclusive to any other combination, so the probabilities are added. Each block pick is independent of all other picks, so the probabilities can be multiplied. For this scenario there are three possible combinations:

P(2 red blocks and 1 yellow block) = P(red then red then yellow) + P(red then yellow then red) + P(yellow then red then red) =

$(\frac{12}{20} \times \frac{11}{19} \times \frac{8}{18}) + (\frac{12}{20} \times \frac{8}{19} \times \frac{11}{18}) + (\frac{8}{20} \times \frac{12}{19} \times \frac{11}{18}) =$

$\frac{3\ x\ 12\ x\ 11\ x\ 8}{20\ x\ 19\ x\ 18} = \frac{44}{95}$

**Question 527: C**

Multiply through by 15: $3(3x + 5) + 5(2x - 2) = 18\ x\ 15$

Thus: $9x + 15 + 10x - 10 = 270$

$9x + 10x = 270 - 15 + 10$

$19x = 265$

$x = 13.95$

**Question 528: C**

This is a rare case where you need to factorise a complex polynomial:

(3x  )(x  ) = 0, possible pairs: 2 x 10, 10 x 2, 4 x 5, 5 x 4

(3x - 4)(x + 5) = 0

3x - 4 = 0, so x = $\frac{4}{3}$

x + 5 = 0, so x = -5

**Question 529: C**

$\frac{5(x-4)}{(x+2)(x-4)} + \frac{3\ (x+2)}{(x+2)(x-4)}$

$= \frac{5x-20+3x+6}{(x+2)(x-4)} = \frac{8x-14}{(x+2)(x-4)}$

**Question 530: E**

p $\alpha$ $\sqrt[3]{q}$, so p = k $\sqrt[3]{q}$

p = 12 when q = 27 gives 12 = k $\sqrt[3]{27}$, so 12 = 3k and k = 4

so, p = 4 $\sqrt[3]{q}$

Now p = 24:

24 = 4$\sqrt[3]{q}$, so 6 = $\sqrt[3]{q}$ and q = 6$^3$ = 216

**Question 531: A**

It is easiest to do this calculation in 2 stages – remember, $x^4 = (x^2)^2$

$(\sqrt{7} - 2)(\sqrt{7} - 2) = 7 + 4 - 2\sqrt{7} - 2\sqrt{7} = 11 - 4\sqrt{7}$

Square this value again:

$(11 - 4\sqrt{7})(11 - 4\sqrt{7}) = 121 + (16 \times 7) - 44\sqrt{7} - 44\sqrt{7}$

$= 233 - 88\sqrt{7}$

So, the answer is A.

**Question 532: C**

Note that $1.151 \times 2 = 2.302$.

Thus: $\frac{2 \times 10^5 + 2 \times 10^2}{10^{10}} = 2 \times 10^{-5} + 2 \times 10^{-8}$

$= 0.00002 + 0.00000002 = 0.00002002$

**Question 533: E**

$y^2 + ay + b$

$= (y + 2)^2 - 5 = y^2 + 4y + 4 - 5$

$= y^2 + 4y + 4 - 5 = y^2 + 4y - 1$

So a = 4 and y = -1

**Question 534: E**

Take $5(m + 4n)$ as a common factor to give: $\frac{4(m+4n)}{5(m+4n)} + \frac{5(m-2n)}{5(m+4n)}$

Simplify to give: $\frac{4m+16n+5m-10n}{5(m+4n)} = \frac{9m+6n}{5(m+4n)} = \frac{3(3m+2n)}{5(m+4n)}$

**Question 535: C**

$A \, \alpha \, \frac{1}{\sqrt{B}}$. Thus, $= \frac{k}{\sqrt{B}}$.

Substitute the values in to give: $4 = \frac{k}{\sqrt{25}}$.

Thus, $k = 20$.

Therefore, $A = \frac{20}{\sqrt{B}}$.

When B = 16, $A = \frac{20}{\sqrt{16}} = \frac{20}{4} = 5$

**Question 536: D**

Angles SVU and STU are opposites and must therefore add up to 180°. Thus, STU must be 91°.

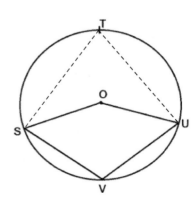

The angle at the centre of a circle is twice the angle at the circumference so the reflex / larger angle of SOU must be: $91 \times 2 = 182°$.

Both angles around SOU must add to 360, so the smaller angle: $360 - 182 = 178°$

## Question 537: E

The surface area of an open cylinder $A = 2\pi rh$. Cylinder B is an enlargement of A, so the increases in radius (r) and height (h) will be proportional: $\frac{r_A}{r_B} = \frac{h_A}{h_B}$. Let us call the proportion coefficient n, where $n = \frac{r_A}{r_B} = \frac{h_A}{h_B}$.

So $\frac{Area\ A}{Area\ B} = \frac{2\pi r_A h_A}{2\pi r_B h_B} = n\ x\ n = n^2$. $\frac{Area\ A}{Area\ B} = \frac{32\pi}{8\pi} = 4$, so, n = 2.

The proportion coefficient n = 2 also applies to their volumes, where the third dimension (also radius, i.e. the $r^2$ in $V = \pi r^2 h$) is equally subject to this constant of proportionality. The cylinders' volumes are related by $n^3 = 8$. If the smaller cylinder has volume $2\pi$ cm³, then the larger will have volume $2\pi$ x $n^3 = 2\pi$ x 8 = 16π cm³.

## Question 538: E

$$= \frac{8}{x(3-x)} - \frac{6(3-x)}{x(3-x)}$$
$$= \frac{8 - 18 + 6x}{x(3-x)}$$
$$= \frac{6x - 10}{x(3-x)}$$

## Question 539: B

For the black ball to be drawn in the last round, white balls must be drawn every round. Thus the probability is given by

$$P = \frac{9}{10} \text{ x } \frac{8}{9} \text{ x } \frac{7}{8} \text{ x } \frac{6}{7} \text{ x } \frac{5}{6} \text{ x } \frac{4}{5} \text{ x } \frac{3}{4} \text{ x } \frac{2}{3} \text{ x } \frac{1}{2}$$
$$= \frac{9 \text{ x } 8 \text{ x } 7 \text{ x } 6 \text{ x } 5 \text{ x } 4 \text{ x } 3 \text{ x } 2 \text{ x } 1}{10 \text{ x } 9 \text{ x } 8 \text{ x } 7 \text{ x } 6 \text{ x } 5 \text{ x } 4 \text{ x } 3 \text{ x } 2 \text{ x } 1} = \frac{1}{10}$$

## Question 540: C

The probability of getting a king the first time is $\frac{4}{52} = \frac{1}{13}$, and the probability of getting a king the second time is $\frac{3}{51}$. These are independent events; thus, the probability of drawing two kings is $\frac{1}{13} x \frac{3}{51} = \frac{3}{663} = \frac{1}{221}$

## Question 541: B

The probabilities of all outcomes must sum to one, so if the probability of rolling a 1 is $x$, then: $x + x + x + x + 2x = 1$. Therefore, $x = \frac{1}{7}$.

The probability of obtaining two sixes $P_{12} = \frac{2}{7} x \frac{2}{7} = \frac{4}{49}$

## Question 542: B

There are plenty of ways of counting, however the easiest is as follows: 0 is divisible by both 2 and 3. Half of the numbers from 1 to 36 are even (i.e. 18 of them). 3, 9, 15, 21, 27, 33 are the only numbers divisible by 3 that we've missed. There are 25 outcomes divisible by 2 or 3, out of 37.

## Question 543: C

List the six ways of achieving this outcome: HHTT, HTHT, HTTH, and TTHH, THTH, THHT. There are $2^4$ possible outcomes for 4 consecutive coin flips, so the probability of two heads and two tails is: $6 \text{ x } \frac{1}{2^4} = \frac{6}{16} = \frac{5}{8}$

## Question 544: D

Count the number of ways to get a 5, 6 or 7 (draw the square if helpful). The ways to get a 5 are: 1, 4; 2, 3; 3, 2; 4, 1. The ways to get a 6 are: 1, 5; 2, 4; 3, 3; 4, 2; 5, 1. The ways to get a 7 are: 1, 6; 2, 5; 3, 4; 4, 3; 5, 2; 6, 1. That is 15 out of 36 possible outcomes.

| | 1 | 2 | 3 | 4 | 5 | 6 |
|---|---|---|---|---|---|---|
| 1 | 2 | 3 | 4 | 5 | 6 | 7 |
| 2 | 3 | 4 | 5 | 6 | 7 | 8 |
| 3 | 4 | 5 | 6 | 7 | 8 | 9 |
| 4 | 5 | 6 | 7 | 8 | 9 | 10 |
| 5 | 6 | 7 | 8 | 9 | 10 | 11 |
| 6 | 7 | 8 | 9 | 10 | 11 | 12 |

## Question 545: C

There are x+y+z balls in the bag, and the probability of picking a red ball is $\frac{x}{(x+y+z)}$ and the probability of picking a green ball is $\frac{z}{(x+y+z)}$. These are independent events, so the probability of picking red then green is $\frac{xz}{(x+y+z)^2}$ and the probability of picking green then red is the same. These outcomes are mutually exclusive, so are added.

## Question 546: B

There are two ways of doing it, pulling out a red ball then a blue ball, or pulling out a blue ball and then a red ball. Let us work out the probability of the first: $\frac{x}{(x+y+z)} \times \frac{y}{x+y+z-1}$, and the probability of the second option will be the same. These are mutually exclusive options, so the probabilities may be summed.

## Question 547: A

[x: Player 1 wins point, y: Player 2 wins point]
Player 1 wins in five rounds if we get: yxxxx, xyxxx, xxyxx, xxxyx.
(Note the case of xxxxy would lead to player 1 winning in 4 rounds, which the question forbids.)
Each of these have a probability of $p^4(1-p)$. Thus, the solution is $4p^4(1-p)$.

## Question 548: A

$y = 2(\frac{x}{4} - 7)^2 - 5$

$\frac{y+5}{2} = (\frac{x}{4} - 7)^2$

$\sqrt{\frac{y+5}{2}} = \frac{x}{4} - 7$

$7 \pm \sqrt{\frac{y+5}{2}} = \frac{x}{4}$

$28 \pm 4\sqrt{\frac{y+5}{2}} = x$

**Question 549: D**

$$r^3 = \frac{3V}{4\pi}$$

Thus, $r = \left(\frac{3V}{4\pi}\right)^{1/3}$

Therefore, S $= 4\pi \left[\left(\frac{3V}{4\pi}\right)^{\frac{1}{3}}\right]^2 = 4\pi \left(\frac{3V}{4\pi}\right)^{\frac{2}{3}}$

$= \frac{4\pi(3V)^{\frac{2}{3}}}{(4\pi)^{\frac{2}{3}}} = (3V)^{\frac{2}{3}} \times \frac{(4\pi)^1}{(4\pi)^{\frac{2}{3}}}$

$= (3V)^{\frac{2}{3}}(4\pi)^{1-\frac{2}{3}} = (4\pi)^{\frac{1}{3}}(3V)^{\frac{2}{3}}$

**Question 550: A**

Let each unit length be x.

Thus, $S = 6x^2$. Therefore, $x = \left(\frac{S}{6}\right)^{\frac{1}{2}}$

V = x³. Thus, $V = \left[\left(\frac{S}{6}\right)^{\frac{1}{2}}\right]^3$ so $V = \left(\frac{S}{6}\right)^{\frac{3}{2}}$

**Question 551: B**

Multiplying the second equation by 2 we get $4x + 16y = 24$.

Subtracting the first equation from this we get $13y = 17$, so $y = \frac{17}{13}$.

Then solving for $x$ we get $x = \frac{10}{13}$.

You could also try substituting possible solutions one by one, although given that the equations are both linear and contain easy numbers, it is quicker to solve them algebraically.

**Question 552: A**

Multiply by the denominator to give: $(7x + 10) = (3y^2 + 2)(9x + 5)$

Partially expand brackets on right side: $(7x + 10) = 9x(3y^2 + 2) + 5(3y^2 + 2)$

Take x terms across to left side: $7x - 9x(3y^2 + 2) = 5(3y^2 + 2) - 10$

Take x outside the brackets: $x[7 - 9(3y^2 + 2)] = 5(3y^2 + 2) - 10$

Thus: $x = \frac{5(3y^2 + 2) - 10}{7 - 9(3y^2 + 2)}$

Simplify to give: $x = \frac{(15y^2)}{(7 - 9(3y^2 + 2))}$

**Question 553: E**

$$3x\left(\frac{3x^7}{x^{\frac{1}{3}}}\right)^3 = 3x\left(\frac{3^3 x^{21}}{x^{\frac{3}{3}}}\right)$$

$$= 3x\,\frac{27x^{21}}{x} = 81x^{21}$$

**Question 554: D**

$$2x[2^{\frac{7}{14}} x^{\frac{7}{14}}] = 2x[2^{\frac{1}{2}} x^{\frac{1}{2}}]$$
$$= 2x(\sqrt{2}\sqrt{x}) = 2\left[\sqrt{x}\sqrt{x}\right][\sqrt{2}\sqrt{x}]$$
$$= 2\sqrt{2x^3}$$

**Question 555: A**

$A = \pi r^2$, therefore $10\pi = \pi r^2$

Thus, $r = \sqrt{10}$

Therefore, the circumference is $2\pi\sqrt{10}$

**Question 556: D**

$3.4 = 12 + (3+4) = 19$

$19.5 = 95 + (19+5) = 119$

**Question 557: D**

$$2.3 = \frac{2^3}{2} = 4$$
$$4.2 = \frac{4^2}{4} = 4$$

**Question 558: E**

This is a tricky question that requires you to know how to 'complete the square':

$(x + 1.5)(x + 1.5) = x^2 + 3x + 2.25$

Thus, $(x + 1.5)^2 - 7.25 = x^2 + 3x - 5 = 0$

Therefore, $(x + 1.5)^2 = 7.25 = \frac{29}{4}$

Thus, $x + 1.5 = \sqrt{\frac{29}{4}}$

Thus $x = -\frac{3}{2} \pm \sqrt{\frac{29}{4}} = -\frac{3}{2} \pm \frac{\sqrt{29}}{2}$

**Question 559: B**

Whilst you definitely need to solve this graphically, it is necessary to complete the square for the first equation to allow you to draw it more easily:

$(x + 2)^2 = x^2 + 4x + 4$

Thus, $y = (x + 2)^2 + 10 = x^2 + 4x + 14$

This is now an easy curve to draw ($y = x^2$ that has moved 2 units left and 10 units up). The turning point of this quadratic is to the left and well above anything in $x^3$, so the **only** solution is the first intersection of the two curves in the upper right quadrant around (3.4, 39).

There is only one solution → answer is B.

**Question 560: C**

By far the easiest way to solve this is to sketch them (don't waste time solving them algebraically). As soon as you've done this, it'll be very obvious that y = 2 and y = 1-x² don't intersect, since the latter has its turning point at (0, 1) and zero points at x = -1 and 1. y = x and y = x² intersect at the origin and (1, 1), and y = 2 runs through both.

**Question 561: B**

Notice that you're not required to get the actual values to solve this – just the number's magnitude. Thus, 897653 can be approximated to 900,000 and 0.009764 to 0.01. Therefore, 900,000 x 0.01 = 9,000

**Question 562: C**

Multiply through by 70: $7(7x + 3) + 10(3x + 1) = 14 \times 70$

Simplify: $49x + 21 + 30x + 10 = 980$

$79x + 31 = 980$

$x = \dfrac{949}{79}$

**Question 563: A**

Split the equilateral triangle into 2 right-angled triangles and apply Pythagoras' theorem:

$x^2 = \left(\dfrac{x}{2}\right)^2 + height^2$ . Thus $h^2 = \dfrac{3}{4}x^2$ (where $h$ = height)

$h = \sqrt{\dfrac{3x^2}{4}} = \dfrac{\sqrt{3x^2}}{2}$

The area of a triangle = ½ x base x height = $\dfrac{1}{2}x\dfrac{\sqrt{3x^2}}{2}$

Simplifying gives: $x\dfrac{\sqrt{3x^2}}{4} = x\dfrac{\sqrt{3}\sqrt{x^2}}{4} = \dfrac{x^2\sqrt{3}}{4}$

**Question 564: A**

This is a question testing your ability to spot 'the difference between two squares'.

Factorise to give: $3 - \dfrac{7x(5x - 1)(5x+1)}{(7x)^2(5x+1)}$

Cancel out: $3 - \dfrac{(5x - 1)}{7x}$

**Question 565: C**

The easiest way to do this is to 'complete the square':

$(x - 5)^2 = x^2 - 10x + 25$

Thus, $(x - 5)^2 - 125 = x^2 - 10x - 100 = 0$

Therefore, $(x - 5)^2 = 125$

$x - 5 = \pm\sqrt{125} = \pm\sqrt{25}\sqrt{5} = \pm5\sqrt{5}$

$x = 5 \pm 5\sqrt{5}$

**Question 566: B**

Factorise by completing the square:

$x^2 - 4x + 7 = (x - 2)^2 + 3$

Simplify: $(x - 2)^2 = y^3 + 2 - 3$

$x - 2 = \pm\sqrt{y^3 - 1}$

$x = 2 \pm \sqrt{y^3 - 1}$

**Question 567: D**

Square both sides to give: $(3x + 2)^2 = 7x^2 + 2x + y$

Thus: $y = (3x + 2)^2 - 7x^2 - 2x = (9x^2 + 12x + 4) - 7x^2 - 2x$

$y = 2x^2 + 10x + 4$

**Question 568: C**

Each sweet picked is mutually exclusive to any other sweet picked as they cannot happen at the same time. When dealing with the 3 sweet combinations, the probabilities are multiplied, as the combination is independent of all other combinations. This is the and rule of probability.

In this scenario, there are 3 possible combinations for the first, second and third pick of sweets:

H, H, T

H, T, H

T, H, H

$\left(\frac{4}{12} \times \frac{3}{11} \times \frac{2}{10}\right) + \left(\frac{2}{12} \times \frac{4}{11} \times \frac{3}{10}\right) + \left(\frac{4}{12} \times \frac{2}{11} \times \frac{3}{10}\right) = 3\left(\frac{4}{12} \times \frac{3}{11} \times \frac{2}{10}\right)$

This gives us $\frac{72}{1320}$ (which, of course, could be simplified further, but this is already one of the options given so the step of simplification is unnecessary in this question).

**Question 569: A**

Let the width of the television be 4x and the height of the television be 3x.

Then by Pythagoras: $(4x)^2 + (3x)^2 = 50^2$

Simplify: $25x^2 = 2500$

Thus: $x = 10$. Therefore: the screen is 30 inches by 40 inches, i.e. the area is 1,200 inches².

**Question 570: C**

Square both sides to give: $1 + \frac{3}{x^2} = (y^5 + 1)^2$

Multiply out: $\frac{3}{x^2} = (y^{10} + 2y^5 + 1) - 1$

Thus: $x^2 = \frac{3}{y^{10} + 2y^5}$

Therefore: $x = \sqrt{\frac{3}{y^{10} + 2y^5}}$

**Question 571: C**

The easiest way is to double the first equation and triple the second to get:

$6x - 10y = 20$ $and$ $6x + 6y = 39$.

Subtract the first from the second to give: $16y = 19$,

Therefore, $y = \frac{19}{16}$.

Substitute back into the first equation to give $x = \frac{85}{16}$.

**Question 572: C**
This is fairly straightforward; the first inequality is the easier one to work with: **B** and **D** and **E** violate it, so we just need to check **A** and **C** in the second inequality.
**C**: $1^3 - 2^2 < 3$, but **A**: $2^3 - 1^2 > 3$

**Question 573: B**
Whilst this can be done graphically, it's quicker to do algebraically (because the second graph is not as easy to sketch). Intersections occur where the curves have the same coordinates.
Thus: $x + 4 = 4x^2 + 5x + 5$
Simplify: $4x^2 + 4x + 1 = 0$
Factorise: $(2x + 1)(2x + 1) = 0$
Thus, the two graphs only intersect once at $x = -\frac{1}{2}$

**Question 574: D**
It's better to do this algebraically as the equations are easy to work with and you would need to sketch very accurately to get the answer. Intersections occur where the curves have the same coordinates. Thus: $x^3 = x$
$x^3 - x = 0$
Thus: $x(x^2 - 1) = 0$
Spot the 'difference between two squares': $x(x + 1)(x - 1) = 0$
Thus, there are 3 intersections: at $x = 0, 1 \ and -1$

**Question 575: E**
Note that the line is the hypotenuse of a right-angled triangle with one side unit length and one side of length ½.
By Pythagoras, $\left(\frac{1}{2}\right)^2 + 1^2 = x^2$
Thus, $x^2 = \frac{1}{4} + 1 = \frac{5}{4}$
$x = \sqrt{\frac{5}{4}} = \frac{\sqrt{5}}{\sqrt{4}} = \frac{\sqrt{5}}{2}$

**Question 576: D**
In this question, we take the indices ($-\frac{1}{3}$ and 3) and multiply them. Remember to also cube the 2!
$5x(2x^{-\frac{1}{3}})^3 = 5x(8x^{-1}) = 40$

**Question 577: D**
This is one of the easier maths questions. Take 3a as a factor to give:
$3a(a^2 - 10a + 25)$    $= 3a(a - 5)(a - 5) = 3a(a - 5)^2$

**Question 578: B**

Note that 12 is the Lowest Common Multiple of 3 and 4. Thus:

| | |
|---|---|
| -3 (4x + 3y) = -3 (48) | Multiply each side by -3 |
| 4 (3x + 2y) = 4 (34) | Multiply each side by 4 |
| -12x – 9y = -144 | |
| 12x + 8y = 136 | Add together |

$$-y = -8$$
$$y = 8$$

Substitute y back in:

$$4x + 3y = 48$$
$$4x + 3(8) = 48$$
$$4x + 24 = 48$$
$$4x = 24$$
$$x = 6$$

**Question 579: E**

Don't be fooled, this is an easy question, just obey BODMAS and don't skip steps.

$$\frac{-(25-28)^2}{-36+14} = \frac{-(-3)^2}{-22}$$

This gives: $\frac{-(9)}{-22} = \frac{9}{22}$

**Question 580: E**

Since there are 26 possible letters for each of the 3 letters in the license plate, and there are 10 possible numbers (0-9) for each of the 3 numbers in the same plate, then the number of license plates would be:

$(26) \times (26) \times (26) \times (10) \times (10) \times (10) = 17,576,000$

**Question 581: B**

Expand the brackets to give: $4x^2 - 12x + 9 = 0$.

Factorise: $(2x - 3)(2x - 3) = 0$.

Thus, only one solution exists, x = 1.5.

Note that you could also use the fact that the discriminant, $b^2 - 4ac = 0$ to get the answer.

**Question 582: C**

$$= \left(x^{\frac{1}{2}}\right)^{\frac{1}{2}} (y^{-3})^{\frac{1}{2}}$$

$$= x^{\frac{1}{4}} y^{-\frac{3}{2}} = \frac{x^{\frac{1}{4}}}{y^{\frac{3}{2}}}$$

**Question 583: A**

To answer this question, convert 4 and 16 to $2^2$ and $2^4$.

$$2^{2x} \times 2^{4y} = 2^z$$
$$2x + 4y = z$$

**Question 584: C**

Following BODMAS:

$$= 5 \left[ 5(6^2 - 5 \times 3) + 400^{\frac{1}{2}} \right]^{1/3} + 7$$

$$= 5 \left[ 5(36 - 15) + 20 \right]^{\frac{1}{3}} + 7$$

$$= 5 \left[ 5(21) + 20 \right]^{\frac{1}{3}} + 7$$

$$= 5 \left( 105 + 20 \right)^{\frac{1}{3}} + 7$$

$$= 5 \left( 125 \right)^{\frac{1}{3}} + 7$$

$$= 5 \left( 5 \right) + 7$$

$$= 25 + 7 = 32$$

**Question 585: B**

Consider a triangle formed by joining the centre to two adjacent vertices. Six similar triangles can be made around the centre – thus, the central angle is 60 degrees. Since the two lines forming the triangle are of equal length, we have 6 identical equilateral triangles in the hexagon.

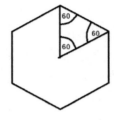

Now split the triangle in half and apply Pythagoras' theorem:

$$1^2 = 0.5^2 + h^2$$

Thus, $h = \sqrt{\frac{3}{4}} = \frac{\sqrt{3}}{2}$

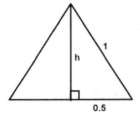

Thus, the area of the triangle is: $\frac{1}{2}bh = \frac{1}{2} \times 1 \times \frac{\sqrt{3}}{2} = \frac{\sqrt{3}}{4}$

Therefore, the area of the hexagon is: $\frac{\sqrt{3}}{4} \times 6 = \frac{3\sqrt{3}}{2}$

**Question 586: B**

Let x be the width and x+19 be the length.

Thus, the area of a rectangle is $x(x + 19) = 780$.

Therefore:

$$x^2 + 19x - 780 = 0$$

$$(x - 20)(x + 39)$$

$$x - 20 = 0 \text{ or } x + 39 = 0$$

$$x = 20 \text{ or } x = -39$$

Since length can never be a negative number, we disregard $x = -39$ and use $x = 20$ instead.

Thus, the width is **20 metres** and the length is **39 metres**.

**Question 587: B**

The quickest way to solve is by trial and error, substituting the provided options. However, if you're keen to do this algebraically, you can do the following:

Start by setting up the equations: perimeter = 2L + 2W = 34

Thus: L + W = 17

Using Pythagoras: $L^2 + W^2 = 13^2$

Since L + W = 17, W = 17 - L

Therefore: $L^2 + (17 - L)^2 = 169$

$L^2 + 289 - 34L + L^2 = 169$

$2L^2 - 34L + 120 = 0$

$L^2 - 17L + 60 = 0$

$(L - 5)(L - 12) = 0$

Thus: L = 5 and L = 12

And: W = 12 and W = 5

**Question 588: C**

Multiply both sides by 8:  $4(3x - 5) + 2(x + 5) = 8(x + 1)$

Remove brackets:     $12x - 20 + 2x + 10 = 8x + 8$

Simplify:         $14x - 10 = 8x + 8$

Add 10:          $14x = 8x + 18$

Subtract 8x:       $6x = 18$

Therefore:        $x = 3$

**Question 589: C**

Recognise that 1.742 x 3 is 5.226. Now, the original equation simplifies to: $= \frac{3 \times 10^6 + 3 \times 10^5}{10^{10}}$

$= 3 \times 10^{-4} + 3 \times 10^{-5} = 3.3 \times 10^{-4}$

**Question 590:  A**

$Area = \frac{(2 + \sqrt{2})(4 - \sqrt{2})}{2}$

$= \frac{8 - 2\sqrt{2} + 4\sqrt{2} - 2}{2}$

$= \frac{6 + 2\sqrt{2}}{2}$

$= 3 + \sqrt{2}$

**Question 591: C**

Square both sides: $\frac{4}{x} + 9 = (y - 2)^2$

$\frac{4}{x} = (y - 2)^2 - 9$

Cross Multiply: $\frac{x}{4} = \frac{1}{(y-2)^2 - 9}$

$x = \frac{4}{y^2 - 4y + 4 - 9}$

Factorise: $x = \frac{4}{y^2 - 4y - 5}$

$x = \frac{4}{(y+1)(y-5)}$

**Question 592: D**

Set up the equation: $5x - 5 = 0.5(6x + 2)$

$10x - 10 = 6x + 2$

$4x = 12$

$x = 3$

**Question 593: C**

Round numbers appropriately: $\dfrac{55 + (\frac{9}{4})^2}{\sqrt{900}} = \dfrac{55 + \frac{81}{16}}{30}$

81 rounds to 80 to give: $\dfrac{55 + 5}{30} = \dfrac{60}{30} = 2$

**Question 594: D**

There are three outcomes from choosing the type of cheese in the crust. For each of the additional toppings to possibly add, there are 2 outcomes: 1 to include and another not to include a certain topping, for each of the 7 toppings

Thus, the number of different kinds of pizza is: $3 \times 2 \times 2 \times 2 \times 2 \times 2 \times 2 \times 2 = 3 \times 2^7$

$= 3 \times 128 = 384$

**Question 595: A**

Although it is possible to do this algebraically, by far the easiest way is via trial and error. The clue that you shouldn't attempt it algebraically is the fact that rearranging the first equation to make x or y the subject leaves you with a difficult equation to work with (e.g. $x = \sqrt{1 - y^2}$) when you try to substitute in the second.

An exceptionally good student might notice that the equations are symmetric in x and y, i.e. the solution is when $x = y$. Thus $2x^2 = 1$ and $2x = \sqrt{2}$ which gives $\dfrac{\sqrt{2}}{2}$ as the answer.

**Question 596: C**

If two shapes are congruent, then they are the same size and shape: corresponding sides and angles are equal. Thus, congruent objects can be rotations and mirror images of each other. The two triangles in E are indeed congruent (SAS).

**Question 597: B**

Rearrange the equation: $x^2 + x - 6 \geq 0$

Factorise: $(x + 3)(x - 2) \geq 0$

Remember that this is a quadratic inequality so requires a quick sketch to ensure you don't make a silly mistake with which way the sign is.

Thus, $y = 0$ when $x = 2$ and $x = -3$. $y > 0$ when $x > 2$ or $x < -3$.

Thus, the solution is: $x \leq -3 \ and \ x \geq 2$.

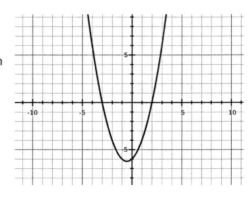

**Question 598: B**

Using Pythagoras: $a^2 + b^2 = x^2$

Since the triangle is isosceles: $a = b$, so $2a^2 = x^2$

Area $= \frac{1}{2} base \; x \; height = \frac{1}{2}a^2$. From above, $a^2 = \frac{x^2}{2}$

Thus, the area $= \frac{1}{2}x\frac{x^2}{2} = \frac{x^2}{4}$

**Question 599: A**

If X and Y are doubled, the value of Q increases by 4. Halving the value of A reduces this to 2. Finally, tripling the value of B reduces this to ⅔, i.e. the value decreases by ⅓.

**Question 600: C**

The quickest way to do this is to sketch the curves. This requires you to factorise both equations by completing the square:

$x^2 - 2x + 3 = (x-1)^2 + 2$

$x^2 - 6x - 10 = (x-3)^2 - 19$ Thus, the first equation has a turning point at (1, 2) and doesn't cross the x-axis. The second equation has a turning point at (3, -19) and crosses the x-axis twice

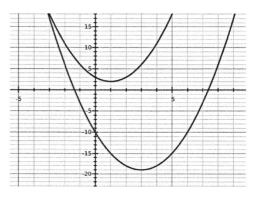

# MOCK PAPER A

## SECTION 1

**Question 1:**
A square sheet of paper is 20cm long. How many times must it be folded in half before it covers an area of 12.5cm$^2$?

A. 3        B. 4        C. 5        D. 6        E. 7

**Question 2:**
Mountain climbing is viewed by some as an extreme sport, while for others it is simply an exhilarating pastime that offers the ultimate challenge of strength, endurance, and sacrifice. It can be highly dangerous, even fatal, especially when the climber is out of his or her depth, or simply gets overwhelmed by weather, terrain, ice, or other dangers of the mountain. Inexperience, poor planning, and inadequate equipment can all contribute to injury or death, so knowing what to do right matters.

Despite all the negatives, when done right, mountain climbing is an exciting, exhilarating, and rewarding experience. This article is an overview beginner's guide and outlines the initial basics to learn. Each step is deserving of an article in its own right, and entire tomes have been written on climbing mountains, so you're advised to spend a good deal of your beginner's learning immersed in reading widely. This basic overview will give you an idea of what is involved in a climb.

Which statement best summarises this paragraph?
A.  Mountain climbing is an extreme sport fraught with dangers.
B.  Without extensive experience embarking on a mountain climb is fatal.
C.  A comprehensive literature search is the key to enjoying mountain climbing.
D.  Mountain climbing is difficult and is a skill that matures with age if pursued.
    The terrain is the biggest unknown when climbing a mountain and therefore presents the biggest danger.

**Question 3:**
50% of an isolated population contract a new strain of resistant Malaria. Only 20% are symptomatic, of which 10% are female. What percentage of the total population do symptomatic males represent?

A.  1%        B.  9%        C.  10%        D.  80%

**Question 4:**

John is a UK citizen who is looking to buy a holiday home in the South of France. He is purchasing his new home through an agency. Unlike a normal estate agent, they offer monthly discount sales of up to 30%. As a French company, the agency sells in Euros. John decides to hold off on his purchase until the sale in the interest of saving money.  What is the major assumption made in doing this?

A.  The house he likes will not be bought in the meantime.

B.  The agency will not be declared bankrupt.

C.  The value of the pound will fall more than 30%.

D.  The value of the pound will fall less than 30%.

E.  The value of the euro may increase by up to 35% in the coming weeks.

**Question 5:**

In childcare professions, by law, there must be an adult to child ratio of no more than 1:4. Child minders are hired on a salary of £8.50 an hour. What is the maximum number of children that can be continually supervised for a period of 24 hours on a budget of £1,000?

A.  1                B.  8                C.  12                D.  16                E.  468

**Question 6:**

A table of admission prices for the local cinema is shown below:

|            | Peak | Off-peak |
|------------|------|----------|
| **Adult**      | £11  | £9.50    |
| **Child**      | £7   | £5.50    |
| **Concession** | £7   | £5.50    |
| **Student**    | £5   | £5       |

How much would a group of 3 adults, 5 children, a concession and 4 students save by visiting at an off-peak time rather than a peak time?

A.  £11.50          B.  £13.50          C.  £15.50          D.  £17.50          E.  £18.50

**Question 7:**

All musicians play instruments. All oboe players are musicians. Oboes and pianos are instruments. Karen is a musician. Which statement is true?

A.  Karen plays two instruments.

B.  All musicians are oboe players.

C.  All instruments are pianos or oboes.

D.  Karen is an oboe player.

E.  None of the above.

**Question 8:**
Flow mediated dilatation is a method used to assess vascular function within the body. It essentially adopts the use of an ultrasound scan to measure the percentage increase in the width of an artery before and after occlusion with a blood pressure cuff. Ultrasound scans are taken by one sonographer, and the average lumen diameter is then measured by an analyst. What is a potential flaw in the methodology of this technique?

A. Results will not be comparable within an individual if different arteries start at different diameters.
B. Results will not be comparable between individuals if they have different baseline arterial diameters.
C. Ultrasound is an outdated technique with no use in modern medicine.
D. This methodology is subject to human error.
E. This methodology is not repeatable.

**Question 9:**
If it takes 20 minutes to board an aeroplane, 15 minutes to disembark and the flight lasts two and a half hours. In the event of a delay, it is not uncommon to add 20 minutes to the flight time. Megan is catching the flight in question as she needs to attend a meeting at 5pm. The location of the meeting is 15 minutes from the airport without traffic; or 25 minutes with traffic. Which of the following statements is valid considering this information?

A. If Megan wants to be on time for her meeting, given all possibilities described, the latest she can begin boarding at the departure airport is 1.30pm.
B. If Megan starts boarding at 1.40pm she will certainly be late.
C. If Megan aims to start boarding at 1.10pm she will arrive in time whether the plane is delayed or not.
D. If Megan wishes to be on time, she doesn't have to worry about the plane being delayed as she can make up the time during the transport time from the arrival airport to the meeting.

**Question 10:**
A cask of whiskey holds a total volume of 500L. Every two and a half minutes half of the total volume is collected and discarded. How many minutes will it take for the entire cask to be emptied?

A. 80           B. 160           C. 200           D. 240           E. ∞

**Question 11:**
The keypad to a safe comprises the digits 1 - 9. The code itself can be of indeterminate length. The code is therefore set by choosing a reference number so that when a code is entered the average of all the different numbers entered must equal the chosen reference number.

Which of the following is true?
A. If the reference number was set greater than 9, the safe would be locked forever.
B. This safe is extremely insecure as if random digits were pressed for long enough it would average out at the correct reference number.
C. More than one number is always required to achieve the reference number.
D. All of the above are true.
E. None of the above are true.

**Question 12:**

The use of antibiotics is one of the major paradoxes in modern medicine. Antibiotics themselves provide a selection pressure to drive the evolution of antibiotic resistant strains of bacteria. This is largely due to the rapid growth rate of bacterial colonies and asexual cell division. As such, a widespread initiative is in place to limit the prescription of antibiotics.

Which of the following is a fair assumption?

A. Antibiotic resistance is impossible to avoid as it is driven by evolution.

B. If bacteria reproduced at a slower rate antibiotic resistance would not be such an issue.

C. Medicine always creates more problems than it solves.

D. In the past antibiotics were used frivolously.

E. All of the above could be possible.

**Question 13:**

At a society meeting, 1000 people are entitled to vote in the elections for Chairperson with a one-person-one-vote system. The election rules state if no candidate obtains more than 50% of the votes cast in the first ballot, a second ballot must be held between the top two candidates. 350 votes were cast for a particular candidate in the first ballot. Then a second ballot took place.

Under these circumstances which one of the following is possible?

A. The candidate won the election, came second, or came third.

B. The candidate either won the election or came second.

C. The candidate came second or third, but did not win.

D. The candidate came third.

E. The candidate definitely won the election.

**Question 14:**

Ever since Uranus was discovered, astronomers have believed there may be more planets in the Solar System. Small deviations in the orbits of Uranus and Neptune suggest another planet might exist. Astronomers have named this hypothetical undiscovered planet 'Planet X'. These deviations in orbit can also be explained by incorrect predictions. Since Uranus and Neptune take many decades to circle the sun, astronomers rely on old data to calculate their orbits. As this data is likely to be inaccurate, the calculated orbits are probably wrong, and so Uranus and Neptune will deviate from them even if there is no 'Planet X'.

Which one of the following best expresses the main conclusion of the above argument?

A. The use of old and inaccurate data indicates that Planet X cannot exist.

B. Astronomers are right to think that there must be an undiscovered planet.

C. The deviations in the orbits of Uranus and Neptune cannot tell us whether Planet X exists.

D. The calculations of the orbits of Uranus and Neptune are probably wrong.

E. Uranus and Neptune will deviate from the predicted orbits whether or not Planet X exists.

**Question 15:**

One in four deaths caused by road accidents involving commercial vehicles is caused by the driver falling asleep at the wheel. The problem even affects police officers, who are now more likely to die while driving when tired than from physical attacks. Evidence at the scene (such as tyre marks) can tell investigators how quickly the car driver braked. Late breaking indicates a lack of concentration which might be caused by tiredness. The problem with this evidence is that it is not conclusive, whereas conclusive evidence can be offered for other offences such as drink driving.

Which of the following can be drawn as a conclusion of the passage above?

A. Accidents caused by drivers falling asleep at the wheel are a greater problem than drink driving.

B. Commercial vehicle drivers and the police are more prone to falling asleep at the wheel because of the long hours they work.

C. The number of hours per day that commercial drivers should be allowed to drive should be reduced.

D. It will not be as easy to prosecute drivers for falling asleep at the wheel as it is for drink driving.

E. It would be unfair to prosecute people for falling asleep at the wheel.

**Question 16:**

A study involving a brain-training exercise was carried out on more than a thousand adults aged 65 and over, some of whom later developed dementia. Results showed that the benefits of the five-week mental agility course undertaken by some of the adults lasted for at least five years. This led to an improvement in everyday activities such as money management and the ability to do housework. If those with trained brains developed dementia, they did so later than those in the control group. The results also showed that, for those people in the study who developed dementia, following their diagnosis, their mental decline occurred faster than for those who had undertaken the training.

Which one of the following can be drawn as a conclusion from the above passage?

A. People do a decreasing amount of housework as they grow older.

B. It is preferable to have swift mental decline once dementia develops.

C. Older people do not perform mentally challenging tasks unless forced to do so.

D. Keeping the mind active delays the onset of dementia.

E. All over-65s who undertake brain training live for at least five years afterwards.

**Question 17:**

According to the current mainstream scientific view, Near Death Experiences (NDEs) are explicable in purely physiological terms. Specifically, they are caused by cerebral anoxia (oxygen deficiency in brain tissue), which occurs in a dying brain. On the other hand, recent research on hundreds of successfully resuscitated cardiac patients found that only twenty per cent reported NDEs. If NDEs had purely medical causes then most of the patients should have experienced them, since they had all been clinically dead and experienced cerebral anoxia. NDEs therefore do not have purely physiological causes.

Which one of the following best expresses the main conclusion of the above passage?

A.  Not all successfully resuscitated cardiac patients have NDEs.

B.  Not all clinically dead patients have NDEs.

C.  NDEs are caused by oxygen deficiency in the brain.

D.  NDEs are not necessarily caused by physical events alone.

E.  NDEs are a physical property of the human brain

**Question 18:**

A study on identical twins concluded that genetics contribute roughly half of the attributes we need to be happy. People often find such studies scary, seeing something sinister about us being mere puppets of our biology. However, put in non-scientific terms, it sounds like common sense. Parents frequently notice their children have different personality traits from a very young age. Perhaps it is nicer to think this is caused by something 'fluffy' like a soul. Even if this were true, why is it more reassuring than the thought that genes are responsible? Either way, you are born as you are.

Which one of the following statements is best supported as the conclusion of the passage above?

A.  Roughly half of what we need to be happy is decided by our genetic make-up.

B.  We may as well accept the idea that our potential for happiness in life is to some extent decided at birth.

C.  Whether or not you are happy in life is either determined by your soul or your genes.

D.  Whether or not you are happy in life is not something over which you yourself have any control.

E.  The person you are at birth is the person you will be throughout your life.

**Question 19:**

Horrific images of the earthquake in Haiti were seen immediately all over the world, and by the next day the full extent of the damage was seen by the entire world. Clearly, the main problem was moving aid from the airport to distant areas, and with the roads largely blocked, the only practical method was to use helicopters. The great nations of the world should be ashamed that food was not getting to the people who needed it, and that even a week later, their relief still depended on the ability of courageous and skilful drivers to reach them in trucks.

Which one of the following is an underlying assumption of the argument above?

A.  The relief agencies were able to import trucks to Haiti but not helicopters.

B.  The great nations of the world had helicopters at their disposal which could reach Haiti within a week.

C.  There was enough food in Haiti to supply all the people in the weeks after the earthquake.

D.  The images failed to prompt the great nations of the world into relief operations after the earthquake.

E.  The people of Haiti were able to clear their roads within a week of the earthquake.

**Question 20:**

A company sells custom design t-shirts. A breakdown of their costs is shown below:

| Number of Items | Cost per Item | |
| --- | --- | --- |
| | **Black and white** | **Colour** |
| 0 – 99 | £3.00 | £5.00 |
| 100 - 499 | £2.50 | £4.50 |
| 500 - 999 | £2.00 | £4.00 |
| 1000+ | £1.00 | £3.00 |

Customers with a never-before-printed design must also pay a surcharge of £50 to cover the cost of building a jig. What is the total cost for an order of unique stag-do t-shirts: 50 in colour, and 200 in black and white?

A.  £650          B.  £700          C.  £750          D.  £800          E.  £850

**Question 21:**

The Scouts is a movement for young people first established by Lord Baden Powell. As the founder he was the first chief scout of the association. Since his initial appointment there have been a number of notable chief scouts including Peter Duncan and Bear Grylls. Some of the first camping trips conducted by Lord Powell's scout troop were on Brown Sea Island.

Now the Scout movement is a worldwide global phenomenon giving children from all backgrounds the opportunity not only to embark upon adventure but also to engage in the understanding and teaching of foreign culture. Traditionally religion formed the backbone of the scouting movement which was reflected in the scouts promise: "I promise to do my duty to God and to the Queen".

Which of the following applies to the scout movement?

A.  Scouts work for the Queen.
B.  The scout network is aimed at adventurous individuals.
C.  Chief scout is appointed by the Queen.
D.  You have to be religious to be a scout.
E.  None of the above.

**Question 22:**

Three rats are placed in a maze that is in the shape of an equilateral triangle. They pick a direction at random and walk along the side of a triangle. Sophie thinks they are less likely to collide than not. Is she correct?

A.  Yes, because mice naturally keep away from each other.
B.  No, they are more likely to collide than not.
C.  No, they are equally likely to collide than not collide.
D.  Yes, because the probability they collide is 0.25.
E.  None of the above.

**Question 23:**
The use of human cadavers in the teaching of anatomy is hotly debated. Whilst many argue that it is an invaluable teaching resource, demonstrating far more than a textbook can, others argue that it is an outdated method, which puts unfair stress on an already bereaved family. One of the biggest pros for using human tissue in anatomical teaching is the variation that it displays. Whilst textbooks demonstrate a standard model averaged over many 100s of specimens, many argue that it is the variation between cadavers that really reinforces anatomical knowledge.

The opposition argues that it is a cruel process that damages the grieving process of the affected family since the use of the cadaver often occupies a period of up to 12 months. As such the relative in question is returned to the bereaved family for burial around the time it would be expected that they were recovering as described in the grieving model.

Does the article support or reject the use of cadavers in anatomical teaching?
A. Supports the use
B. Rejects the use
C. Impartial
D. Can't tell
E. None of the above

**Question 24:**
A ferry is carrying its full capacity. At the time of departure (7am) the travel time to the nearest hour is announced as 13 hours. What is the latest that the ferry could arrive at its destination?

A. 08.29          B. 20.00          C. 20.29          D. 20.30          E. 20.59

**Question 25:**
A game is played using a circle of 55 stepping-stones. A die is rolled showing the numbers 1 - 6. The number on the die tells you how many steps you may take during your go. The only rule is that during your go you must take your steps in the routine two steps forward, 1 step back. The winner is the first person to move around the full circle of stepping-stones.

What is the minimum number of rolls required to win?
A. 17          B. 18          C. 19          D. 32          E. 55

**Question 26:**
On a racetrack there are 3 cars recording lap times of 40 seconds, 60 seconds, and 70 seconds. They all started simultaneously 4 minutes ago. How much longer will the race need to continue for them to all cross the start line again at the same time?

A. 4 minutes          C. 14 minutes          E. 1 hour 12 minutes
B. 10 minutes          D. 32 minutes

**Question 27:**

A class of 60 2nd year medical students are conducting an experiment to measure the velocity of nerve conduction along their radial arteries. This work builds on a previous result obtained demonstrating the effects of how right-handed men have faster nerve conduction velocities than gender matched left-handed individuals. 60% of the class are female of which 3% were unable to take part due to underlying heart conditions. 2 of the male members of the class were also unable to take part. On average the female cohort had faster nerve conduction velocities than men in their dominant arm.

Right-handed women have the fastest nerve conduction velocities.

A.  True                          B.  False                          C.  Can't tell

**Question 28:**

Mark is making a double tetrahedron dice by joining two square based pyramids together at their bases. Each square based pyramid is 5cm wide and 8cm tall. What area of card would have been required to produce the nets for the whole die?

A.  150cm$^2$          B.  180 cm$^2$          C.  210 cm$^2$          D.  240 cm$^2$          E.  270 cm$^2$

**Question 29:**

A serial dilution is performed by lining up 10 wells and filling each one with 9ml of distilled water. 1 ml of a concentrated solvent is then added to the first well and mixed. 1 ml of this new solution is drawn from the first well and added to the second and mixed. The process is repeated until all 10 wells have been used.

If the solvent starts off at concentration x, what will its final concentration be after 10 wells of serial dilution?

A.  $x/10^9$          B.  $x/10^{10}$          C.  $x/10^{11}$          D.  $x/10^{12}$          E.  $x/10^{13}$

**Question 30:**

A student decides to measure the volume of all the blood in his body. He does this by injecting a known quantity of substrate into his arm, waiting a period of 20 minutes, then drawing a blood sample and measuring the concentration of the substrate in his blood. What assumption has he made here?

A.  The substrate is only soluble in blood.          D.  The substrate is not degraded.

B.  The substrate is not bioavailable.               E.  All of the above.

C.  The substrate is not excreted.

**Question 31:**

Jason is ordering a buffet for a party. The buffet company can provide a basic spread at £10 per head. However more luxurious items carry a surcharge. Jason is particularly interested in cupcakes and shell fish. With these items included the buffet company provides a new quote of £10 per head. In addition to simply ordering the food Jason must also purchase cutlery and plates. Plates come in packs of 20 for £8 whilst cutlery is sold in bundles of 60 sets for £10.

With a budget of £2,300 (to the nearest 10 people) what is the maximum number of people Jason can provide food on a plate for?

A.  180                B.  190                C.  209                D.  210                E.  220

**Question 32:**

What were once methods of hunting have now become popular sports. Examples include archery, the javelin throw, the discus throw and even throwing a boomerang. Why such dangerous hobbies have begun to thrive is now being investigated by social scientists. One such explanation is that it is because they are dangerous that we find them appealing in the first place. Others argue that it is a 'throwback' to our ancestral heritage, where, as a hunter gatherer, being a proficient hunter was something to show off and flaunt. Whilst this may be the case, it is well observed that many find the chase of a hunt exciting if not controversial.

Sports like archery provide excitement analogous to that of the chase during a hunter gatherer hunt.
A.  True
B.  False
C.  Can't tell

**END OF SECTION**

# SECTION 2

**Question 1:**
A crocodile's tail weighs 30kg. Its head weighs as much as the tail and one half of the body and legs. The body and legs together weigh as much as the tail and head combined.

What is the total weight of the crocodile?
A. 220kg      B. 240kg      C. 260kg      D. 280kg      E. 300kg

**Question 2:**
A body is travelling at $x$ ms$^{-1}$ with $y$ J of kinetic energy. After a period of retardation the kinetic energy of the body is $1/16y$. Assuming that the mass of the body has remained constant what is its new velocity?

A. $1/196x$      B. $1/16x$      C. $1/8x$      D. $1/4x$      E. $4x$

**Question 3:**
Which of the following cannot be classified as an organ?
1. Blood      3. Larynx      5. Prostate      7. Skin
2. Bone      4. Pituitary Gland      6. Skeletal Muscle

A. 1 and 6      B. 2 and 3      C. 5 and 7      D. 1 and 5      E. 1,4, 5 and 6

**Question 4:**
An increase in aerobic respiratory rate could be associated with which of the following physiological changes?
1. A larger percentage of water vapour in expired air
2. Increased expired $CO_2$
3. Increased inspired $O_2$
4. Perspiration
5. Vasodilatation

A. 3 only      C. 1, 2 and 3 only      E. All of the above
B. 1 and 2 only      D. 2, 3 and 5

**Question 5:**
The nephron is to the kidney, as the _____ is to striated muscle:

A. Actin filament      C. Myofibril      E. Vein
B. Artery      D. Sarcomere

**Question 6:**

A diabetic patient's glucagon and insulin levels are measured over 12 hours.

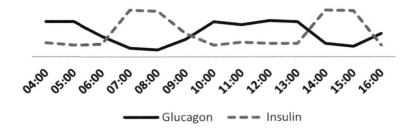

——— Glucagon    - - - Insulin

During this time the patient is given two large boli of glucose. A graphical representation of this is shown above.

At which times would you expect the patients' blood glucose to be greatest?

A.  05:00 and 12:00
B.  07:00 and 14.00

C.  08:00 and 15:00
D.  10:00 and 13:00

E.  06:00, 10:00 and 16:00

**Question 7:**

In addition to the A, B or O classification, blood groups can also be distinguished by the presence of Rhesus antigen (Rh). Care must be taken in blood transfusion as once blood types are mixed a Rh -ve individual will mount an immune response against Rh +ve blood. This is particularly well exemplified in haemolytic disease of the newborn – where a Rh-ve mother carries a Rh+ve foetus.

Applying what is written here and your knowledge of the human immune system, explain why the mother's first child would be relatively safe and unaffected, yet further offspring would be at high risk.

A.  The first pregnancy is always such a shock to the body it compromises the immune system.
B.  Antibodies take longer than 9 months to produce and mature to an active state.
C.  First born children are immunologically privileged.
D.  There is a high risk of haemorrhage to both mother and child during birth.
E.  Plasma T cells require time to multiply to lethal levels.

**Question 8:**

Which of the following is NOT present in the Bowman's capsule?

A.  Urea
B.  Glucose

C.  Sodium
D.  Water

E.  Haemoglobin

**Question 9:**
At present a large effort is being made to produce tailored patient care. One of the ultimate goals of this is to be able to grow personal, genetically identical organs for those with end stage organ failure. This process will first require the harbouring of what cell type?

A. Cells from the organ that is failing
B. Haematopoietic stem cells
C. Embryonic stem cells

D. Adult stem cells
E. All of the above

**Question 10:**
Below are three statements about electromagnetic radiation. Which is / are correct?

1. For identical amplitude, waves with the smallest wavelength transfer the most energy.
2. The speed of electromagnetic waves is directly proportional to their wavelength.
3. Microwaves can be dangerous because they can be easily absorbed by water molecules.

A. 1 only
B. 2 only

C. 3 only
D. 1 and 2

E. 1 and 3
F. None of the above

**Question 11:**
From which of the following elemental groups are you most likely to find a catalyst?

A. Alkali Metals
B. Transition metals

C. Alkaline Earth Metals
D. Noble Gases

E. Halogens

**Question 12:**
1.338kg of francium is mixed in a reaction vessel with an excess of distilled water. What volume will the hydrogen produced occupy at room temperature and pressure? Mr of Francium = 223

A. 20.4dm³       B. 36dm³       C. 40.8dm³       D. 60.12dm³       E. 72dm³

**Question 13:**
The composition by mass of a compound is Carbon 53%, Hydrogen 11%, and Oxygen 36%, to the nearest percentage.
What is the empirical formula of this compound?

A. $CH_2O$
B. $C_2 H_6O_2$

C. $C_2H_6O$
D. $CHO$

E. $C_3H_5O_2$

**Question 14:**
What is the actual molecular formula of the compound in question 13 if the $M_r$ is 45?

A. $C_2H_6O$
B. $C_4H_{12}O_2$

C. $C_3H_8O$
D. $C_4H_8O_2$

E. More information needed

**Question 15:**

$1.2 \times 10^{10}$ kg of sugar is dissolved in $4 \times 10^{12}$L of distilled water. What is the concentration?

A. $3 \times 10^{-2}$ g/dL        C. $3 \times 10^{1}$ g/dL        E. $3 \times 10^{3}$ g/dL
B. $3 \times 10^{-1}$ g/dL        D. $3 \times 10^{2}$ g/dL

**Question 16:**

Which of the following is not essential for the progression of an exothermic chemical reaction?

A. Presence of a catalyst
B. Increase in entropy
C. Achieving activation energy
D. Attaining an electron configuration more closely resembling that of a noble gas
E. None of the above

**Question 17:**

Which of the following combinations are commonly used in the treatment of drinking water?

A. $F_2$ and $Cl_2$        C. $F^-$ and $Cl^-$        E. $H^+$ and $Cl^-$
B. $H_2$ and $Cl_2$        D. $F^-$ and $H^+$

**Question 18:**

Which of the following is a unit equivalent to the Volt?

A. $A.\Omega^{-1}$      B. $J.C^{-1}$      C. $W.s^{-1}$      D. $C.s$      E. $W.C.\Omega$

**Question 19:**

Complete the sentence below:

A voltmeter is connected in _____ and therefore has _____ resistance; whereas an ammeter is connected in _____ and has _____ resistance.

A. Parallel, zero, parallel, infinite        D. Series, zero, parallel, infinite
B. Parallel, zero, series, infinite        E. Series, infinite, parallel, zero
C. Parallel, infinite, series, zero

**Question 20:**

A body "A" of mass 12kg travelling at 15m/s undergoes inelastic collision with a fixed, stationary object "B" of mass 20kg over a period of 0.5 seconds. After the collision body A has a new velocity of 3m/s. What force must have been dissipated during the collision?

A. 288N      B. 298N      C. 308N      D. 318N      E. 328N

**Question 21:**

What process is illustrated here: $^{14}_{6}C \rightarrow {}^{14}_{7}N + x$

A. Thermal decomposition
B. Alpha decay

C. Beta decay
D. Gamma decay

**Question 22:**

A radio dish is broadcasting messages into deep space on a 20 Hz radio frequency of wavelength 3km. With every hour how much further does the signal travel into deep space?

A. 200,000 km
B. 216,000 km

C. 232,000 km
D. 248,000 km

E. 264,000 km

**Question 23:**

A formula: $\sqrt[3]{\dfrac{z(x+y)(l+m-n)}{3}}$ is given. Which of the following options would you expect this formula to calculate?

A. A length
B. An area

C. A volume
D. A volume of rotation

E. A geometric average

**Question 24:**

Evaluate the following: $(4.2 \times 10^{10}) - (4.2 \times 10^{6})$

A. 415,800,000
B. 415,800

C. 41,995,800,000
D. 419,958,000

E. 4,242,000,000

**Question 25:**

Calculate $a - b$

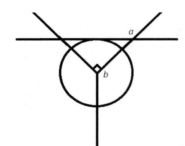

A. 0°
B. 5°
C. 10°
D. 15°
E. 20°

**Question 26:**

Jack has a bag with a complete set of snooker balls (15 red, 1 yellow, 1 green, 1 brown, 1 blue, 1 pink and 1 black ball) within it. Blindfolded, Jack draws two balls from the bag without replacing them.
What is the probability that he draws a blue and a black ball in any order?

A. 2/41        B. 2/210        C. 1/210        D. 1/105        E. 2/441

**Question 27:**

An experiment is repeated using an identical methodology and upon further review it is proven to demonstrate identical scientific practice. If the result obtained is different to the first, this would be due to:

A. Calibration Bias
B. Systematic Bias
C. Random Chance
D. Serial dilution
E. Inaccuracies in the methodology

**END OF SECTION**

# SECTION 3

1) *Doctors should wear white coats, as it helps to create a placebo effect, rendering the treatment more effective.*

Explain what is meant by this statement. Argue to the contrary. To what extent do you agree with the statement? What points can you see that contradict this statement?

2) *"Medicine is a science of uncertainty and an art of probability."*

*William Osler*

Explain what this statement means. Argue to the contrary. To what extent do you agree with the statement?

3) *"The New England Journal of Medicine reports that 9 out of 10 doctors agree that 1 out of 10 doctors is an idiot."*

*Jay Leno*

What do you understand by this statement? Explain why the assumption above may be inaccurate and argue to the contrary.

4) *"My father was a research scientist in tropical medicine, so I always assumed I would be a scientist, too. I felt that medicine was too vague and inexact, so I chose physics."*

*Stephen Hawking*

Explain what this statement means. Argue to the contrary. To what extent do you agree with the statement?

**END OF PAPER**

# MOCK PAPER B

## SECTION 1

**Question 1:**
"If vaccinations are now compulsory because society has decided that they should be forced, then society should pay for them." Which of the following statements would weaken this argument the most statement?

A. Many people disagree that vaccinations should be compulsory.
B. The cost of vaccinations is too high to be funded locally.
C. Vaccinations are supported by many local communities and GPs.
D. Healthcare workers do not want vaccinations.
E. None of the above

**Question 2:**
Josh is painting the outside walls of his house. The paint he has chosen is sold only in 10L tins. Each tin costs £4.99. Assuming a litre of paint covers an area of 5m², and the total surface area of Josh's outside walls is 1050m²; what is the total cost of the paint required if Josh wants to apply 3 coats?

A.  £104.79          B.  £209.58          C.  £314.37          D.  £419.16          E.  £523.95

**Question 3:**
The stars of the night sky have remained unchanged for many hundreds of years, which allows sailors to navigate using the North Star. However, this only applies within the Northern Hemisphere as the populations of the Southern Hemisphere are subject to an alternative night sky.

An asterism can be used to locate the North Star, which comes by many names including the plough, the saucepan, and the big dipper. Whilst the North Star's position remains fixed in the sky (allowing it to point north reliably always) the rest of the stars traverse around the North Star in a singular motion. In a very long time, the North Star will one day move from its location due to the movement of the Earth.

Which of the following is **NOT** an assumption made in this argument?
A. The Earth is rotating on its axis.
B. Sailors still need to navigate using the stars.
C. An analogous southern star is used to navigate in the Southern hemisphere.
D. The plough is not the only method of locating the North Star.
E. None of the above.

**Question 4:**

John wishes to deposit a cheque. The bank's opening times are 9am until 5pm Monday to Friday, 10am until 4pm on Saturdays, and the bank is closed on Sundays. It takes on average 42 bank hours for the money from a cheque to become available.

If John wishes to have the money by 8pm on Tuesday, what is the latest he can cash the cheque?

A.  5pm the Saturday before
B.  5pm the Friday before
C.  1pm the Thursday before

D.  1pm the Wednesday before
E.  9am the Tuesday before

**Question 5:**

How many different squares can be visualised in the image shown to the right?

A.  25         C.  48         E.  63
B.  32         D.  58

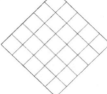

**Question 6:**

In 4 years, I will be one third of the age that my brother will be next year.  In 20 years' time he will be double my age. How old am I?

A.  4          B.  9          C.  15          D.  17          E.  23

**Question 7:**

Aneurysmal disease has been proven to induce systemic inflammatory effects, reaching far beyond the site of the aneurysm. The inflammatory mediator responsible for these processes remains unknown, however the effects of systemic inflammation have been well categorised and observed experimentally in pig models.

This inflammation induces an aberration of endothelial function within the innermost layer of blood vessel walls. The endothelium not only represents the lining of blood vessels but also acts as a transducer converting the haemodynamic forces of blood into a biological response. An example of this is the NO pathway, which uses the shear stress induced by increased blood flow to drive the formation of NO. NO diffuses from the endothelium into the smooth muscle surrounding blood vessels to promote vasodilatation and therefore acts to reduce blood flow.

Failure of this process induces high risk of vascular damage and therefore cardiovascular diseases such as thrombosis and atherosclerosis.

What is a valid conclusion from the text above?
A.  Aneurysmal disease does not affect the NO pathway.
B.  Aneurysms directly increase the likelihood of cardiovascular disease.
C.  Aneurysms are the opposite of transducers.
D.  Observations of this kind should be made in humans to see if the results can be replicated.
E.  Aneurysms induce high blood flow.

**Question 8:**

A traffic surveyor is stood at a T-junction between a main road and a side street. He is only interested in traffic leaving the side street. He logs the class of vehicle, the colour and the direction of travel once on the main road. During an 8-hour period he observes a total of 346 vehicles including bikes, of which 200 were travelling west whilst the rest travelled east. The overwhelming majority of vehicles seen were cars, at 90%, with bikes, vans and articulated lorries together comprising the remaining 10%. Red was the most common colour observed whilst green was the least. Black and white vehicles were seen in equal quantities.

Which of the following is an accurate inference based on his survey?

A.  Global sales are highest for those vehicles which are coloured red.

B.  Cars are the most popular vehicle on all roads.

C.  Green vehicles are less popular than red vehicles in the area that the surveyor was based.

D.  The daily average rate of traffic out of a T junction in Britain is 346 vehicles over 8 hours.

E.  To the east of the junction is a dead end.

**Question 9:**

William, Xavier, and Yolanda race in a 100m race. All of them run at a constant speed during the race. William beats Xavier by 20m. Xavier beats Yolanda by 20m. By how many metres does William beat Yolanda?

A.  30m          B.  36m          C.  40m          D.  60m          E.  64m

**Question 10:**

A television is delivered in a box that has volume 60% larger than that of the television. The television is 150cm x 100cm x 10cm. How much surplus volume is there?

A.  0.09m³          B.  0.9 m³          C.  9 m³          D.  90 m³          E.  900 m³

**Question 11:**

Matthew and David are deciding where they would like to go camping from Friday to Sunday. Upon completing their research, they discover the following:

- Whitmore Bay charges £5.50 per night and does not require a booking. The site provides showers, washing up facilities and easy access to a beach

- Port Eynon charges £5 per night and a booking is compulsory. However, the site does not provide showers but does have 240V sockets free of charge

- Jackson Bay charges £7 per night and is billed as a luxury site with compulsory booking, private showers, toilets, mobile phone charging facilities and kitchens.

David presents the following suggestion:

As Port Eynon is the farthest distance to travel the benefit of its cheap nightly rate is negated by the cost of petrol. Instead, he recommends they visit Jackson Bay as it is the shortest distance to travel and will therefore be the cheapest.

Which of the following best illustrates a flaw in this argument?

A. Whitmore bay may be only a few miles further which means the total cost would be less than visiting Jackson Bay.
B. With kitchen facilities available they will be tempted to buy more food, increasing the cost.
C. The campsite may be fully booked.
D. There may be a booking fee driving the cost up above that of the other campsites.
E. All of the above.

**Question 12:**
The manufacture of any new pharmaceutical is not permitted without scrupulous testing and analysis. This has led to the widespread, and controversial use of animal models in science. Whilst it is possible to test cytotoxicity on simple cell cultures, to truly predict the effect of a drug within a physiological system it must be trialled in a whole organism. With animals being cheap to maintain, readily available, rapidly reproducing, and not subject to the same strict ethical laws, they have become an invaluable component of modern scientific practice.
Which of the following best illustrates the main conclusion of this argument?

A. New pharmaceuticals cannot be approved without animal experimentation.
B. Cell culture experiments are unhelpful.
C. Modern medicine would not have achieved its current standard without animal experimentation.
D. Logistically animals are easier to keep than humans for mandatory experiments.
E. All of the above.

**Question 13:**
After looking at interviews conducted with a number of adult learners, our research suggested that the learners who felt they were most successful were all highly motivated. We noticed that early success had heightened motivation in some cases and saw that both success and motivation may be due to a special aptitude for learning. We also noticed that many of those who felt they were most motivated were also learning in favourable conditions or for fun, which meant they may have become motivated since starting their classes. Though these conditions seem persuasive, the results led us to the same conclusion. It's impossible to learn anything without motivation.

Which one of the following is **NOT** a flaw in the above argument?

A. It assumes that those who felt they were successful actually were.
B. It assumes that those who felt they were motivated actually were.
C. The research does not establish that there are no successful learners who lacked motivation.
D. The research is only concerned with adult learners.
E. It assumes that in order to be motivated you may have to have a special aptitude for learning.

**Question 14:**

A nationwide survey showed that the majority of people would not be willing to give up their car in favour of public transport. However, in a recent survey of people living in an area with heavy traffic problems, 76% stated that they would prefer to travel to work by public transport if the system was made more reliable. This shows that the previous findings were wrong. We should therefore restrict car use and start a programme to improve the nation's public transport network as soon as possible.

Which one of the following is the best statement of the flaw in the argument above?
A. It fails to specify which types of public transport are to be improved.
B. The counter arguments are not explained in detail.
C. The statistic presented may not be representative of the whole population.
D. It does not consider the 24% who would not prefer to use public transport.
E. It fails to explain how the public transport system can be improved.

**Question 15:**

A restaurant owner makes 100 burgers and 50 hotdogs at the start of the day, to sell that day. The burgers are priced at £8.00, and the hotdogs are priced at £6.00.
By the end of lunchtime, there are 20 burgers and 15 hotdogs left, and the prices for these are halved for sale in the afternoon.
At the end of the day, there are still 2 burgers and 3 hotdogs left, which are disposed of.

Each burger costs £2.50 to make, and each hotdog costs £1.50 to make.

How much profit does the restaurant make from the sales of burgers and hotdogs on this day?

A. £958          B. £633          C. £1,283          D. £1,066          E. £741

**Question 16:**

A train driver runs a service between Cardiff and Merthyr. On average a one-way trip takes 40 minutes to drive but he requires 5 minutes to unload passengers and a further 5 minutes to pick up new ones. The distance between Cardiff and Merthyr is 22 miles.

Assuming he works an 8-hour shift with two 20-minute breaks, and when he arrives to work the first train is already loaded with passengers how far does he travel (in miles)?

A. 132          B. 143          C. 154          D. 176          E. 198

**Question 17:**

The massive volume of traffic that travels down the M4 corridor regularly leads to congestion at peak times. A case is being made by local councils in congested areas to introduce relief lanes thus widening the motorway in an attempt to relieve the congestion. This would involve introducing either a new 2 or 4 lanes to the motorway on average costing 1 million pounds per lane per 10 miles.

Many conservationist groups are concerned as this will involve the destruction of large areas of countryside either side of the motorway. They argue that the side of a motorway is a unique habitat with many rare species residing there.

The local councils argue that with many hundreds if not thousands of cars sitting idle on the motorway pumping pollutants out into the surrounding areas, it is better for the wildlife if the congestion is eased and traffic can flow through. The councils have also remarked that if congestion is eased there would be less money needed to repair the roads from car incidents with could in theory be given to the conservationist groups as a grant.

Which of the following is assumed in this passage?

A. Wildlife living on the side of the motorway cannot be re-homed.
B. Congestion causes car incidents.
C. Relief lanes have been proven to improve traffic jams.
D. A and B.
E. B and C.
F. All of the above.
G. None of the above.

**Question 18:**

Apples and oranges are sold in packs of 5 for the price of £1 and £1.25 respectively. Alternatively, apples can be purchased individually for 30p, and oranges can be purchased individually for 50p. Helen is making a fruit salad, and she remarks that her order would have cost her an extra £6.25 if she had purchased the fruit individually.

Which of the following could have been her order?

A. 15 apples 10 oranges
B. 15 apples 15 oranges
C. 25 apples 10 oranges
D. 25 apples, 15 oranges
E. 30 apples, 30 oranges

**Question 19:**

Laura is blowing up balloons for a birthday party. The average volume of a balloon is $300cm^3$ and Laura's maximum forced expiratory rate in a single breath is 4.5L/min. What is the fastest Laura could inflate 25 balloons assuming it takes her 0.5 secs to breathe in per balloon, and somebody else ties the balloons for her?

A. 112.5 seconds
B. 122.5 seconds
C. 132.5 seconds
D. 142.5 seconds
E. 152.5 seconds

**Question 20:**

George reasons that A is equal to B which is not equal to C. In which case C is equal to D which is equal to E.

Which of the following, if true, would most *weaken* George's argument?

A. A does not equal D.

B. B is equal to E.

C. A and C are not equal.

D. C is equal to 0.

E. None of the above

**Question 21:**

In a single day how many times do the hour, minute and second hands of an analogue clock all point to the same number?

A. 12

B. 24

C. 36

D. 48

E. 72

**Question 22:**

"People who practice extreme sports should have to buy private health insurance."

Which of the following statements most strongly supports this argument?

A. Exercise is healthy and private insurance offers better reward schemes.

B. Extreme sports have a higher likelihood of injury.

C. Healthcare should be free for all.

D. People that practice extreme sports are more likely to be wealthy.

**Question 23:**

Explorers in the US in the 18th Century had to contest with a great variety of obstacles ranging from natural to man-made. Natural obstacles included the very nature and set up of the land, presenting explorers with the sheer size of the land mass, the lack of reliable mapping as well as the lack of paths and bridges. On a human level, challenges included the threat from outlaws and other hostile groups. Due to the nature of the settling situation, availability of medical assistance was sparse and there was a constant threat of diseases and fatal results of injuries.

Which of the following statements is correct with regards to the above text?

A. Medical supply was good in the US in the 18th Century.

B. The land was easy to navigate.

C. There were few outlaws threatening the individual.

D. Crossing rivers could be difficult.

E. All the above.

**Question 24:**

The statement "The human race is not dependent on electricity" assumes what?

A. We have no other energy resource.

B. Electricity is cheap.

C. Electrical appliances dominate our lives.

D. Electricity is now the accepted energy source and is therefore the only one available.

E. All of the above.

**Question 25:**

Wine is sold in cases of 6 bottles. A bottle of wine holds 70cl of fluid whereas a wine glass holds 175ml. Cases of wine are currently on offer for £42 a case buy one get one free. If Elin is hosting a 3-course dinner party for 27 of her friends, and she would like to provide everyone with a glass of wine per course, how much will the wine cost her?

A. £42

B. £84

C. £126

D. £168

E. £210

**Question 26:**

Hannah buys a television series in boxset. It contains a full 7 series with each series comprising 12 episodes. Rounded to the nearest 10 each episode lasts 40 minutes.

What is the shortest amount of time it could possibly take to watch all the episodes back-to-back?

A. 49 hours

B. 51 hours

C. 53 hours

D. 56 hours

E. 60 hours

**Question 27:**

Many are familiar with the story that aided in the discovery of the "germ". Semmelweis worked in a hospital where maternal death rates during labour were astronomically high. He noticed that medical students often went straight from dissection of cadavers to the maternity wards. As an experiment Semmelweis split the student cohort in half. Half did their maternity rotation instead before dissection whereas the other half maintained their traditional routine. In the new routine, maternity ward before dissection, Semmelweis recorded an enormous reduction in maternal deaths and thus the concept of the pathogen was born.

What is best exemplified by this passage?

A. Science is a process of trial and error.

B. Great discoveries come from pattern recognition.

C. Provision of healthcare is closely associated with technological advancements.

D. Experiments always require a control.

E. All of the above.

**Question 28:**

Jack sits at a table opposite a stranger. The stranger says here I have 3 precious jewels: a diamond, a sapphire, and an emerald. He tells Jack that if he makes a truthful statement Jack will get one of the stones, if he lies he will get nothing.

What must Jack say to ensure he gets the sapphire?

A. Tell the stranger his name.

B. Tell the stranger he must give him the sapphire.

C. Tell the stranger he wants the emerald.

D. Tell the stranger he does not want the emerald or the diamond.

E. Tell the stranger he will not give him the emerald or the diamond.

**Question 29:**

Simon invests 100 pounds in a savings account that awards compound interest on a 6-monthly basis at 50%. Simon's current account awards compound interest on a yearly basis at 90%.

After 2 years will Simon's investment in the savings account yield more money than it would have in the current account?

A. Yes

B. No

C. Can't tell

**Question 30:**

My mobile phone has a 4-number pin code using the values $1 - 9$. To determine this, I use a standard algorithm of multiplying the first two numbers, subtracting the third and then dividing by the fourth. I change the code by changing the answer to this algorithm – I call this the key. What is the largest possible key?

A. 42    B. 55    C. 70    D. 80    E. 81

**Question 31:**

A group of scientists is investigating the role of different nutrients after exercise. They set up two groups of averagely fit individuals, consisting of the same number of both males and females aged 20 – 25, and weighing between 70 and 85 kilos. Each group will conduct the same 1hr exercise routine of resistance training, consisting of various weighted movements. After the workout they will receive a shake with vanilla flavour that has identical consistency and colour in all cases. Group A will receive a shake containing 50 g of protein and 50g of carbohydrates. Group B will receive a shake containing 100 g of protein and 50 g of carbohydrates. All participants have their lean body mass measured before starting the experiment.

Which of the following statements is correct?
A.  The experiment compares the response of men and women to endurance training.
B.  The experiment is flawed as it does not take into consideration that men and women respond differently to exercise.
C.  The experiment does not consider age.
D.  The experiment mainly looks at the role of protein after exercise.
E.  None of the above.

**Question 32:**

A child weighs 35kg and is 120cm tall. Using the equation, $BMI = \dfrac{weight/kg}{(height/m)^2}$, what is the BMI of the child to the nearest two decimal places?

A.  0.0024          B.  0.29          C.  24.31          D.  29.17          E.  1020

**END OF SECTION**

# SECTION 2

## Question 1:

GLUT2 is an essential and ATP independent mediator in the liver's uptake of plasma glucose. This is an example of:

A. Active transport

B. Diffusion

C. Exocytosis

D. Facilitated Diffusion

E. Osmosis

## Question 2:

The molecular weight of glucose is 180 g/mol. 5.76Kg of glucose is split evenly between two cell cultures under anaerobic conditions. One cell culture is taken from human cardiac muscle, whilst the other is a yeast culture. What will be the difference (in moles) between the amount of $CO_2$ produced between the two cultures?

A. 0 mol

B. 4 mol

C. 8 mol

D. 12 mol

E. 16 mol

## Question 3:

Which of the following cell types does not contain DNA?

A. Kidney cells

B. Liver cells

C. Nerve cells

D. Red blood cells

E. None of the above

## Question 4:

Which of the following is a function of the cardiovascular system?

A. Distribution of heat

B. Oxygenation of blood

C. Removal of waste products from the body

D. All of the above

E. None of the above

**Question 5:**

Pepsin and trypsin are both digestive enzymes. Pepsin acts in the stomach whereas trypsin is secreted by the pancreas. Which graph below (trypsin in black and pepsin in grey) would most accurately demonstrate their relative activity against pH?

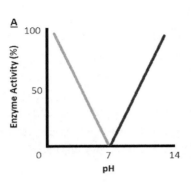

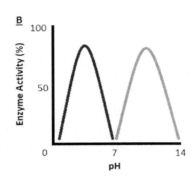

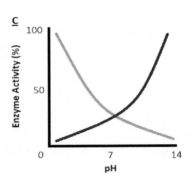

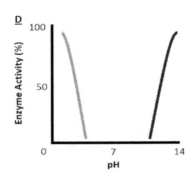

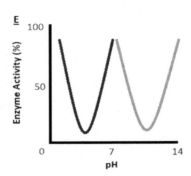

**Question 6:**

MRSA is a strain of Staphylococcus aureus that is resistant to an antibiotic called methicillin. It is responsible for several difficult-to-treat infections in humans. The fact that MRSA exists is a direct consequence of which of the following processes?

A. Natural selection

B. Genetic engineering

C. Sexual reproduction

D. Lamarckism

E. Co-dominance

**Question 7:**

What is the electron configuration of magnesium in $MgCl_2$?

A. 2,8          B. 2,8,2          C. 2,8,4          D. 2,8,8          E. None of the above

**Question 8:**

A calcium sample is run in a mass spectrometer. It is later discovered that the sample was contaminated with the most abundant isotope of chromium. A section of the trace is shown below. What was the actual abundance of the most common calcium isotope?

A.  1/9              B.  6/17              C.  1/2              D.  11/19              E.  17/19

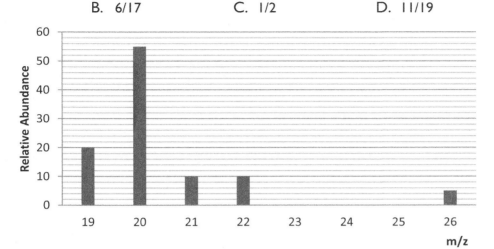

**Question 9:**

A warehouse receives 15 tonnes of arsenic in bulk. Assuming that the sample is at least 80% pure, what is the minimum amount, in moles, of arsenic that they have obtained? (Mr of arsenic = 75).

A.  $1.6 \times 10^5$        B.  $2 \times 10^5$        C.  $1.6 \times 10^6$        D.  $2 \times 10^6$        E.  $1.6 \times 10^7$

**Question 10:**

A sample of silicon is run in a mass spectrometer. The resultant trace shows m/z peaks at 26 and 30 with relative abundance 60% and 30% respectively. What other isotope of silicon must have been in the sample to give an average atomic mass of 28?

A.  28              B.  30              C.  32              D.  34              E.  36

**Question 11:**

72.9g of pure magnesium ribbon is mixed in a reaction vessel with the equivalent of 54g of steam. The ensuing reaction produces $72dm^3$ of hydrogen. Which of the following statements is true?

A.  This is a complete reaction
B.  This is a partial reaction
C.  There is an excess of steam

D.  There is an excess of magnesium
E.  Magnesium hydroxide is a product

**Question 12:**

Which species acts as the reducing agent in the following equation?:
$3Cu^{2+} + 3S^{2-} + 8H^+ + 8NO_3^- \rightarrow 3Cu^{2+} + 3SO_4^{2-} + 8NO + 4H_2O$

A.  $Cu^{2+}$        B.  $S^{2-}$        C.  $H^+$        D.  $NO_3^-$        E.  $H_2O$

**Question 13:**
Which of the following is **not** true of alkanes?

A. They have the homologous formula $C_nH2_{n+2}$
B. They are saturated
C. They are reactive
D. They produce only $CO_2$ and water when burnt in an excess of oxygen
E. None of the above

**Question 14:**
A rubber balloon is inflated and rubbed against a sample of animal fur for a period of 15 seconds. At the end of this process the balloon is carrying a charge of -5 coulombs. What magnitude of current must have been induced during the process of rubbing the balloon against the animal fur; and in which direction was it flowing?

A. 0.33A into the balloon
B. 0.33A into the fur
C. 0.33A in no net direction
D. 75A into the balloon
E. 75A into the fur

**Question 15:**
Which of the following is a unit equivalent to the Amp?

A. $V.\Omega$
B. $(W.V)/s$
C. $C.\Omega$
D. $(J.s^{-1})/V$
E. $C.s$

**Question 16:**
The output of a step-down transformer is measured at 24V and 10A. Given that the transformer is 80% efficient what must the initial power input have been?

A. 240W
B. 260W
C. 280W
D. 300W
E. 320W

**Question 17:**
An electric winch system hoists a mass of 20kg 30 metres into the air over a period of 20 seconds. What is the power output of the winch assuming the system is 100% efficient?

A. 100W
B. 200W
C. 300W
D. 400W
E. 500W

**Question 18:**
On day 1 of an experiment, a sample is tested and has a count rate of 130Bq.
The same sample is tested on day 7, and the count rate is now 40Bq.
Given that the background radiation count rate is 10Bq, on what day of the experiment will the count rate of the sample be 25Bq?

A. Day 8
B. Day 9
C. Day 10
D. Day 11
E. More information needed

**Question 19:**

An 80W filament bulb draws 0.5A of household electricity. Using the information that household electricity is available in the UK at 240V, determine the efficiency of the bulb.

A.  25%          B.  33%          C.  50%          D.  66%          E.  75%

**Question 20:**

Rearrange the following equation in terms of t: $x = \frac{\sqrt{b^3 - 9st}}{13j} + \int_{-z}^{z} 9a - 7$

A.  $t = \frac{(13jx - \int_{-z}^{z} 9a - 7)^2 - b^3}{9s}$

B.  $t = \frac{13jx^2}{b^3 - 9s} - \int_{-z}^{z} 9a - 7$

C.  $t = x - \frac{\sqrt{b^3 - 9s}}{13j} - \int_{-z}^{z} 9a - 7$

D.  $t = \frac{x^2}{\frac{b^3 - 9s}{13j} + \int_{-z}^{z} 9a - 7}$

E.  $t = \frac{[13j(x - \int_{-z}^{z} 9a - 7)]^2 - b^3}{-9s}$

**Question 21:**

An investment of £500 is made in a compound interest account. At the end of 2 years the balance reads £1125. What is the interest rate?

A.  20%          B.  35%          C.  50%          D.  65%          E.  80%

**Question 22:**

What is the equation of the line of best fit for the scatter graph below?

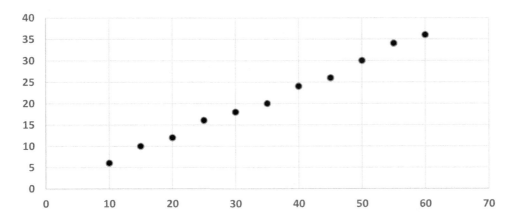

A.  y = 0.2x + 0.35          C.  y = 0.4x + 0.35          E.  y = 0.6x + 0.35
B.  y = 0.2x − 0.35          D.  y = 0.4x − 0.35

**Question 23:**

Simplify: $m = \sqrt{\dfrac{9xy^3z^5}{3x^9yz^4}} - m$

A.  $m = \sqrt{\dfrac{3y^2z}{x^8}} - m$

B.  $m^2 = \dfrac{3y^2z}{x^8} - m$

C.  $2m = \sqrt{\dfrac{3y^2z}{x^8}}$

D.  $2m^2 = 3x^{-8}y^2z$

E.  $4m^2 = 3x^{-8}y^2z$

**Question 24:**

Which of the following is a suitable descriptive statistic for non-normally distributed data?

A.  Mean

B.  Normal range

C.  Confidence interval

D.  Interquartile range

E.  Mode

**Question 25:**

Which of the following best describes the purpose of statistics?
A.  Evaluate acceptable scientific practice.
B.  Reduce the ability of others to criticise the data.
C.  To quickly analyse data.
D.  Calculate values representative of the population from a subset sample.
E.  To allow for universal comparison of scientific methods.

**Question 26:**

A rotating disc has two wells, in which bacteria are cultured. The first well is 10 cm from the centre whereas the second well is 20 cm from the centre. If the inner well completes a revolution in 1 second, how much faster is the outer well travelling?

A.  0.314m/s

B.  0.628m/s

C.  0.942m/s

D.  1.256m/s

E.  1.590m/s

**Question 27:**

Which is the equivalent function to: $y = 9x^{-\frac{1}{3}}$?

A.  $y = \dfrac{1}{x}$

B.  $y = \sqrt[3]{9x}$

C.  $y = \dfrac{1}{\sqrt[3]{9x}}$

D.  $y = \dfrac{9}{\sqrt[3]{x}}$

E.  $y = \dfrac{3}{\sqrt[3]{x}}$

**END OF SECTION**

# SECTION 3

1) *"Progress is made by trial and failure; the failures are generally a hundred times more numerous than the successes; yet they are usually left unchronicled."*

*Williams Ramsey*

Explain what this statement means. Argue to the contrary. To what extent do you agree with the statement?

2) *"He who studies medicine without books sails an uncharted sea, but he who studies medicine without patients does not go to sea at all."*

*William Osler*

Explain what this statement means. Argue to the contrary. To what extent do you agree with the statement?

3) *"'Medicine is the restoration of discordant elements; sickness is the discord of the elements infused into the living body"*

*Leonardo da Vinci*

Explain what this statement means. Argue to the contrary. To what extent do you think this simplification holds true within modern medicine?

4) *"Modern medicine is a negation of health. It isn't organized to serve human health, but only itself, as an institution. It makes more people sick than it heals."*

*Ivan Illich*

What does this statement mean? Argue to the contrary, that the primary duty of a doctor is not to prolong life. To what extent do you agree with this statement?

**END OF PAPER**

# MOCK PAPER C

## SECTION 1

**Question 1:**

Adam, Beth and Charlie are going on holiday together. A single room costs £60 per night, a double room costs £105 per night and a four-person room costs £215 per night. It is possible to opt out from the cleaning service and to pay £12 less each night per room.

What is the minimum amount the three friends could pay for their holiday for a three-night stay at the hotel?

A.  £122          B.  £144          C.  £203          D.  £423          E.  £432

**Question 2:**

I have two 96ml glasses of squash. The first is comprised of $\frac{1}{6}$ squash and $\frac{5}{6}$ water. The second is comprised of $\frac{1}{4}$ water and $\frac{3}{4}$ squash. The contents of both glasses are fully mixed. I take 48ml from the first glass and add it to glass two. I then take 72ml from glass two and add it to glass one.

How much squash is now in each glass?

A.  16ml squash in glass one and 72ml squash in glass two.
B.  40ml squash in glass one and 32ml squash in glass two.
C.  48ml squash in glass one and 32ml squash in glass two.
D.  48ml squash in glass one and 40ml squash in glass two.
E.  80ml squash in glass one and 40ml squash in glass two.

**Question 3:**

It may amount to millions of pounds each year of taxpayers' money; however, it is strongly advisable for the HPV vaccination in schools to continue. The vaccine, given to teenage girls, has the potential to significantly reduce cervical cancer deaths and furthermore, the vaccines will decrease the requirement for biopsies and invasive procedures related to the follow-up tests. Extensive clinical trials and continued monitoring suggest that both Gardasil and Cervarix are safe and tolerated well by recipients. Moreover, studies demonstrate that a large majority of teenage girls and their parents are in support of the vaccine.

Which of the following is the conclusion of the above argument?

A.  HPV vaccines are safe and well tolerated.
B.  It is strongly advisable for the HPV vaccination in schools to remain.
C.  The HPV vaccine amounts to millions of pounds each year of taxpayers' money.
D.  The vaccine has the potential to significantly reduce cervical cancer deaths.
E.  Vaccinations are vital to disease prevention across the population.

**Question 4:**

Anna cycles to school, which takes 30 minutes. James takes the bus, which leaves from the same place as Anna, but 6 minutes later and gets to school at the same time as Anna. It takes the bus 12 minutes to get to the post office, which is 3km away. The speed of the bus is $\frac{5}{4}$ the speed of the bike. One day Anna leaves 4 minutes late.

How far does she get before she is overtaken by the bus?

A.  1.5km          B.  2km          C.  3km          D.  4km          E.  6k

**Question 5:**

In a school year, there are 2 separate maths sets, and each student is assigned to one of them. Set 1 is the 'top set', where students tackled more difficult questions than in Set 2, which is the lower set.

The maths teacher is trying to work out who needs to be moved up from Set 2 to Set 1, and who to award a certificate at the end of term. The students must fulfil certain criteria:

| Reward | Criteria |
|---|---|
| Move to Set 1 | Attendance over 95% |
|  | Average test mark over 92 |
|  | Less than 5% homework handed in late |
| Awarded a Certificate | Absences below 4% |
|  | Average test mark over 89 |
|  | At least 98% homework handed in on time |

|  | Terry | Alex | Bahara | Lucy | Shiv |
|---|---|---|---|---|---|
| **Attendance %** | 97 | 92 | 97 | 100 | 98 |
| **Average test mark %** | 89 | 93 | 94 | 95 | 86 |
| **Homework handed in on time %** | 96 | 92 | 100 | 96 | 98 |

Who would move from Set 2 to Set 1, and who would receive a certificate?

A.  Bahara would move up from Set 2 to Set 1 and receive a certificate.
B.  Bahara and Lucy would move up from Set 2 to Set 1 and Bahara would receive a certificate.
C.  Bahara, Terry and Lucy would move up from Set 2 to Set 1 and Bahara and Shiv would receive a certificate.
D.  Lucy would move up from Set 2 to Set 1 and Bahara would receive a certificate.
E.  Lucy would move up from Set 2 to Set 1 and Bahara and Terry would receive a certificate.

**Question 6:**

18 years ago, A was 25 years younger than B is now. In 21 years time, A will be 28 years older than B was 14 years ago. How old is A now if A is $\frac{5}{6}$B?

A.  27          B.  28          C.  35          D.  42          E.  46

**Question 7:**

The time now is 10.45am. I am preparing a meal for 16 guests who will arrive tomorrow for afternoon tea. I want to make 3 scones for each guest, which can be baked in batches of 6. Each batch takes 35 minutes to prepare and 25 minutes to cook in the oven and I can start the next batch while the previous batch is in the oven. I also want to make 2 cupcakes for each guest, which can be baked in batches of 8. It takes 15 minutes to prepare the mixture for each batch and 20 minutes to cook them in the oven. I will also make 3 cucumber sandwiches for each guest. 6 cucumber sandwiches take 5 minutes to prepare.

Assuming I can only work on one component of the meal at a time, what will the time be when I finish making all the food for tomorrow?

A.  4:35pm          B.  5.55pm                C.  6:00pm              D.  6:05pm              E.  7:20pm

**Question 8:**

| Pyramid | Base edge (m) | Volume (m$^3$) |
|---------|---------------|----------------|
| 1 | 3 | 33 |
| 2 | 4 | 64 |
| 3 | 2 | 8 |
| 4 | 6 | 120 |
| 5 | 2 | 8 |
| 6 | 6 | 120 |
| 7 | 4 | 64 |

What is the difference between the height of the smallest and tallest pyramids?

A.  1m               B.  5m                    C.  4m                  D.  6m                  E.  8m

**Question 9:**

The wage of Employees at Star Bakery is calculated as: £210 + (Age x 1.2) – 0.8 (100 - % attendance). Jessica is 35 and her attendance is 96%. Samira is 65 and her attendance is 89%.

What is the difference between their wages?

A.  £30.40                    C.  £248.80                      E.  £279.20

B.  £60.50                    D.  £263.20

**Question 10:**

It is important that research universities demonstrate convincing support of teaching. Undergraduates comprise an overwhelming proportion of all students and universities should make an effort to cater to the requirements of the majority of their student body. After all, many of these students may choose to pursue a path involving research and a strong education would provide students with skills equipped towards a career in research.

What is the conclusion of the above argument?

A. Undergraduates comprise an overwhelming proportion of all students.
B. A strong education would provide a strong foundation and skills equipped towards a career in research.
C. Research universities should strongly support teaching.
D. Institutions should provide undergraduates with a high-quality learning experience.
E. Research has a greater impact than teaching and limited funds should mainly be invested in research.

**Question 11:**

American football has reached a level of violence that puts its players at too high a level of risk. It has been suggested that the NFL, the governing body for American football, should dispose of the use of the iconic helmets. The hard-plastic helmets all must meet minimum impact-resistance standards intended to enhance safety, however in reality they give players a false sense of security that only results in harder collisions. Some players now suffer from early onset dementia, mood swings and depression. The proposal to ban helmets for good should be supported. Moreover, it would prevent costly legal settlements involving the NFL and ex-players suffering from head trauma.

What is the conclusion of the above argument?

A. Sports players should not be exposed to unnecessary danger.
B. Helmets give players a false sense of security.
C. Players can suffer from early onset dementia, mood swings and depression.
D. The proposal to ban helmets should be supported.
E. American football is too violent and puts its players at risk.

**Question 12:**

At the final stop (stop 6), 10 people get off the tube. At the previous stop (stop 5) $\frac{1}{2}$ of the passengers got off. At stop 4, $\frac{3}{5}$ of the passengers got off. At stop 3, $\frac{1}{3}$ of the passengers got off and at stops 1 and 2, $\frac{1}{6}$ of the passengers got off.

How many passengers got on at the first stop?

A. 10          B. 36          C. 90          D. 108          E. 3600

**Question 13:**
Everyone likes English. Some students born in spring like maths and some like biology. All students born in winter like music and some like art. Of those born in autumn, no one likes biology, and everyone likes art.

Which of the following is true?
A. Some students born in spring like both biology and maths.
B. Students born in spring, winter, and autumn all like art.
C. No one born in winter or autumn likes biology.
D. No one who likes biology also likes art.
E. Some students born in winter like 3 subjects.

**Question 14:**
Until the twentieth century, the whole purpose of art was to create beautiful, flawless works. Artists attained a level of skill and craft that took decades to perfect and could not be mirrored by those who had not taken great pains to master it. The serenity and beauty produced from movements such as impressionism has however culminated in repulsive and horrific displays of rotting carcasses designed to provoke an emotional response rather than admiration. These works cannot be described as beautiful by either the public or art critics. While these works may be engaging on an intellectual or academic level, they no longer constitute art.

Which of the following is an assumption of the above argument?
A. Beauty is a defining property of art.
B. All modern art is ugly.
C. Twenty first century artists do not study for decades.
D. The impressionist movement created beautiful works of art.
E. Some modern art provokes an emotional response.

**Question 15:**
The cost of sunglasses is reduced over the bank holiday weekend. On Saturday, the price of the sunglasses is reduced by 10%, compared to the price on Friday. On Sunday the price of the sunglasses is reduced again by 10%, compared to the price on Saturday. On Monday, the price of the sunglasses is reduced by a further 10%, compared to the price on Sunday. What percentage of the price on Friday is the price of the sunglasses on Monday?

A. 55.12%    B. 59.10%    C. 63.80%    D. 70.34%    E. 72.9%

**Question 16:**
Putting the digit 7 on the right-hand side of a two-digit number causes the number to increase by 565. What is the value of the two-digit number?

A. 27    B. 52    C. 62    D. 66    E. 627

## Question 17:

When folded, which box can be made from the net shown below?

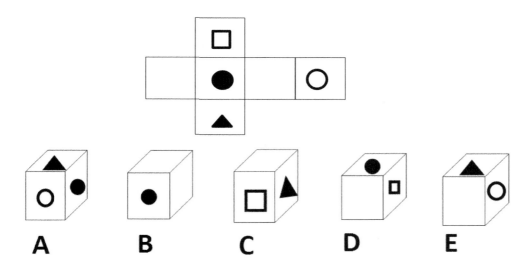

## Question 18:

The grid below is comprised of 49 squares. The shaded area is 588cm². What is its perimeter in cm?

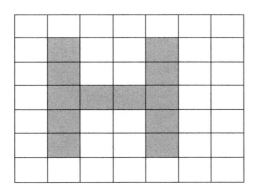

A.  26          B.  49          C.  84          D.  126          E.  182

**Question 19:**

The UK energy market is highly competitive. In an effort to attract more business and increase revenue, the company EnergyFirst has invested significant funds into its publicity. Last month, they doubled their advertising expenditures, becoming the energy company to invest the largest proportion of investment into advertising. As a result, it is expected that EnergyFirst will expand its customer base at a rate exceeding its competitors in the ensuing months. Other energy companies are likely to follow by example.

Which of the following, if true, is most likely to weaken the above argument?

A.  Other companies invest more money into good customer service.

B.  Research into the energy industry demonstrates a low correlation between advertising investment and new customers.

C.  The UK energy market is not highly competitive.

D.  EnergyFirst currently has the smallest customer base.

E.  Visual advertising heavily influences customers.

**Question 20:**

The consumption of large quantities of red meat is suggested to have negative health ramifications. Carnitine is a compound present in red meat and a link has been discovered between carnitine and the development of atherosclerosis, involving the hardening and narrowing of arteries. Intestinal bacteria convert carnitine to trimethylamine-N-oxide, which has properties that are damaging to the heart. Moreover, red meat consumption has been associated with a reduced life expectancy. It may be that charring meat generates toxins that elevate the chance of developing stomach cancer. If people want to be healthy, a vegetarian diet is preferable to a diet including meat. Vegetarians often have lower cholesterol and blood pressure and a reduced risk of heart disease.

Which of the following is an assumption of the above argument?

A.  Diet is essential to health, and we should all want to be healthy.

B.  Vegetarians do the same amount of exercise as meat eaters.

C.  Meat has no health benefits.

D.  People who eat red meat die earlier.

E.  Red meat is the best source of iron.

**Question 21:**

Auckland is 11 hours ahead of London. Calgary is 7 hours behind London. Boston is 5 hours behind London. The flight from Auckland to London is 22 hours, but the plane must stop for 2 hours in Hong Kong. The flight from London to Calgary is 8 hours 30 minutes. The flight from Calgary to Boston is 6 hours 30 minutes. Sam leaves Auckland at 10am for London. On arrival to London, he waits 3 hours then gets the plane to Calgary. Once in Calgary, he waits 1.5 hours and gets the plane to Boston. What time is it when Sam arrives in Boston?

A.  13:30pm          B.  22.30pm          C.  01:00am          D.  01:30am          E.  03:30am

**Question 22:**

Light A flashes every 18 seconds, light B flashes every 33 seconds and light C flashes every 27 seconds. The three lights all flashed at the same time 5 minutes ago.

How long will it be until they next all flash simultaneously?

A.  33 seconds            C.  300 seconds            E.  594 seconds

B.  294 seconds           D.  333 seconds

**Question 23:**

Drivers in the age group 17-19 comprise 1.5% of all drivers; however, 12% of all collisions involve young drivers in this age category. The RAC Foundation wants a graduated licensing system with a 1-year probationary period with restrictions on what new drivers can do on roads. Additionally, driving instructors need to emphasise the dangers of driving too fast and driving tests should be designed to make new drivers more focused on noticing potential hazards. These changes are essential and could stop 4,500 injuries on an annual basis.

What is the assumption of the above argument?

A. Young drivers are more likely to have more passengers than other age groups.

B. Young drivers spend more hours driving than older drivers.

C. Young drivers are responsible for the collisions.

D. The cars that young people drive are unsafe.

E. Most young drivers involved in accidents are male.

**Question 24:**

Many countries spent billions on vaccines in response to advice that a virus had the potential to kill millions. These countries are now trying to sell the stockpiles of vaccines which they do not need. There is concern that advice given by officials may have been influenced by pharmaceutical companies. Clearly such companies would have an interest in making sure that governments spend large sums of money on vaccines. It is essential that an investigation into this matter takes place as soon as possible so that those responsible can be held to account.

Which one of the following is an assumption on which this argument depends?

A. The pharmaceutical companies influenced the advice given by officials.

B. The advice given by officials was not appropriate.

C. It will not be possible for the stockpiles of vaccines to be sold.

D. The pharmaceutical companies misjudged the dangers of the virus.

E. Groups with financial interests do not advise officials in other areas of decision making.

**Question 25:**

Consider the following statements:

| **1** There are fewer rats than people. | **2** There are not more people than rats. | **3** There are at least as many rats as people. | **4** There are not more rats than people. |
|---|---|---|---|

Which two of the above statements are equivalent?

A. 1 and 3    B. 1 and 4    C. 2 and 3    D. 2 and 4    E. 3 and 4

**Question 26:**

A significant social trend in the 20<sup>th</sup> century was that people moved away from their place of birth in order to access education and work. This gave individuals more opportunities and helped the economy by producing mobility within the workforce. The negative side of this is now being felt as more and more elderly people face the problems of old age without family members nearby to care for them. This has negative effects on the economy as well as on the individual, as more and more state funding for care is needed.

Which one of the following could be drawn as a conclusion of the above passage?

A. The benefits of a mobile workforce have to be compared with the costs to elderly people and the economy.
B. Elderly people are expecting the state to provide care for them rather than relying on their children.
C. People should try to find education and work close to their place of birth.
D. The state should provide care for elderly people to make mobility of the workforce possible.
E. People should make caring for their elderly parents a priority over choice of work opportunities.

**Question 27:**

Any company that wishes to sell a new drug must provide the government with details of research about its safety and possible side effects. At present, this information is confidential, but there are plans to make it available to the public. While patients are surely entitled to more information about the drugs they are prescribed, this will also inevitably make public vital details about the ingredients of certain drugs and how they are manufactured. Drug companies are naturally reluctant to release this information to their competitors. Therefore, through fear of imitators, drug companies will no longer introduce new and important drugs into the country.

Which one of the following, if true, would most weaken the above argument?

A. There are sufficient drugs already on the market and so there is no need to introduce new ones.
B. The drug industry is a very competitive business and secrecy is vital if companies are to survive.
C. People may be reluctant to use certain drugs when they have fuller information about them.
D. People are better informed about the side effects of drugs abroad than they are in this country.
E. Strong patent laws prevent companies from using the information to create rival drugs.

**Question 28:**

There are an increasing number of historical and significant buildings in the UK which are said to be 'At Risk'. Without a change in the law most of these buildings are doomed to crumble to the ground. This is because these buildings are no longer structurally sound. The existing strict renovation laws mean that they are too expensive or impractical for private individuals or developers to renovate and repair. There are certainly people out there who would be willing to maintain these buildings if they could use more modern and less expensive techniques and materials. Surely it is better to sacrifice some of the original building's character than lose the entire structure?

Which one of the following best expresses the main conclusion of the above argument?

A. There is nothing wrong with changing the character of historic buildings.
B. 'At Risk' buildings need to be renovated according to strict rules.
C. A change in the law is needed if we hope to preserve more 'At Risk' buildings.
D. Existing laws make 'At Risk' buildings too expensive for most developers.
E. Historians can learn more from buildings which have not been modernised by modern developers.

**Question 29:**

Many people believe that foreign travel broadens the mind and that there is an inherent benefit in spending some time in a culture different from your own. Many students are taking 'gap' years where they spend time in another country. Whilst this may offer some benefits in terms of confidence and independence, it is wrong to assume that foreign travel alone can provide this. Global travel can have negative impacts on local cultures and the environment. Home country based 'gap' year projects are often seen as unglamorous, but the benefit of working with different groups of people and different cultures within our own society can be equally rewarding.

Which one of the following is the main conclusion of the above passage?

A) Foreign gap year projects must have an element of community work for them to be worthwhile.
B) Foreign travel is not the only way to gain confidence and independence.
C) Projects within our own society can be as rewarding as foreign travel.
D) There is inherent benefit in spending some time abroad.
E) It is important that gap year students consider the impact of their travel on the communities they work in.

**Question 30:**

"Sugar should be taxed like alcohol and cigarettes."

Which of the following statements, if true, most supports this claim?

A. Sugar can cause diabetes.
B. Sugar has high addictive potential and is associated with various health concerns.
C. High sugar diets increase obesity.
D. People that eat a lot of sugar are more likely to start abusing alcohol.
E. None of the above.

**Question 31:**

There is no empirical evidence that human activities directly result in global warming, and this is used as a reason against decreasing carbon emissions. However, many scientists believe that human activity is highly likely to cause global warming since higher levels of greenhouse gases cause the atmosphere to thicken, retaining heat. It therefore seems sensible that we should not wait for proof considering the catastrophic effects of climate change, regardless of subsequent findings. Similarly, if a tree branch had a significant chance of falling on you, it would be sensible to move away immediately.

What is the main conclusion?

A. Many scientists believe that human activity is highly likely to cause global warming.
B. We should not wait for proof of climate change.
C. If a tree branch had a significant chance of falling on you, it would be sensible to move away immediately.
D. The effects of climate change are catastrophic.
E. There is no empirical evidence that human activities directly result in global warming, so we should not reduce carbon emissions.

**Question 32:**

"Unpaid national service is a good way for young people to prepare themselves to become productive members of a democratic society"

Which of the following most closely parallels the reasoning of the above argument?

A.  Young people should undertake work experience to prepare themselves for adulthood.
B.  Voting should only be extended to those who contribute to society.
C.  Internships are a good way for employers to learn which graduates are worth hiring.
D.  Unpaid internships are a good way to learn how to become a productive employee.
E.  Unemployed people should contribute to society through work schemes if they can't find jobs.

**END OF SECTION**

# SECTION 2

**Question 1:**

Which of the following is / are **not** involved in the carbon cycle?

1. Lipid molecules in an animal cell
2. Plasmids in a bacterial species
3. Proteins made by a plant cell

A.  1 and 2                    C.  1 only                    E.  None of the above
B.  1 and 3                    D.  2 only

**Question 2:**

Which of the following statements regarding enzymes are correct?

1.  Enzymes are denatured at high temperatures or extreme pH values.
2.  Amylase is produced in the salivary glands only and converts starch to sugars.
3.  Lipases catalyse the breakdown of oils and fats into glycerol and fatty acids. This takes place in the small intestine.
4.  Bile is stored in the pancreas and travels down the bile duct to neutralise stomach acid.

A.  1 and 3 only              C.  1, 2 and 3 only            E.  3 and 4 only
B.  1, 3 and 4 only           D.  2 and 4 only

**Question 3:**

Which of the following describes the role of the colon?

A.  Food is combined with bile and digestive enzymes.
B.  Storage of faeces.
C.  Reabsorption of water.
D.  Faeces leave the alimentary canal.
E.  Any digested food is absorbed into the lymph and blood.

**Question 4:**

Which of the following statements regarding transmission of signals in the nervous system are true?

1.  The signal is transmitted across the synapse by diffusion.
2.  Transmitter molecules are stored in the pre-synaptic neuron.
3.  Transmitter molecules bind to specific receptors on the post-synaptic membrane.

A.  1 and 3 only              C.  1, 2 and 3 only            E.  2 only
B.  1 and 2 only              D.  2 and 3 only

## Question 5:
Which of the following statements are true regarding the transition elements?

1. Iron (II) compounds are light green.
2. Transition elements are neither malleable nor ductile.
3. Transition metal carbonates may undergo thermal decomposition.
4. Transition metal hydroxides are soluble in water.
5. When $Cu^{2+}$ ions are mixed with sodium hydroxide solution, a blue precipitate is formed.

A. 1 and 2        B. 1 and 3        C. 1, 3 and 5        D. 3 and 5        E. 5 only

## Question 6:
What is the value of C when the equation is balanced?

$\underline{5}$ PhCH$_3$ + $\underline{A}$ KMnO$_4$ + $\underline{9}$ H$_2$SO$_4$ = $\underline{5}$ PhCOOH + $\underline{B}$ K$_2$SO$_4$ + $\underline{C}$ MnSO$_4$ + $\underline{14}$ H$_2$O

A. 3        B. 4        C. 5        D. 7        E. 9

## Question 7:
Tongue-rolling is controlled by the dominant allele T, while non-rolling is controlled by the recessive allele, t.
Red-green colour blindness is controlled by a sex-linked gene on the X chromosome. Normal colour vision is controlled by dominant allele B, while red-green colour blindness is controlled by the recessive allele, b.
The mother of a family is colour blind and heterozygous for tongue-rolling, while the father has normal colour vision and is a non-roller.

Which of the following statement(s) is / are correct?

1. More males than females in a population are red-green colour blind.
2. 50% of children will be non-rollers.
3. All the male children will be colour-blind.

A. 1 and 2 only        C. 2 only        E. 3 only
B. 1, 2 and 3          D. 2 and 3 only

## Question 8:
Make y the subject of the formula: $\frac{y+x}{x} = \frac{x}{a} + \frac{a}{x}$

A. $y = \frac{x^2}{a} + a$

B. $y = \frac{x^2+a^2-ax}{a}$

C. $y = \frac{-ax}{x^2+a^2}$

D. $y = \frac{x^2}{ax} + a - x$

E. $y = a^2 - ax$

**Question 9:**

What is the mass in grams of calcium chloride, $CaCl_2$, in 25cm³ of a solution with a concentration of 0.1 mol.l⁻¹? (Ar of Ca is 40 and Ar of Cl is 35)

A. 0.28g          B. 0.46g          C. 0.48g          D. 0.72g          E. 1.28g

**Question 10:**

Consider the equations: A: $y = 3x$ and B: $y = \frac{6}{x} - 7$. At what values of x do the two equations intersect?

A. x=2 and x=9          C. x=6 and x=27          E. x=18
B. x=3 and x=6          D. x=6

**Question 11:**

Which of the following statement(s) regarding the circulatory system is / are correct?

1. The pulmonary artery carries oxygenated blood from the right ventricle to the lungs.
2. The aorta has a high content of elastic tissue and carries oxygenated blood from the left ventricle around the body.
3. The mitral valve is between the pulmonary vein and the left atrium.
4. The vena cava carries deoxygenated blood from the body to the right atrium.

A. 1 and 3          B. 1 and 2          C. 2 only          D. 2 and 4          E. 3 only

**Question 12:**

A compound with a molar mass of 120 g.mol⁻¹ contains 12g of carbon, 2g of hydrogen and 16g oxygen. What is the molecular formula of the compound? (Ar C = 12, Ar H = 1, Ar O = 16).

A. $CH_2O$          B. $C_2H_4O_2$          C. $C_4H_2O$          D. $C_4H_8O_4$          E. $C_8H_{16}O_8$

**Question 13:**

Rupert plays one game of tennis and one game of squash.

The probability that he will win the tennis game is $\frac{3}{4}$

The probability that he will win the squash game is $\frac{1}{3}$

What is the probability that he will win one game only?

A. $\frac{3}{12}$          B. $\frac{7}{12}$          C. $\frac{4}{5}$          D. $\frac{13}{12}$          E. $\frac{7}{6}$

**Question 14:**

What is the median of the following numbers:

$\frac{7}{36}$ ; $0.\dot{3}$ ; $\frac{11}{18}$ ; $0.25$; $0.75$; $\frac{62}{72}$ ; $\frac{7}{7}$

A. $\frac{7}{36}$          B. $0.\dot{3}$          C. $\frac{11}{18}$          D. $\frac{62}{72}$          E. 0.75

**Question 15:**
16.4g of nitrobenzene is produced from 13g of benzene in excess nitric acid: $C_6H_6 + HNO_3 \rightarrow C_6H_5NO_2 + H_2O$

What is the percentage yield of nitrobenzene ($C_6H_5NO_2$)? (Ar C = 12, Ar N = 14, Ar H = 1, Ar O = 16)

A.  65%        B.  67%        C.  72%        D.  78%        E.  80%

**Question 16:**
Which of the following points regarding electromagnetic waves are correct?

1.  Radiowaves have the longest wavelength and the lowest frequency.
2.  Infrared radiation has a shorter wavelength than visible light and is used in optical fibre communication, and heater and night vision equipment.
3.  All of the waves from gamma to radio waves travel at the speed of light (about 300,000,000 m/s).
4.  Infrared radiation is used to sterilise food and to kill cancer cells.
5.  Darker skins absorb more UV light, so less ultraviolet radiation reaches the deeper tissues.

A.  1 and 2        B.  1 and 3        C.  1, 3 and 5        D.  2 and 3        E.  2 and 4

**Question 17:**
Two carriages of a train collide and then start moving together in the same direction. Carriage 1 has mass 12,000 kg and moves at 5ms⁻¹ before the collision. Carriage 2 has mass 8,000 kg and is stationary before the collision. What is the velocity of the two carriages after the collision?

A.  2 ms⁻¹        B.  3 ms⁻¹        C.  4 ms⁻¹        D.  4.5 ms⁻¹        E.  5 ms⁻¹

**Question 18:**
Which of the following statements are true?

1.  Control rods are used to absorb electrons in a nuclear reactor to control the chain reaction.
2.  Nuclear fusion is commonly used as an energy source.
3.  An alpha particle is comprised of two protons and two neutrons and is the same as a helium nucleus.
4.  When $^{14}_{6}C$ undergoes beta decay, an electron and $^{14}_{7}N$ are produced.
5.  Beta particles are less ionising than gamma rays and more ionising than alpha particles.

A.  1 and 2        C.  3 and 4        E.  None of the statements are true
B.  1 and 3        D.  3, 4 and 5

**Question 19:**
Simplify fully:  $\dfrac{(3x^{½})^3}{3x^2}$

A.  $\dfrac{3x}{\sqrt{x}}$        B.  $\dfrac{9}{x}$        C.  $3x^{½}$        D.  $3x\sqrt{x}$        E.  $\dfrac{9}{\sqrt{x}}$

**Question 20:**

Which of the following are true?

1. Lightning, as well as nitrogen-fixing bacteria, converts nitrogen gas to nitrate compounds.
2. Decomposers return nitrogen to the soil as ammonia.
3. The shells of marine animals contain calcium carbonate, which is derived from dietary carbon.
4. Nitrogen is used to make the amino acids found in proteins.

A. 1 only
B. 1 and 2

C. 2 and 3
D. 2, 3 and 4

E. They are all true

**Question 21:**

Write $\frac{\sqrt{20}-2}{\sqrt{5}+3}$ in the form: $p\sqrt{5} + q$

A. $2\sqrt{5} - 4$
B. $3\sqrt{5} - 4$
C. $3\sqrt{5} - 5$
D. $4\sqrt{5} - 6$
E. $5\sqrt{5} + 4$

**Question 22:**

Which of the following statements is / are false?

1. Simple molecules do not conduct electricity because there are no free electrons and there is no overall charge.
2. The carbon and silicon atoms in silica are arranged in a giant lattice structure and it has a very high melting point.
3. Ionic compounds do not conduct electricity when dissolved in water or when melted because the ions are too far apart.
4. Alloys are harder than pure metals.

A. 1 and 2
B. 1, 2 and 4

C. 1, 2, 3 and 4
D. 2 and 4

E. 3 only

**Question 23:**

The graph below shows a circle with radius 5 and centre (0,0).

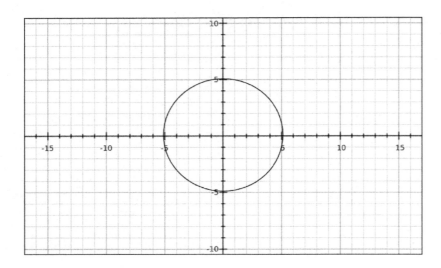

What are the values of x when the line $y = 3x - 5$ meets the circle?

A.  $x = 0$ or $x = 3$

B.  $x = 0$ or $x = 3.5$

C.  $x = 1$ or $x = 3.5$

D.  $x = 1.5$ or $x = -3$

E.  $x = 1.5$ or $x = -2$

**Question 24:**

Which if the following statements regarding heat transfer is / are correct?

1.  In liquids and gases, heat energy is transferred from hotter to colder places by conduction because particles in liquid and gases move more quickly when heated.
2.  Liquid and gas particles in hot areas are less dense than in cold areas.
3.  Heat transfer via radiation does not need particles to travel.
4.  Dull surfaces are good at absorbing and poor at reflecting infrared radiation, whereas shiny surfaces are poor at absorbing, but good at reflecting infrared radiation.

A.  1 and 2

B.  1, 2 and 4

C.  2 and 3

D.  2 and 4

E.  4 only

**Question 25:**

The following points refer to the halogens:

1.  Iodine is a grey solid and can be used to sterilise wounds. It forms a purple vapour when warmed.
2.  The melting and boiling points increase as you go up the group.
3.  Fluorine is very dangerous and reacts instantly with iron wool, whereas iodine must be strongly heated as well as the iron wool for a reaction to occur and the reaction is slow.
4.  When bromine is added to sodium chloride, the bromine displaces chlorine from sodium chloride.
5.  The hydrogen atom and chlorine atom in hydrogen chloride are joined by a covalent bond.

Which of the above statements is / are false?

A.  1, 3 and 5          C.  2 and 4          E.  3, 4 and 5
B.  1, 2 and 3          D.  3 only

**Question 26:**

Consider the triangle to the right where BE=4cm, EC=2cm and AC=9cm.

What is the length of side DE?

A.  4cm
B.  5.5cm
C.  6cm
D.  7.5cm
E.  8cm

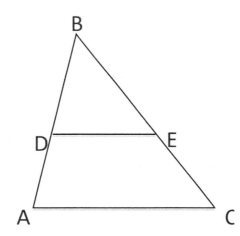

**Question 27:**

A ball is projected vertically upwards with an initial speed of 40 ms$^{-1}$. What is the maximum height reached? (Take gravity to be 10 ms$^{-2}$ and assume negligible air resistance).

A.  25m          B.  45m          C.  60m          D.  75m          E.  80m

**END OF SECTION**

# SECTION 3

1) *'The NHS should not treat obese patients'*

Explain what this statement means. Argue to the contrary, that we **should** treat obese patients. To what extent do you agree with this statement?

2) *'We should all become vegetarian'*

Explain what this statement means. Argue to the contrary, that we **should not** all become vegetarian. To what extent do you agree with this statement?

3) *'Certain vaccines should be mandatory'*

Explain what this statement means. Argue to the contrary, that vaccines **should not** be mandatory. To what extent do you agree with this statement?

4) *'Compassion is the most important quality of a healthcare professional'*

Explain what this statement means. Argue to the contrary, that there are more important qualities than compassion for health professionals. To what extent do you agree with this statement?

**END OF PAPER**

# ANSWER KEY

| | Paper A | | | | Paper B | | | | Paper C | | |
|---|---|---|---|---|---|---|---|---|---|---|---|
| Section 1 | | Section 2 | | Section 1 | | Section 2 | | Section 1 | | Section 2 | |
| 1 | C | 1 | B | 1 | A | 1 | D | 1 | D | 1 | D |
| 2 | D | 2 | D | 2 | C | 2 | E | 2 | D | 2 | C |
| 3 | B | 3 | A | 3 | C | 3 | E | 3 | B | 3 | C |
| 4 | D | 4 | E | 4 | D | 4 | E | 4 | B | 4 | C |
| 5 | D | 5 | D | 5 | D | 5 | D | 5 | B | 5 | C |
| 6 | B | 6 | B | 6 | B | 6 | A | 6 | C | 6 | E |
| 7 | A | 7 | D | 7 | D | 7 | A | 7 | D | 7 | B |
| 8 | D | 8 | E | 8 | C | 8 | D | 8 | D | 8 | B |
| 9 | C | 9 | D | 9 | B | 9 | A | 9 | A | 9 | A |
| 10 | E | 10 | C | 10 | A | 10 | D | 10 | C | 10 | A |
| 11 | A | 11 | B | 11 | E | 11 | A | 11 | D | 11 | D |
| 12 | D | 12 | E | 12 | D | 12 | B | 12 | D | 12 | D |
| 13 | B | 13 | D | 13 | E | 13 | C | 13 | E | 13 | F |
| 14 | C | 14 | C | 14 | C | 14 | A | 14 | A | 14 | C |
| 15 | D | 15 | B | 15 | B | 15 | D | 15 | E | 15 | E |
| 16 | D | 16 | A | 16 | E | 16 | D | 16 | C | 16 | C |
| 17 | D | 17 | E | 17 | E | 17 | C | 17 | E | 17 | B |
| 18 | B | 18 | B | 18 | D | 18 | D | 18 | E | 18 | C |
| 19 | B | 19 | C | 19 | A | 19 | D | 19 | B | 19 | E |
| 20 | D | 20 | A | 20 | B | 20 | E | 20 | A | 20 | E |
| 21 | E | 21 | C | 21 | B | 21 | E | 21 | A | 21 | A |
| 22 | B | 22 | B | 22 | B | 22 | E | 22 | B | 22 | E |
| 23 | C | 23 | C | 23 | D | 23 | E | 23 | C | 23 | A |
| 24 | C | 24 | B | 24 | C | 24 | D | 24 | B | 24 | D |
| 25 | B | 25 | A | 25 | B | 25 | D | 25 | C | 25 | C |
| 26 | B | 26 | B | 26 | E | 26 | B | 26 | A | 26 | C |
| 27 | C | 27 | C | 27 | E | 27 | C | 27 | E | 27 | E |
| 28 | C | | | 28 | C | | | 28 | C | | |
| 29 | B | | | 29 | A | | | 29 | C | | |
| 30 | E | | | 30 | D | | | 30 | B | | |
| 31 | D | | | 31 | D | | | 31 | B | | |
| 32 | A | | | 32 | C | | | 32 | D | | |

# RAW TO SCALED SCORES

| Section 1 | | | | | | | | | Section 2 | | | | | | | |
|---|---|---|---|---|---|---|---|---|---|---|---|---|---|---|---|---|
| 1 | 1 | 11 | 2.8 | 21 | 5.4 | 31 | 8.3 | | 1 | 1 | 11 | 3.5 | 21 | 6.6 |
| 2 | 1 | 12 | 3.0 | 22 | 5.7 | 32 | 9.0 | | 2 | 1 | 12 | 3.7 | 22 | 6.9 |
| 3 | 1 | 13 | 3.2 | 23 | 6.0 | | | | 3 | 1.3 | 13 | 4 | 23 | 7.3 |
| 4 | 1 | 14 | 3.5 | 24 | 6.3 | | | | 4 | 1.6 | 14 | 4.3 | 24 | 7.6 |
| 5 | 1.2 | 15 | 3.7 | 25 | 6.6 | | | | 5 | 1.9 | 15 | 4.6 | 25 | 8 |
| 6 | 1.5 | 16 | 4.0 | 26 | 6.9 | | | | 6 | 2.2 | 16 | 5 | 26 | 8.5 |
| 7 | 1.8 | 17 | 4.2 | 27 | 7.1 | | | | 7 | 2.5 | 17 | 5.3 | 27 | 9 |
| 8 | 2.0 | 18 | 4.5 | 28 | 7.4 | | | | 8 | 2.8 | 18 | 5.6 | | |
| 9 | 2.3 | 19 | 4.8 | 29 | 7.7 | | | | 9 | 3.0 | 19 | 5.9 | | |
| 10 | 2.5 | 20 | 5.1 | 30 | 8.0 | | | | 10 | 3.2 | 20 | 6.2 | | |

# MOCK PAPER A ANSWERS

## SECTION 1

**Question 1: C**
The simplest solution is to calculate the total area at the start as 20 x 20 = 400cm². Then recognise that with every fold the area will be reduced by half therefore the area will decrease as follows: 400, 200, 100, 50, 25, 12.5 – requiring a total of 5 folds.

**Question 2: D**
This is the correct option, as it is the only statement that doesn't categorically state a fact that was discussed in conditional tense in the paragraph.

**Question 3: B**
Of the 50% carrying the parasite 20% are symptomatic. Therefore 0.5 x 0.2 = 10% of the total population are infected and symptomatic. Of which 0.1 x 0.9 = 9% are male.

**Question 4: D**
The most important part of the question to note is the figure of 30% reduction during sale time. Although A and B are possible the question asks specifically regarding cost. Therefore, it is only worth waiting for the sale period if the sterling to euro exchange rate does not depreciate more than the magnitude of the sale. As such solution D is the only correct answer as it describes anticipating a loss in sterling value less than 30% against the euro.

**Question 5: D**
Begin by calculating the number of childminders that can be hired for a 24-hour period as 24 x 8.5 = 204. Therefore, a total of 4 childminders can be hired continually for 24 hours with £184 left over – as the question states the hire has to be for a whole 24-hour period and therefore the remainder £184 cannot be used. As such D is the correct answer of 4 x 4 = 16.

**Question 6: B**
The simplest way to approach this question is to recognise that there is a difference of £1.50 between peak and off-peak prices for all individuals except students.
The total savings can therefore be calculated as (3 + 5 + 1) x 1.5 = 9 x 1.5 = 13.5.

**Question 7: E**
**A – incorrect** – Karen is a musician, so she must play an instrument, but we do not know how many instruments she plays.
**B – incorrect** – although all oboe players are musicians, it does not mean all musicians play the oboe.
**C – incorrect** – although oboes and pianos are instruments, they are not necessarily the only instruments.
**D – incorrect** – Karen is a musician, but that merely means that she plays an instrument, we do not know if it is the oboe.
All of the possible answers A – D are incorrect, so option **E** is correct.

## Question 8: D

Answers A and B are simply incorrect as the measurement taken is a percentage increase (/decrease) which will normalise baseline diameters therefore allowing for comparison over multiple time points. You should be aware from your studies that ultrasound is an invaluable technique in distinguishing between adjacent tissue types. Any methodology is repeatable if it is correctly chronicled and followed therefore leaving the correct answer of D.

## Question 9: C

If both the flight and travel from the airport are delayed this will be the longest the journey could possible take – producing a total journey time of 20 + 15 + 150 + 20 + 25 = 230 minutes or 3 hours 50 minutes. Therefore, given all possible eventualities, to arrive at 5pm, boarding should begin at 13.10pm.

**A and B – incorrect** – use all of the 'best case scenarios' to work out this question! If she begins boarding at **1:40pm,** she will have finished boarding at **2:00pm.** Add 2.5hrs for the flight time and another 15 minutes for disembarking, to bring us to **4:45pm.** Assume there is no delay. Assume there is no traffic, so it takes 15 minutes to get from the airport to the meeting location. This means Megan could arrive at the meeting for **5:00pm.** This working proves **A** and **B** are both **incorrect.**

**D – incorrect** – a delayed plan would add 20 minutes to the journey whilst the transport to the meeting at the other end takes a minimum of 15 minutes – even if Megan could teleport instantaneously from the airport to the meeting, she would be 5 minutes later than if there wasn't a plane delay.

## Question 10: E

This is almost a trick question and simply an application of exponential decay. Recall that an exponential decay is asymptotic to 0 as no matter how small the volume within the cask becomes, only half of it is ever removed. It could be argued that this process cannot continue once a single molecule of whiskey is left – and when splitting that single molecule in half it is no longer whiskey. However, the question does not ask "how long till all the whiskey is gone" but rather "how many minutes will it take for the entire cask to be emptied" and therefore the process can continue infinitely – even if the only thing left in the cask is a collection of quarks … or half that.

## Question 11: A

As the largest digit on the number pad is 9, even if 9 was pressed for an infinitely long time the average for all of the numbers entered would still average out at no larger than 9! Therefore, it would be impossible to achieve a reference number larger than 9. Indeed, this is an extremely insecure safe but not for the reason described in B (for if the same incorrect number was pressed indefinitely, it would never average out as the correct one) but rather because the safe could in theory be opened with a single digit.

## Question 12: D

**A** is **incorrect** as it ignores the section of the text that states the evolution of resistant strains is driven by the presence of antibiotics themselves. The text states that the rate of bacterial reproduction is a large contributing factor and therefore not wholly responsible – hence **B** is **incorrect.** Since this is just one example (and only the information in the text should be considered for these questions) for C to make such a general statement is complete unjustified. Hence, **C** is **incorrect.**

## Question 13: B

The candidate must have won or come second to be in the second ballot.

**A, D** and **C – incorrect** – if they came third, they would not have been in the second ballot.

**E – incorrect** – we cannot know if the candidate won the election.

## Question 14: C

**A** and **D – incorrect** – poor orbit calculations do not disprove the existence of planet X.

**B – incorrect** – it is not certain whether planet X must exist or not.

**E – incorrect** – it does not follow from the evidence. C is the argument expressed in the conclusion.

## Question 15: D

This passage details drivers falling asleep behind the wheel and how this may be determined by the police in crash sites. It concludes that unlike drink driving offences where conclusive evidence can be drawn, it is difficult to determine if a driver had fallen asleep behind the wheel – D. A and B cannot be concluded from the passage. C is not an assumption made in the passage. E is not a conclusion.

## Question 16: D

This passage details the impact of mental exercises on health. It concludes that keeping mentally active delays dementia onset – **D** is **correct**.

**A** and **B** are not conclusions. **C** cannot be drawn from this passage. **E** cannot be concluded.

## Question 17: D

This argument discusses the cause of NDE in resuscitated patients.

**D – correct** – the conclusion drawn is that NDEs are not only caused by physical event.

**A – incorrect** – this is simply a fact that we are told in the passage, rather than a conclusion about the passage.

**B – incorrect** – again, this is simply a fact stated in the passage, not a conclusion.

**C – incorrect** – this is an explanation of what NDEs are, not a conclusion.

**E – incorrect** – this is neither a conclusion nor a correct explanation.

## Question 18: B

This argument discusses the role genes play in an individual's happiness experienced throughout life. The argument concludes that the idea that our potential for happiness in life is to some extent decided at birth – **B** is **correct**.

**A** is an argument but not a conclusion. **C, D** and **E** cannot be concluded – the argument does not imply that the person you are at birth is the person you will be throughout your life, but that one should accept the role genes have in one's happiness.

## Question 19: B

This argument seeks to explain the cause of delayed food delivery to rural regions during the Haiti earthquake. It concludes that great nations should be ashamed, and that they are to blame. The assumption is that the great nations' resources would have been faster and more efficient than local resources available – **B** is **correct**. **A** is not assumed, there is no mention of relief agencies. **C, D,** and **E** are not assumed.

**Question 20: D**
Due to the quantities colour t-shirts are priced at £5 and black and white at £2.50. Therefore, the order will incur a total cost of 50 + (50 x 5) + (200 x 2.5) = £800.

**Question 21: E**
**A – incorrect** – although the passage mentions the scouts promise, which include 'do (their) duty to God and to the Queen', this does not mean that scouts are working **for** the Queen.
**B – incorrect** – the scout network does give children the opportunity to embark upon adventure, but it is also to give them the opportunity to 'engage in the understanding and teaching of foreign culture'.
**C – incorrect** – this information is not mentioned in the passage, so it cannot be inferred from the passage.
**D – incorrect** – there is no mention of having to be religious to join the scouts, it merely informs us that religion traditionally formed the backbone of the scouting movement.

We cannot reliably conclude from the passage that any of the statements A-D apply to the scout movement, thus **E** is the **correct** answer.

**Question 22: B**
There are two directions: clockwise and anticlockwise and rats will only collide if they pick opposing directions.
Rat A - clockwise, Rat B - clockwise, Rat C - clockwise = 0.5 x 0.5 x 0.5 = 0.125.
Rat A - anticlockwise, Rat B - anticlockwise, Rat C - anticlockwise = 0.5 x 0.5 x 0.5 = 0.125.
0.125 + 0.125 = 0.25. So, the probability they do **not** collide is 0.25, and the probability that they do collide is 0.75. They are more likely to collide than not, so option **B** is **correct.**

**Question 23: C**
The article seen here is a particularly good effort at a discursive text as it is completely impartial. Note that the article simply states the facts from either side in equal measure. Nowhere does the author present their opinion on the matter nor do they insinuate their beliefs in anyway.

**Question 24: C**
The journey time is rounded to the nearest hour (13). Therefore, the longest it could possibly be is 13 hours 29 minutes or it would be round up to 8 hours. Therefore, the latest the ferry will arrive, assuming the travel time estimate is accurate, is given as 20.29.
If it were 13 hours 30 minutes, this would be rounded **up** to the nearest hour, which would give 14 hours, i.e. 21:00 arrival.

**Question 25: C**
The correct answer is 19.
Assume, although very unlikely, that you roll a 5 every single go – you would actually be moving further forwards than if you were roll a 6 every single go, as you would move forward-forward-back-forward-forward, while if rolling a 6 you would have to move back once more. Therefore, rolling a lower number (5) in this case is beneficial, as you move 3 forward on each roll.
Moving forwards 3 each time → 55/3. 54/3 = 18, so $55/3 = 18\frac{1}{3}$, which needs to be rounded up to 19 rolls.

**Question 26: B**
The LCM of 40 and 60 = 120 seconds. The LCM of 120 and 70 = 840 seconds.

840 seconds = 14 minutes, so every 14 minutes, each of the 3 cars crosses the start line again. Since they started 4 minutes ago, they will all cross the start line simultaneously in 10 minutes.

## Question 27: C

A large amount of subtly different data is described here. Of note is the first experiment which describes how nerve conduction is faster in right-handed men than it is in left-handed men. This result is not transferable to women until it is proven! The experiment currently being conducted only considers dominant hand in men vs. women. That could be either hand or not necessarily the females' right hand. For example, all of the females in this experiment could have been left-handed and there is no information in the text to say otherwise, therefore we cannot tell.

## Question 28: C

Recognise that two square based pyramids will comprise 8 triangles of base width 5 and height 8; plus, two 5 x 5 squares. Thus, giving a total area of 8(8/2 x 5) + 2(5 x 5) = 210 cm²

## Question 29: B

In order to approach this question first realise that in the first well 1ml of solvent is being combined with 9ml of distilled water producing 1eq of solute in 10ml – hence the first well produces a dilution by a factor of 10. With each progressive dilution the concentration is reduced by a further factor of 10 – hence by well 10 the concentration is at $x/10^{10}$

## Question 30: E

The compartments of the human body are occupied by numerous fluids, as the student is only interested in measuring the volume of blood, it is essential he chooses a solute that will only dissolve in blood. So as his known quantity of solute remains no, it must be neither removed nor added during its time in the body. Hence all of the written assumptions must be made and many more.

## Question 31: D

The fastest way to approach this question is by calculating the total price per head for the cheapest option as 10 + (8/20) + (10/60) = 10.567. To make the maths simpler this can be rounded safely to £11 a head at this stage. 2,300/11 is approximately equal to 209 which when rounded to the nearest 10 is 210 people.

## Question 32: A

Whilst this passage is attempting to weigh up two sides of an argument, it has a clear one-sided approach focussing heavily on the excitement of dangerous sports. It even states that hunting is recognised as exciting by some. Since the previous sentence discussed the link between archery and hunting, the statement is a fair extrapolation to make.

**END OF SECTION**

# SECTION 2

### Question 1: B

Let tail = T, body and legs = B and head = H.

As described in the question H = T + 0.5B and B = T + H.

We have already been told that T = 30Kg.

Therefore, substitute the second equation into the first as H = 30 + 0.5(30 + H).

Re-arranging reveals that -0.5H = 45Kg and therefore the weight of the head is 90Kg, the body and legs 120Kg and as we were told the tail weighs 30Kg. Thus, giving a total weight of 240Kg

### Question 2: D

Recall that kinetic energy can be calculated as $E = 0.5mv^2$. Therefore, if mass remains constant it is the $v^2$ term that must be reduced to a sixteenth. In other words, $v^2 = 1/16$ and therefore the correct velocity is $1/4x$.

### Question 3: A

An organ is defined as comprising multiple tissue types. As blood and skeletal muscle are themselves tissues they cannot be classified as organs.

### Question 4: E

This question is best considered in terms of the aerobic respiration equation. With that in mind it becomes apparent that increased forward drive through the reaction will produce large amounts of water and $CO_2$ whilst demanding an increased supply of $O_2$. Further from this equation we realise that aerobic respiration produces large amounts of heat, and as such it is expected – in the interest of thermoregulation – that the body will both perspire and vasodilate in attempt to increase heat loss. Therefore, E is the correct answer.

### Question 5: D

Recall that the nephron is the smallest functional unit of the kidney. The question therefore is asking you what is the smallest basic functional unit of striated muscle? To which the answer is the sarcomere. Note that a myofibril is a collection of many sarcomeres and is therefore not the correct answer.

### Question 6: B

Insulin is a polypeptide hormone released by the pancreas in response to elevated plasma glucose levels. Therefore, it can be expected that plasma glucose concentration will be proportional to the concentration of insulin in the blood. Furthermore, recall that glucagon also released by the pancreas mobilises glucose stores. Therefore, the greatest concentration of plasma glucose would be expected at the time when glucagon is highest during a period of elevated insulin.

### Question 7: D

Answers A and C are both nonsense and can be eliminated straight away. You will know from your study of the immune system that it is plasma B cells that produce antibodies and that plasma T cells do not exist. Also recall that an immune response can be mounted as quickly as within a fortnight which leaves the only correct answer, D. The passage states that only once blood types are mixed is the immune response initiated, therefore answer D provides an explanation as to how this happens but also why the first-born child is unaffected.

**Question 8: E**

Urea, glucose, sodium and water are all present in the Bowman's capsule, as they can cross the endothelial cells and glomerular basement membrane, to enter the Bowman's capsule.

Haemoglobin is found in red blood cells, and these are too large to pass the endothelial cells and glomerular basement membrane, so are not found in the Bowman's capsule (unless in diseased patients!).

**Question 9: D**

An organ consists of many cell types which once differentiated are committed to that single cell line. Therefore, a totipotent stem cell is required to produce the multiple cell types required. In order to ensure that the organ is an exact genetic match, stem cells from the individual in question must be used. Unless that individual is an embryo, adult stem cells must be used.

**Question 10: E**

1 – correct – energy increases with frequency and consequently decreases with wavelength, so waves with the shortest wavelengths transfer the most energy.

2 – incorrect – for waves, $v = f \times \lambda$, and the speed is the constant for this relationship. Frequency and wavelength are inversely proportional.

3 – correct – microwaves get absorbed by water molecules and can cause heating of human tissue (remember, humans are 60-70% water!).

**Question 11: B**

The transition metals are the most abundant catalysts – presumably due to their ability to achieve a variable number of stable states. Therefore, the correct answer is the d-block elements.

**Question 12: E**

Begin by writing down the balanced equation that describes the reaction of francium with water: $2Fr + 2H_2O \rightarrow 2FrOH + H_2$. Next calculate the moles of francium entering the reaction as 1338/223 = 6. We therefore know from the stoichiometry of the equation that this reaction will produce 3 moles of hydrogen. Recall that 1 mole of gas at room temperature and pressure occupies $24dm^3$. Therefore, the hydrogen produced in this reaction will occupy $3 \times 24 = 72dm^3$.

**Question 13: C**

This question is likely to be easiest to answer by going through all of the options available.

**A – incorrect** – mass of C = 12, mass of H = 2, mass of O = 16 – we can see immediately that this is not correct as the mass of O is greater than the mass of C, which is not reflected by the composition by ass (53% C, 36% H).

**B – incorrect** – mass of C = 24, mass of H = 6, mass of O = 32 – again, we can see immediately that the mass of O exceeds the mass of C, so we can rule this option out.

**C – correct** – mass of C = 24, mass of H = 6, mass of O = 16. In the composition, mass of O is roughly 3 times that of H, which is reflected in the composition by mass ($11 \times 3 \approx 36$). Additionally, the mass of C is 1.5 times the mass of O, which is reflected in the composition by mass ($36 \times 1.5 \approx 53$). Thus, this is the correct answer!

**D – incorrect** – mass of C = 12, mass of H = 1, mass of O = 16 – the mass of O exceeds the mass of C, so we can rule this option out.

**E – incorrect** – mass of C = 36, mass of H = 5, mass of O = 32. The mass of C is roughly 7 times (35/5) the mass of H in this compound, which is not reflected in the composition by mass, where the mass of C is roughly

5 times the mass of H. Also, the masses of O and C are too similar in this option. So, we can rule this option out.

### Question 14: A

This question requires you to have a correct answer from the previous question, although these questions are unfair in the fact that this current question cannot be answered without success in the first part – there are always one or two of these per paper.

Simply calculate the Mr of your empirical formula: $2(12) + 5(1) + 1(16) = 24 + 5 + 16 = 45$.

Then divide the Mr of the compound by the Mr of the empirical formula $= 45 / 45 = 1$.

So, the empirical formula is equal to the Mr of the compound – so the actual molecular formula is also $C_2H_6O$.

### Question 15: B

The calculation in this question is simple: concentration = mass/volume, what this question is really testing is the manipulation of unorthodox units. Begin by noting the use of g/dL in the final answers and therefore begin by converting the quantities in the question into these units. $1.2 \times 10^{10}$ kg $= 1.2 \times 10^{13}$ grams and with 10 decilitres in a litre, $4 \times 10^{12}$ L $= 4 \times 10^{13}$ dL. $\frac{(1.2 \times 10^{13})}{(4 \times 10^{13})} = 3 \times 10^{-1}$ g/dL.

### Question 16: A

**A – correct** – a catalyst is not essential for the progression of a chemical reaction, it only acts to lower the activation energy and therefore increase the likelihood and rate of reaction.

**B – incorrect** – in exothermic reactions, H is negative, and S (entropy) is positive, so there is an increase in entropy (disorder). So, an increase in entropy **is essential** for the progression of an exothermic reaction.

**C – incorrect** – the activation energy is the minimum energy required for a reaction to occur, therefore achieving activation energy **is essential** for the progression of an exothermic chemical reaction.

**D – incorrect** – the electron configuration of noble gases is the most stable, so exothermic reactions, which have more stable products than reactants, do attain an electron configuration that more closely resembles that of a noble gas.

**E – incorrect** – as A is correct.

### Question 17: C

Chloride and fluoride **ions** are used in the treatment of drinking water – so **C** is **correct**.

### Question 18: B

Recall that V = E/Q; therefore, when substituting SI units into these equations it is discovered that:
$V = J/C = JC^{-1}$.

### Question 19: C

Recall that voltmeters are always connected in parallel – and so that they don't draw any current from the circuit have an infinite resistance. Ammeters on the other hand are connected in series and therefore must not perturb the flow of given, meaning they have zero resistance.

### Question 20: A

Much of the information in this question is not needed and is simply put there to distract you. This question can be most quickly solved using the equation F=ma or force = mass x acceleration. As object A is the only things moving in this scenario it is the only source of energy to be considered. Its mass will be the same before and after the collision and so we need only calculate the magnitude of retardation. Given as $(15 - 3)/0.5 = 24ms^{-2}$. Therefore, when plugging into the first equation we realise that $F = 12 \times 24 = 288N$ of force dissipated. Alternatively, this question could be solved by calculating the rate of change of momentum.

## Question 21: C

Note the atomic masses and numbers in the equation. Whilst the atomic mass has remained constant the atomic number has increased by one and hence the element has changed. The only explanation for this is that a neutron has turned into a proton (and an electron which is represented by $x$). Therefore, the correct answer is C – beta radioactive decay.

## Question 22: B

Begin by calculating the velocity of the wave as speed = wavelength x frequency = $3 \times 20 = 60km/s$. Which in a time period of one hour (3600s) would equate to a total distance of $60 \times 3600 = 216,000km$.

## Question 23: C

The numerator of the fraction consists of 3 distinct terms or 3 distinct dimensions. As all other functions within the equation are constants one would consider this the volume of a complex 3D shape.

## Question 24: B

$4.2 \times 10^{10} = 42,000,000,000$

$4.2 \times 10^{6} = 4,200,000$

Now we have a simple subtraction: $42,000,000,000 - 4,200,000 = 41,995,800,000$

## Question 25: A

Note the triangle formed by the right-angle lines and the tangent. Recall that as this is a right-angle triangle then the other two angles must be 45°. As angles along a straight line add up to 180° a must equal $180 - 45 = 135°$. Angles around the origin must add up to 360° and therefore b = $(360 - 90)/2 = 135°$. Therefore, the correct answer is A.

## Question 26: C

The probability of drawing a blue ball (1/21) and then a black ball (1/20) is $1/21 \times 1/20 = 1/420$. However, note that it is also possible that these balls could also be drawn out in the opposite order, which has a probability of $1/21 \times 1/20 = 1/420$.

Therefore, using the *or* rule of probability, we add the 2 probabilities to give us 2/420. This simplifies to 1/210.

## Question 27: C

The question states that the repeat experiment is identical to the first in all aspects apart from the result. Therefore, although a number of the options may be true like calibration bias, it would have been applied to both experiments and therefore should not affect the result. As such the difference in results is simply due to random chance.

**END OF SECTION**

# SECTION 3

*Doctors should wear white coats, as it helps to create a placebo effect, rendering the treatment more effective.*

- This statement addresses the role of the patient's personal experience in his/her cure or treatment of their disease. It is an interesting topic since the role of psychological factors in the treatment of disease is largely unexplored. There is a growing body of evidence that supports the effectiveness of placebo treatments for some diseases when it comes to managing patient symptoms, but there is very little that addresses the role of attire and visual appearance of doctors.

- It is also important to immediately question the truth of the statement. There is some evidence to suggest that there is such a thing as a "white coat effect" that influences patient's behaviour and the perception of their problems when they are faced with a doctor. Questioning the statement is very important as it demonstrates that you reflect on the issue.

- When answering this question, there are several factors to consider. There is the role that clothing plays in the definition of professions. How does the attire of an individual influence the way he or she is perceived by those receiving his/her service? Some examples here are police officers or judges where the uniforms are heavily tied to the public perception of their profession. Police officers are a particularly good non-medical example, since there are uniformed and non-uniformed officers that play different roles playing on the different public perception of uniform and civilian clothing and the fact that without the uniform the police officer is not recognisable. Then the question arises if this should apply for doctors too. Does it make a difference if doctors have clothing that visually separate them from other people in the hospital and does this have an influence on the patient's experience of treatment. Other points to consider when addressing the role of attire is the depiction of doctors in the public sphere. This includes TV shows, books, news etc.

- Arguing against the statement is more difficult than it seems simply because you should make sure that you provide a diverse answer that addresses several aspects. On one hand, there is the connection of a specific attire to a specific professional role as described above. On the other hand, there is the question whether attire is relevant to influence the patient's experience to improve health outcome. The whole point of a placebo effect in this context is that it improves the outcome.

- Another point to consider when arguing against this statement is the power distribution that comes with the uniforms and whether that is something that is beneficial for the patient-doctor relationship.

- Arguing to the contrary, you can look at situations where a professionalization of the doctor-patient relationship can be beneficial. Now, to be clear, the relationship between doctor and patients should always be professional, but in the context of this question, you can use the role of attire and its role in establishing this professionalization. Examples for this include conversations about life-style changes and the role the patient can play in improving his/her own health, especially if this involves giving something up. In this case, attire can give the doctor legitimacy and a certain degree of authority.

*"Medicine is a science of uncertainty and an art of probability."*

- This statement addresses the fact that there is no such thing as certainty in medicine. People are different and individual and so is their experience of disease. For this reason, the statement argues that all a doctor can do in terms of approaching a sense of certainty, the doctor should weigh up different probabilities and possibilities of disease. The argument also suggests that weighing up the different options of diagnoses is an art, rather than acquired knowledge. This suggests some degree of natural talent. It also provides a degree of contrast between the aspect of science that provides the theoretical basis for pretty much every decision we make in medicine and the art of the application of knowledge. It also acknowledges that science always contains a degree of uncertainty, even when individuals believe in the absolute truth of their theory/ knowledge.

- Arguing to the contrary basically aims at increasing the perceived role of science and certainty versus that of art and uncertainty or flexibility. The main problem with this statement is the general perception associated with the words "science" and art. They naturally lie on different ends of a spectrum with science being associated with facts and certainty and art being associated with softer skills and an absence of certainty.

- If you choose to go into a more example-oriented direction, there are several points you can raise to write a good and strong essay. One example is the treatment of infectious diseases with antibiotics, especially in severe cases. Often you will find that the disease is treated with a broad-spectrum antibiotic that is likely to target the causative agent based on local experiences and local occurrence of diseases. This is then later adjusted, if necessary, once a precise identification of the causative agent was possible. Other examples include the stratification of disease causes. One example here is smoking and lung cancer. Whilst it is generally accepted that smoking increases the risk of lung cancer, there are still non-smokers that get lung cancer and life-time smokers that do not. This pattern can be applied to a variety of parameters to result in similar results.

- In general, you can keep this essay very philosophical and abstract, or you can aim more at direct examples to illustrate your points. Both options have strengths and weaknesses. A theoretical essay will stay more with the overall style of the statement, whilst a more example-oriented essay will be easier to write and to keep track of. However, it will also be more difficult to find appropriate examples.

- In the conclusion, when you give your opinion, it pays to be very direct on one hand, but also to be very specific. Depending on which route you took for your main body arguments, this may be easier or more difficult. You can also pick up the idea of medicine being art again as this is an interesting point and ties in with the idea that medicine cannot be exclusively learned from books but should also contain a component of patient interaction.

*"The New England Journal of Medicine reports that 9 out of 10 doctors agree that 1 out of 10 doctors is an idiot."*

- This statement addresses how scientific research will never find complete acceptance in the field. It also suggests that no matter what is being published by even the most highly acclaimed scientific journals, there is always a risk of error. In the end, it illustrates that medical research usually is a game of probabilities as there is never complete certainty when it comes to the pattern of diseases or the optimal treatment of disease.

- On a face value level, this question is simple. It is very vague in its assertion, not defining which one of the 10 doctors think that the other is an idiot. Do they all think the same person is an idiot or do they think different persons are idiots? This an important issue to raise when answering this question as it presents a fundamental flaw of the question, especially if one is to apply it to general medical research and research practice. Even in the sometimes uncertain realm of medical research, parameters such as populations of subjects are always clearly defined, which is what gives any form of research value. If this was not the case, research would be completely arbitrary. Coming back to the question then, if all 9 doctors believe that that the one specific one of them is an idiot and they have no prior contact and no connection to each other, then chances are that this single doctor is actually an idiot. If, however, there is no pattern whatsoever to the claim that one doctor is an idiot, then that weakens the claim. Especially if the whole concept is then widened to a population level.

- Arguing to the contrary has different obvious points. You can either stay very close to the actual wording of the question which will lead you down a similar road as I have illustrated above, or you can use the question as a parable for the way we conduct scientific research. This will require you to have a good understanding of scientific method.

- If you decide to go down the scientific method pathway, you will have several things to point of. Firstly, is the definition of populations, as this is completely ignored in the question. In any form of research defining the pool of data you draw from is essential as only this will deliver accurate and usable information. It is all about reducing vagueness as much as possible. Secondly you need to define the research criteria. What exactly is meant by an idiot in this case for example? Only if you formulate a clear-cut goal can you then acquire the data needed to come to a meaningful result. The term 'asking the right questions' comes to mind. Thirdly you need to ensure repeatability. For this you need to define your populations very broadly and in appropriate sizes. You must make sure that there is as little connection between the subjects as possible as this will reduce and bias from personal relationships.

- These two options should help you write a strong essay, especially since they can be combined in essentially any way you choose to create a unique argument.

*"My father was a research scientist in tropical medicine, so I always assumed I would be a scientist, too. I felt that medicine was too vague and inexact, so I chose physics."*

- There are several components to this question that you need to be aware of if you want to write a good essay. On one hand is the person Stephen Hawking himself. Being a world-renowned theoretical physicist, gives the whole quote an almost comical note. This is something you should be aware of, as you will always have to point out problems with the questions. Moving beyond this, there are several other points you should be aware of. One is the vagueness of the statement. This obviously is due to the fact that it is taken from what probably was a whole speech, rather than this single passage. Again, something you should point out. Then there is the subject matter of tropical medicine. Tropical medicine is in part still a very new field and a field which much room for exploration simply because there is such a wealth of different life forms in tropical areas that can cause diseases, some of which may never have been observed before. This necessarily adds to the perceived uncertainty. In addition, keep in mind that Stephen Hawking is now 75 years old, which places his father's professional career to the first half of the 20th century, a lot has happened in medicine since then. Secondly you should address the subject matter of physics. Whilst some fields in physics have very little uncertainty and vagueness, a lot of areas are very precise such as gravity or mechanics. So, it is important to make that distinction as physics is such a broad topic.

- When it comes to arguing to the contrary, there are several perspectives you can take. On one hand, you can argue that tropical medicine is more accurate than Hawking gives it credit for. An easy way to do this is to enlarge it to general medicine as the clear majority of general medical principles will still apply in tropical medicine, what will change will be different pathogens and the environmental factors influencing pathology and healing processes. If we accept that in general medicine is a fairly exact science, we can use that to support the same claims about tropical medicine.

- Another point of attack would be to point out the vagueness of some areas of physics. Easy targets here are String theory and the theory of relativity. Neither of those can be supported by non-mathematical evidence at this point and even the potential discovery of the Higgs boson in the Cern super collider does not provide enough answers to these questions yet. There are many other examples in the field of physics that are vague, that's why they have given rise to completely separate job description: the theoretical physicist.

- Finally, you can also consider Hawking's personal history with medicine. His suffering from ALS for decades and being bound to a wheelchair after far outliving any suggested life expectancy it is understandable that he considers medicine as somewhat vague. This could well have influenced him in this statement.

**END OF PAPER**

# MOCK PAPER B ANSWERS

## SECTION 1

### Question 1: A
If society disagrees that vaccinations should be compulsory, then they will not fund them. So, statement **A** is **correct**. It attacks the conclusion.
Statement B - society does not necessarily mean local so this does not address the argument.
Statement C strengthens, not weakens, the argument for vaccinations.
Statement D – the desires of healthcare workers do not affect whether vaccinations are necessary.

### Question 2: C
Start by calculating the area of wall that may be painted per tin of paint as $10 \times 5 = 50m^2$. Therefore, to paint the whole area $1050/50 = 21$ tins of paint are required per coat. As such to complete 3 coats it will cost Josh $3 \times 21 \times 4.99 = 314.37$.

### Question 3: C
A is a correct assumption as procession is a function of rotational motion. B is a necessary assumption or rather inference of the first sentence. The second sentence only says that an asterism can be used, not that it is the only possible method. Nothing is mentioned of navigating the Southern Hemisphere and therefore C is not a valid assumption.

### Question 4: D
Recognise that "bank hours" refers only to hours that the bank is open – which Mon to Fri is 8 hours whereas it is only 6 hours on a Saturday. Although John needs the money by 8pm the bank closes at 5 and that 3 hours difference cannot be used. Hence working backwards John will need 8 hours on the Tuesday, 8 hours on the Monday, Sunday is closed, 6 hours on the Saturday, 8 hours on Friday and 8 hours on Thursday and 4 hours on the Wednesday. With a closing time of 5pm, the latest John can cash the cheque on Wednesday is 1pm.

### Question 5: D
First thing to recognise here of course is that individual diamonds can be combined to form larger diamonds with the 5 x 5 diamond the biggest of them all. To avoid counting them all and risking losing count, instead deduced the number of triangles per corner and per side; then multiply up by 4.

### Question 6: B
Let my current age = m and my brother's current age = g. The first section of this question can therefore be expressed as $m + 4 = 1/3(g + 1)$ whereas the second half can be represented as $2(m + 20) = g + 20$. Therefore, this problem can be solved as simultaneous equations. Rearranged the second equation reads $m = 1/2g - 10$; when substituted into the first equation we form $1/2g – 10 + 4 = 1/3(g + 1)$. Expand and simplify to $1/2g – 6 = 1/3g + 1/3 \rightarrow 1/6g = 6\frac{1}{3}$ which therefore means my brother's current age $= 6\frac{1}{3} / (1/6) = 114/3 = 38$. Which means that my current age $= 1/2(38) – 10 = 9$.

## Question 7: D

A is categorically wrong as the first two paragraphs discuss how aneurysms produce inflammation which in turn blunts endothelial NO action. B is incorrect as it states aneurysms directly promote CVD, this is not a direct process. It is the blunted NO which directly produces the CVD. C can be ignored as nowhere are aneurysms categorised like this. E is incorrect as the text states that aneurysms reduce NO which will reduce vasodilatation, thus increasing basal vasoconstriction and thus reducing blood flow. Leaving the correct answer of D which is of course true as observations are not transferable between species until tested scientifically.

## Question 8: C

Any statement which refers to national or global figures is instantly incorrect, as the text does not mention any statistical analysis has taken place. In order to produce national statistics from a small sample size such as this requires statistical analysis. Thus, we can rule out **A** and **D**.

Whilst **E** could possibly be true it cannot be stated as there are so many possibilities – perhaps the time of the survey was during rush hour in which case the majority of the traffic would have been travelling in the same direction anyway to reach an industrialised area.

**C** is **correct** – we are told that red is the most common colour seen, and green is the least common. Thus, we can infer from the passage that green vehicles are less popular in the area surveyed.

## Question 9: B

The runners aren't apart at a constant distance; they get further apart as they run. Xavier and Yolanda are less than 20m apart at the time William finishes.

Each runner beats the next runner by the same distance, so they must have the same difference between speeds. When William finishes at 100m and Xavier is at 80m. When Xavier crosses the finish line then Yolanda is at 80m. We need to know where Yolanda is when Xavier is at 80m. William's speed = distance/time = 100/T. Xavier's speed = 80/T. So, Xavier has 80% of William's speed. This makes Yolanda's speed 80% of Xavier's and 64% (80% x 80% = 64%) of William's. So, Yolanda is at 64m when William finishes. 100m - 64m = 36m, thus William beats Yolanda by 36m.

## Question 10: A

First, convert to metres and find the volume of the television → $1.5 \times 1 \times 0.1 = 0.15m^3$
The ratio of the volume of the television to the volume of the box is 1:1.6
So, multiply $0.15m^3$ by 1.6, to give $0.24m^3$.
Subtract → $0.24m^3 - 0.15m^3 = 0.09m^3$ = option A.

## Question 11: E

From the information provided all the flaws listed are valid since David's main point is that he has chosen the cheapest. A could be true as there is an additional cost of £3 for staying at Whitmore, therefore if the vehicle they are using achieves sufficient miles per gallon, then travelling the extra few miles could cost less than £3 in terms of petrol. B again is possible which would argue against it being cheap, as would D. And if C is true then David's argument is flawed altogether.

## Question 12: D

C is irrelevant as nowhere does the passage mention standards of modern medical practice. A may be incorrect as nowhere does the article explicitly say that animal testing is the only accepted method of drug approval. B categorically conflicts with the first sentence of the second paragraph.

## Question 13: E

E is the non-flawed argument; it is obvious that aptitude may be motivational. A and B are subjective beliefs which do not prove anything about the people in question. C and D highlight the limited scope of the study.

## Question 14: C

A-It does not matter which transport is improved. B- Explaining the counter argument is not necessary to prove the point. D and E need not be mentioned, as the argument does not concern these things. C- We do not know how many people were surveyed, only that they experienced congestion.

## Question 15: B

First, calculate the cost of making 100 burgers and 50 hotdogs → $(2.50 \times 100) + (1.50 \times 50)$
$= 250 + 75 = £325$.
Next, calculate the money made from selling 80 burgers and 35 hotdogs at full price:
$(80 \times 8) + (35 \times 6) = 640 + 210 = £850$
Now, calculate the money made from selling 18 burgers and 12 hotdogs at half price:
$(18 \times 4) + (12 \times 3) = 72 + 36 = £108$

Total profit $= 850 + 108 - 325 = £633$

## Question 16: E

First calculate an average complete one-way journey time as $40 + 5 + 5 = 50$ minutes. Deducting his breaks, he works a total of 7 hours 20 or 440 minutes. Since the first train is already loaded his first run will only take 45 minutes leaving 395 minutes to complete his working day. $395/50 = 7$ remainder 45. Note that 45 minutes is not enough to fully unload the train, but it is enough to load the train and drive the distance. Therefore, the driver will complete a total of 9 journeys equalling a distance of 198 miles.

## Question 17: E

A is not actually a valid assumption as we do not know what proposal conservationists might be bringing to the local councils, they have only expressed their concern. They may well be bringing a proposal to ask for funding to rehome all the species in the affected environment. B is essential to the final paragraph whilst C must be assumed otherwise the councils would not be presenting these proposals at all.

## Question 18: D

As there is not really information in the question to calculate the answer quickly. Instead consider each answer in term and calculate the differences to find the correct price difference in the question:
$(3x\ 1) + (2 \times 1.25) - (15 \times 0.3) + (10 \times 0.5)$ etc...

## Question 19: A

$1L = 1000$ cubic centimetres and therefore the total volume of air Laura needs to produce is $25 \times 0.3 = 7.5L$. With a total of 25 balloons, she will take $25 \times 0.5 = 12.5$ seconds breathing in and a further $7.5/4.5 = 1\frac{2}{3}$ minutes inflating the balloons. This yields a total time of 1 minute $40 + 12.5$ seconds $= 1$ minute 52.5 seconds or 112.5 seconds.

## Question 20: B

Quickly represent the question schematically as $(A = B) \neq (C = D = E)$. We can now observe that A in fact supports George's argument, C also supports George's argument and D may well be true, but it would have no effect in disrupting the argument, it would only imply D and E are both also equal to 0. However, as E is equal to C it should therefore not equal B. So, statement **B** would most weaken George's argument.

**Question 21: B**

This question is much less complicated than it sounds. Begin by just considering a single hour. Throughout the hour of 1 the hour hand will be pointing at 1. Only during the 5th minute of that hour will the minute hand point to the 1 whereas every 5th second of the minute the second-hand points to the 1. All these events will only coincide once. As there are 24 hours in a day 00:00 through to 23:59 this event will happen 24 times.

**Question 22: B**

A) Potentially correct, but extreme sports also carry higher risks of injury.

B) True.

C) True, but irrelevant for the question.

D) Potentially correct, but irrelevant to the question.

**Question 23: D**

A) False – we are not told about the healthcare directly but are told that injury and disease posed a threat.

B) False – the terrain was difficult, and mapping was poor.

C) False – outlaws were a significant threat.

D) True – as the text states, there was a marked lack of bridges.

**Question 24: C**

Whilst B may be true it is not a reason for dependence, only a supporting factor. Dependence implies that we have no choice but to use electricity. Hence A is wrong as gas is readily available; hence D is wrong for the same reason. This leaves the correct answer of C which is the only statement which truly describes our absolute necessity for electricity – since electrical appliances by definition only function with electricity.

**Question 25: B**

First note that 27 guests plus Elin herself means that 28 people will be eating the 3 courses which will require a total of 28 x 3 = 84 glasses of wine. This is a total volume of 84 x 175 = 14.7L = 21 bottles. As wine is only sold in cases of 6, Elin will have to buy 24 bottles so as not to run out. Recall the buy one get one free offer so she only pays for 2 cases.

**Question 26: A**

Recognise that when rounded to the nearest 10 the shortest an episode could last is 35 minutes. Hence a total of 7 x 12 = 84 episodes would take a total of 84 x 35 = 2,940 minutes = 49 hours.

**Question 27: E**

Points A and B are the best exemplified through this passage. Often great discoveries come from accidental observations and then exact processes are refined through many experiments in a trial-and-error fashion until the correct methodology is achieved. The passage demonstrates how as our understanding of the world around us advance so too does our ability to provide healthcare. D can be observed in the passage as the 50/50 split.

**Question 28: C**

Whilst A and D are true, they do not force the stranger to give him the sapphire – remember Jack can be given any stone for a truthful statement. B and C are both lies and will earn Jack nothing. Instead, if Jack states E, then the stranger has no choice to hand over the sapphire else it would be a false statement.

## Question 29: A

Despite the enormous interest rate in Simon's current account, it is only awarded twice, whereas in the saver account it is awarded 4 times. Hence earnings from the saver account = $100 \times 1.5^4$ = £506 whereas earnings from the current account would have stood at £361.

## Question 30: D

The largest possible key can be obtained where the first two numbers are at a maximum because they are multiplied together → $9 \times 9 = 81$. Subtract the smallest number to yield $81 - 1 = 80$ and again divide by the smallest number which is 1 hence 80 is the largest possible key.

## Question 31: D

A) Incorrect. The text clearly states that the exercise routine is resistance training based.
B) False. Both groups contain equal numbers of men and women per the text.
C) False. Both groups are age matched in the range of 20 to 25 years.
D) Correct. As the only difference between the two shakes is the protein content.

## Question 32: C

The information provided about the child needs to be inserted into the BMI formula: $BMI = 35 \div 1.2^2$
1.2 squared is equal to 1.44 and it may be easier to work out 3500 divided by 144.
Alternatively, you could rule out the answers which are more obviously incorrect – A, B and E – as they are nowhere near the range of a normal BMI (20 – 25).
Then you can substitute the values 24.31 and 29.17 into the equation and see which works!
From doing this, we can see that 24.31 gives the closest match and is the correct answer.

**END OF SECTION**

# SECTION 2

## Question 1: D

As the question states that GLUT2 is ATP independent then answer A of active transport is instantly incorrect as it is ATP dependent. Osmosis is applicable only to water molecules and is therefore incorrect. Exocytosis refers to the movement of molecules out of a cell and is therefore incorrect. Simple diffusion is incorrect as the question states that GLUT2 is essential for the process. This leaves the correct answer of facilitated diffusion.

## Question 2: E

In order to answer this question, you must recall that anaerobic respiration in humans produces only lactate and energy, whilst in yeast the anaerobic respiratory process yields a molecule of ethanol and $CO_2$ per glucose molecule. Therefore, there will be 0 mol of $CO_2$ produced in the human cell culture and you need only work out the moles of $CO_2$ produced by the yeast cell culture to calculate the difference. There is a total of $5.76/0.18 = 32$ mol of glucose, of which half is supplied to the yeast cell culture. With a stoichiometric ratio of 1:1 in the anaerobic respiration equation a total of 16 mol of $CO_2$ will be produced.

## Question 3: D

This is an easy question – you should know that red blood cells do not contain a nucleus nor any DNA! This is a useful quality, as it means that they can be packed with even more haemoglobin and thus transport more oxygen to peripheral tissues.

## Question 4: A

**A – correct** – distribution of heat around the body is a function of the CVS. Vasoconstriction of vessels near the skin occurs when it is cold, thus preventing heat loss. In contrast, vasodilation of these same vessels occurs in hot temperatures, in order to aid the dissipation of heat and prevent hyperthermia.
**B – incorrect** – this is the function of the respiratory system.
**C – incorrect** – this is the function of the kidneys / renal system.

## Question 5: D

Option D is one of only 2 graphs that demonstrate a quadratic relationship with the peak enzyme activity correctly placed – pepsin from the stomach close to pH 1, and trypsin secreted by the pancreas and therefore alkaline around pH 13. The curves traced in option c however are far too broad over the pH range to represent enzyme activity. As the pH scale is logarithmic, even a change of 1 or 0.5 can be devastating to enzyme activity.

## Question 6: A

This question was taken directly from the BMAT syllabus where many examples are listed for different principles. Reading the BMAT syllabus and highlighting these is a very good idea as well as learning the definitions listed. Natural selection occurs when there is a selective pressure – i.e. the presence of methicillin. Some staphylococcus aurei develop a random mutation which leads to methicillin resistance, so in the presence of methicillin, these are the only bacteria that can survive. They are 'selected' because of their unique property.

## Question 7: A

Initially the electron configuration of Mg is 2,8,2. In binding to two chlorine atoms it is effectively ionised to $Mg^{2+}$ and it loses two electrons to leave a complete outer shell and thus the correct answer is 2,8.

## Question 8: D

The first thing to note in this trace is that the m/z axis has been cut short. From looking up the mass of calcium in the periodic table one would expect to see the x axis centred around 40. However here the trace is only displaying those isotopes with valence 2 (z= 2) hence the values are half the size. Therefore (from the periodic table) when dividing the most abundant isotope of chromium by two, 52/2 = 26, we confirm that the outlier bar on the right is indeed the contaminant. Therefore, to calculate the actual abundance of Mr 40 calcium ignore the chromium like so: 55/95 = 11/19.

## Question 9: A

Begin by converting the total weight of arsenic into grams like so $15 \times 10^6 = 1.5 \times 10^7$. Then divide by the Mr of arsenic which is 75 (2sf) giving $2 \times 10^5$. Don't forget that the sample is at worst 80% pure. Therefore, there will be a minimum of $(2 \times 10^5) \times 0.8 = 1.6 \times 10^5$ moles of pure arsenic.

## Question 10: D

Recall that average atomic mass is calculated as the sum of (isotope mass x relative abundance). Therefore 28 = $(26 \times 0.6) + (30 \times 0.3) + 0.1x$. Rearranging this equation reveals that $0.1x = 3.4$ and that the mystery isotope therefore has an atomic mass of 34.

## Question 11: A

First recall that when a group 2 metal reacts with steam a metal oxide is formed and therefore the following chemical equation can be drawn: $Mg + H_2O_{(g)} \rightarrow MgO + H_2$. Note the stoichiometric ratio which is simply 1. Next calculate that there is 72/24 = 3 mol of hydrogen produced. Therefore, assuming that there is 3 mol of all other reactants and the reaction is complete one would expect $3 \times 24.3 = 72.9g$ of magnesium and $3 \times 18 = 54g$ of steam. This is indeed the case and therefore the reaction is complete.

## Question 12: B

The reducing agent is the species which is itself reduced in this instance from looking at the oxidation states we can see that that species is $S^{2-}$. As after the reaction has taken place it has an oxidation state of +6 which would require a loss of negative charge i.e. electrons.

## Question 13: C

The highly stable bonds between carbon atoms, and between carbon and hydrogen atoms, renders alkanes relatively unreactive. This is important to note as it highlights the major difference between alkanes and alkenes.

## Question 14: A

Recall that current = charge/time. The question provides both charge and time in the correct units and so the calculation is relatively simple with no unit conversions required. Therefore current = 5/15 = 1/3 = 0.33A. As the question states that the balloon has a negative charge it has therefore gained electrons. Given that a current is defined as a net movement of electrons, in this situation the current must be flowing into the balloon.

## Question 15: D

Given that Power = IV it can be deduced that I = P/V. Recall that power given in Watts is a measure of the energy transferred per second and therefore has the alternative units $Js^{-1}$. When substituting these units into the power equation re-arranged for Amps it is revealed that $I = (Js^{-1})/V = A$.

**Question 16: D**

For a transformer that is 100% efficient power in must equal power out, recalling that P=IV. Therefore, the transformer has a power output of 24 x 10 = 240W which is 80% of the initial input. As such the initial power input was (240/80) x 100 = 300W.

**Question 17: C**

Begin by calculating the energy required to hoist the mass, this is calculated using the potential energy equation: mgh. Energy = mass x g x height = 20 x 10 x 30 = 6000N. The power output of the motor is calculated as the joules dissipated per second = 6000/20 = 300W

**Question 18: C**

We know that the count rates of 130Bq and 40Bq are affected by the 10Bq of background radiation.
Removed 10Bq from each → 120Bq and 30Bq, which is 2 half-lives (1 half-life brings 120 to 60, then another brings us to 30).
6 days have gone by as these 2 half-lives have elapsed, so we can calculate that a half-life is 3 days.
25Bq = 15Bq from the sample and 10Bq from background radiation. 15Bq is half of 30Bq, so one more half-life will have elapsed between 30Bq on day 7 and the 15Bq, thus bringing us to **day 10**.

**Question 19: D**

Begin by calculating the wattage that the bulb is receiving as 0.5 x 240 = 120W. Given that the energy rating of the bulb is 80W, we can assume that this bulb is only 80/120 = **66%** efficient.

**Question 20: E**

Begin by subtracting the integral from both sides producing $x - \int_{-z}^{z} 9a - 7 = \frac{\sqrt{b^3 - 9st}}{13j}$. Next multiply both sides by 13j and square, rendering $[13j(x - \int_{-z}^{z} 9a - 7)]^2 = b^3 - 9st$. Finally subtract $b^3$ from both sides and divide by -9s leaving the correct answer: $\frac{[13j(x - \int_{-z}^{z} 9a - 7)]^2 - b^3}{-9s} = t$.

**Question 21: C**

The formula for calculating compound interest can be given as: Investment $\times$ (investment rate$^{years}$).
For this situation → $1125 = 500x^2$, where $x$ = the investment rate.
There are 2 options for solving this question, depending on how confident you are with finding square roots!

You could rearrange the formula to $\sqrt{\frac{1125}{500}} = \sqrt{2.25} = 1.5$ → 1.5 – 1.0 = 0.5 = 50% interest rate.

Alternatively, just plug in the numbers until you find one that fits – this may be quicker if you struggle with these calculations (which is understandable!).

**Question 22: E**

Begin by drawing your line of best fit, remembering not to force it through the origin. Begin fitting the general equation y = mx + c to your line. Calculate the gradient as $\Delta y/\Delta x$ and read the y intercept off your annotated graph.

**Question 23: E**

In order to start rearranging the fraction begin by adding m to both sides and squaring to yield $4m^2 = \frac{9xy^3z^5}{3x^9yz^4}$.
Now it is clear to see that this can be most simply displayed in terms of powers. Therefore, **E** is the correct answer.

### Question 24: D
Non-normally distributed data doesn't demonstrate a 50-50 split of data points either side of the mean. Therefore, standard data analysis techniques like normal range are inappropriate (as the formula for normal range is mean$\pm$ 1.96SD). Instead, the interquartile range is used.

### Question 25: D
Random chance is a major issue particularly in medicine. Clinical trials are inherently flawed as they only consider a very small percentage of the population which is far outweighed by the genetic variation demonstrated within the human genome. Therefore, statistics must be used to transform sample data into data representative of the entire population.

### Question 26: B
Begin by calculating the speed of the innermost well as the circumference of travel over time = 20 x 3.14 = 62.8cm/s.
Calculate the outermost well speed in the same manner = 40 x 3.14 = 125.6cm/s. 125.6 – 62.8 = 62.8cm/s faster, which is equal to 0.628m/s. Thus, answer **B** is correct.

### Question 27: D
The correct answer is D $\rightarrow$ $y = \frac{9}{\sqrt[3]{x}}$

You could start by dividing both sides by 9, to give $\frac{y}{9} = 9x^{-\frac{1}{3}}$

$x^{\frac{1}{3}} = \sqrt[3]{x}$ and $x^{-1} = \frac{1}{x}$

So, combine these, to give $x^{-\frac{1}{3}} = \frac{1}{\sqrt[3]{x}}$ $\rightarrow$ $\frac{y}{9} = \frac{1}{\sqrt[3]{x}}$

Now, multiply both sides by 9 $\rightarrow$ $y = \frac{9}{\sqrt[3]{x}}$

**END OF SECTION**

# SECTION 3

*"Progress is made by trial and failure; the failures are generally a hundred times more numerous than the successes; yet they are usually left unchronicled."*

- This statement takes aim at several aspects of science. On one hand, it aims at scientific method. It demonstrates that science itself is based on trial and error and that to come to the right answer we should test theories repeatedly, adjusting them all the time to become more precise and more in keeping with our results. In the end, it is very rare that a theory survives unchanged. It also stresses that the progress of science is slow and laborious as it requires a constant string of trial-and-error experiments before providing any results. The second component the statement addresses is the way the scientific progress is seen in the public and even amongst scientists. The common perception is that only success counts and if a theory cannot be proven it is a failure. This of course is a problem since every failure provides a new angle to start from on the hunt for success. Failure becomes necessary for success to be possible.

- Since this statement basically has two components, when arguing to the contrary, you will have to demonstrate either that failures stand in a different relationship to success or that the reporting of failures is equal to that of successes. Either is going to be difficult as the question stem itself forms a self-fulfilling prophecy. You cannot disprove it, provided it has some truth to it, since you will not find any evidence for it. So, you will have to focus on a more theoretical level to fund support to argue against the quote.

- You can argue that failures, being part of research, are always reflected to some extent in the presentation of data in research papers. They will also appear in the analysis components of any piece of research as failures are essential for the progress of research as it narrows the field of possible answers.

- Another perspective from which you can approach this topic is to separate the failure and the success. Failure of one theory, even if it had been thought to be correct at some point will lead to evolution of a different idea that builds on the conceptual failures of the previous idea. Thereby, one idea facilitates the other and the failing of one concept will directly result in a new concept that then in turn will either remain a success or become a failure at some point down the line.

- You can also consider the role failure plays in our society. It is generally seen as a bad thing and as something to be avoided. This of course does also apply to the scientific community. But at the same time, failure can also provide a new stepping-stone for future success, provided lessons are learned from the cause of the failure that can then be applied for future projects.

*"He who studies medicine without books sails an uncharted sea, but he who studies medicine without patients does not go to sea at all."*

- This statement aims directly at the connection between science and 'soft skills', when it comes to the practice of medicine. It claims that medicine is more than just a science that can be learned by theories alone but has a large human component that gives the scientific aspect of medicine meaning. Without the application of the theoretical knowledge, the subject studied has no value at all, at least it cannot be called medicine.

- When addressing this statement, there are several tension points you should consider. Firstly, there is the uncharted sea. This symbol has several aspects. On one hand, it is threatening and dangerous as the sailor cannot know where difficult streams and lurking rocks are located. On the other hand, it also has a component of excitement and adventure, just think of the old explores Cook and Columbus etc. Secondly the symbol of not sailing at all. In this again, you can use the sailor metaphor to become fully clear on what he means. Imagine a sailor that has excellent navigational skills but lacks the courage to apply them and so wanders to the harbour every day to stare across the sea. All his skill is wasted as he never sets foot on the waves.

- In order to argue against this quote, you should focus on the first part, the sailing an uncharted sea. This is because the second part holds a deep truth that is difficult to disprove. Even when it comes to medical research, you will have to interact with patients that you draw data from for your research. However, it is simple to argue why books play a vital role in medicine. In this case books are synonymous to all forms of theoretical learning.

- The main focus here should be that of safety of the patients. Without books it is only a matter of time until the doctor makes a mistake, crashing his proverbial ship on a proverbial sandbank. Since the focus of medical treatment is the improvement of the patient's condition or quality of life, uncertainty and adventurism have no role in this. At this point it is essential to keep the text on a general level, as medical progress does also come from ignoring the common wisdom. Remember the theory of 4 humours from the Middle Ages, if it hadn't been for somebody breaking with this common wisdom and basis of teaching, modern medicine would never have been born...

- If you write an essay about this topic, make sure that you have a very clear position that will give you a good basis to argue from. Also make sure you have fully understood the statement. Due to the use of metaphors this can be tricky, but on the other hand, if you have understood the question, you can use similar metaphors and they will tie in nicely with the question. This will then give your whole essay a smoother appearance and make it better to read.

*"'Medicine is the restoration of discordant elements; sickness is the discord of the elements infused into the living body"*

To understand this statement, you have to understand Leonardo da Vinci. Being an Renaissance artist and scientist, artist and architect, he had a very varied background but also lived in the late 15th and early 16th century which will obviously have influenced his perception of medicine. The idea of discordant elements that are infused in the body and that have to be rebalanced is clear evidence of that since it basically rephrases the theory of the 4 humours that was the basis of medicine until the 19th century, when pathogens were discovered and described in their properties to cause disease. In general, however, the statement is to be understood in a sense that disease represents a damaging influence on the body, when the default is health, and the job of medicine is to rectify this influence to restore health.

When arguing against this stamen, there are several possible angles of attack. On one hand, there is the historical aspect of the 4 humours mentioned above. This is pretty straight forward since you can easily demonstrate why da Vinci would be influenced by this theory and how this theory was inherently false. On the other hand, you can attack the idea of corruption through diseases causing influence by a more general discussion of disease patterns. Whilst it is true that infectious diseases are cause by the insertion of pathogens into the healthy organism, there are a vast number of diseases that are not. One good example to use would be a discussion of genetic diseases. Of particular note, genetic diseases that are inherited in a recessive pattern, meaning that parent generations must be carriers and therefore be 'corrupted' as well without displaying the actual disease. If you want to go down the mutation route as well, you can point out that not all change causes negative outcomes since mutations form the basis of evolution and thereby the basis of how we as a species came to be.

The second point of attack to argue against da Vinci here is the role of medicine. Whilst it is generally true that the aim of medicine is to cure the patient, sometimes this is either not possible due to a lack of ability of the medical profession, i.e. we just don't have a cure, or it is not desirable since the risk to the patient if undergoing treatment outweighs the risk of the disease or the benefit of treatment. Good examples here are chemotherapy in the frail and elderly. Another example is that of mutations as the motor of evolution as mentioned above.

To the last part of the question, this statement still holds some truth applicable to modern medicine, for example cancer that can be caused by poisonous external influences such as smoking or radiation, in this case the treatment will involve on one hand the removal of the negative stimulus, if possible, and on the other hand the treatment of the negative impact this stimulus has left.

*"Modern medicine is a negation of health. It isn't organized to serve human health, but only itself, as an institution. It makes more people sick than it heals."*

- With this statement, some background knowledge can be very helpful. Ivan Illich was a Croatian-Austrian Priest and philosopher that lived during the 20th century. He is generally known as a critic of the institutions of Western culture such as schools or in this case modern medicine. Looking at the statement it is clear he suggests that medicine has no interest in curing humans but rather prolongs their suffering to sell them as much treatment as possible to fund its own interests.

- In order to argue against this stamen, it can be helpful to detect components of truth in it that can then be refuted. One point that can be raised in connection to this statement is that of medicalisation. By labelling everything that does not conform 100% with the ideal of health in medical terms produces a population of sick people that then require treatment.

- Another point where the statement holds true is in different health care systems such as the one in the US where maintaining a sick status provides continued income to the doctor and the medical professionals involved in treatment. This is less of an issue in publicly funded environment such as the NHS where there is a stricter regulation of resources and therefore less option for artificial prolongation of treatment requirements.

- Arguing against the statement is fairly easy, especially when arguing from the perspective of the NHS. In the NHS, healthcare is provided free of charge for residents and there are no direct barriers in place to block access to health care. This in itself proves Illich wrong since it would serve the institution to make health care a luxury item that comes with the associated price tag.

- Arguing that the primary duty of the doctor is not to prolong life is more difficult, since two of the ethical pillars of the medical profession call for doctors not to do harm and to act in the patients' best interests, both of which aim at the prolongation of life in the majority of cases. There are some exceptions to the prolonging life idea, and it is probably safest to approach this part of the question from that angle as it will ensure that you stay on the right track and don't end up in a direction you didn't want to go.

- Limitations to the idea of prolonging life are pretty much all the cases falling under palliative care where the idea is to remove suffering and providing symptomatic relief rather than curing the dieses causing the symptoms. Common examples here are cancer in the elderly that are not fit enough to undergo chemotherapy or surgery. Other examples are incurable diseases such as inoperable brain tumours etc.

- In this question again, it helps very much to have a clear idea of what you think about the issue. It will make it easier to structure your answer appropriately and it will ensure that you don't navigate yourself into uncertain waters which is fairly easy with this topic, especially when the idea of prolonging life or not is being introduced.

**END OF PAPER**

# MOCK PAPER C ANSWERS

## SECTION 1

### Question 1: D
There are three different options for staying at the hotel. They could either pay for three single rooms for £180, one single and one double room for £165, or one four-person room for £215.

Subtracting the cleaning cost for one night would leave:
£180-(3x£12) = £144
£165-(2x£12) = £141
£215-£12 = £203

The cheapest option is one single and one double room, and they want to stay three nights, giving £141x3 = £423.

### Question 2: D
Glass one starts with 16ml squash and 80ml water. Glass two starts with 72ml squash and 24ml water. 48ml is half of 96ml so 8ml squash and 40ml water is transferred to glass two. Glass two now contains (8+72 = 80ml squash) and (24+40 = 64ml water). Glass two now has a total of 144ml and half of this is transferred to glass one. Glass one now has (40+8 = 48ml squash) and (32+40 = 72ml water). Therefore, glass one has 48ml squash and glass two has 40ml squash.

### Question 3: B
**B** is the main conclusion of the argument. Options **A** and **D** both contribute reasons to support the main conclusion of the argument that the HPV vaccination should remain in schools. **C** is a counter argument, which is a reason given in opposition to the main conclusion. Option **E** represents a general principle behind the main argument.

## Question 4: B

The speed of the bus can be calculated using the relationship: Speed $=\frac{\text{distance}}{\text{time}}$

$\frac{3\text{ km}}{0.2\text{ h}} = 15\text{ kmh}^{-1}$

The bike speed is therefore ($\frac{4}{5}$ x 15 = 12 kmh$^{-1}$). Considering that the bus leaves 2 minutes after the bike, it is now possible to write an expression, where d is the distance travelled when the bus overtakes the bike:

$$\frac{d\text{ km}}{12\text{ km/h}} = \frac{1}{30}\text{h} + \frac{d\text{ km}}{15\text{ km/h}}$$

This expression can be solved by multiplying each term by (12 kmh$^{-1}$ x 15 kmh$^{-1}$):

15d km = 6 km +12d km

3d km = 6 km

d = 2 km

Therefore, the bus overtakes the bike after travelling 2 km.

## Question 5: B

Firstly, determine who will move up to set one. Terry, Bahara, Lucy and Shiv all have attendance over 95%. Alex, Bahara and Lucy all have an average test mark over 92. Terry, Bahara, Lucy and Shiv all have less than 5% homework handed in late. Therefore, Bahara and Lucy will both move up a set. Secondly, determine who will receive a certificate. Terry, Bahara, Lucy and Shiv have absences below 4%. Alex, Bahara and Lucy have an average test score of over 89. Bahara and Shiv have at least 98% homework handed in on time. Therefore, only Bahara will receive a certificate.

## Question 6: C

Firstly, construct two algebraic equations: A-18=B-25 and A=$\frac{5}{6}$B

Next solve these two equations as simultaneous equations by substituting $\frac{5}{6}$B for A in equation 1:

$\frac{5}{6}$B-18=B-25

7=$\frac{1}{6}$B

B=42

Put B=42 back into equation 2:  A= 42 x $\frac{5}{6}$

A=35

## Question 7: D

I need to make 48 scones, which makes up 8 batches.
8 batches would take: 35+ 7(25+10) +25 = 305 minutes

I need to make 32 cupcakes, which makes up 4 batches.
4 batches would take: 15+ (4x20) =95 minutes

I need to make 48 cucumber sandwiches
This would take (8x5) = 40 minutes

Adding 305, 95 and 40 minutes is 440 minutes in total. 440 minutes is equivalent to 7 hours and 20 minutes. Adding 7 hours and 20 minutes to 10:45am leads to 6:05pm so I will be finished at 6:05pm.

## Question 8: D

The volume of a pyramid is given by the equation:

$v = \frac{a^2h}{3}$  where v=volume, a=base and h=height

Rearrange to work out the height for each pyramid: $h = \frac{3v}{a^2}$

| Pyramid | Base edge (m) | Volume (m³) | Calculation: | Height (m) |
|---|---|---|---|---|
| 1 | 3 | 33 | $\frac{3\times33}{9}$ | 11 |
| 2 | 4 | 64 | $\frac{3\times64}{16}$ | 12 |
| 3 | 2 | 8 | $\frac{3\times8}{4}$ | 6 |
| 4 | 6 | 120 | $\frac{3\times120}{36}$ | 10 |
| 5 | 2 | 8 | $\frac{3\times8}{4}$ | 6 |
| 6 | 6 | 120 | $\frac{3\times120}{36}$ | 10 |
| 7 | 4 | 64 | $\frac{3\times64}{16}$ | 12 |

The tallest pyramid is 12m and the smallest is 6m. Subtracting the height of the tallest pyramid from the height of the smallest pyramid leaves 6m.

## Question 9: A

Work out the two wages by substituting the information provided into the formula:

Jessica's wage is: 210 + 42 - 3.2 = 248.8

Samira's wage is: 210 + 78 - 8.8 = 279.2

(Note, to save time you don't really need to include the 210 values, but they are included here for completeness!).

Subtracting 248.8 from 279.2 leave 30.4 so the difference between their wages is £30.4.

## Question 10: C

The main conclusion is **C**. **A** and **B** both represent reasons to support the main conclusion of the argument. Option **D** represents an assumption that is not stated in the argument but is required to support the main conclusion that research universities should strongly support teaching. Option **E** is a counter argument that provides a reason to oppose the main argument.

## Question 11: D

**D** is the main conclusion of the argument. **A** is a general principle of the argument, but the argument is more specific to the use of helmets rather than the wider concept of danger in sport and the responsibilities of the governing bodies to sports players. Options **B** and **C** are reasons to support the main conclusion. Option **E** is an intermediate conclusion, which acts as support for the next stage of the argument and as a reason to support the main conclusion.

## Question 12: D

There are 10 passengers on the tube at the final stop. At stop 5 there were twice the number of passengers on the tube so 20 passengers were at stop 5. At stop 4, there were $\frac{5}{2}$ times the number of passengers at stop 5 so 50 passengers were present at stop 4. At stop 3, there were $\frac{3}{2}$ times the number of passengers at stop 4 so 75 passengers were on the tube. At stop 2, there were $\frac{6}{5}$ times the number of passengers at stop 3 so 90 passengers were present at stop 2. Similarly, at stop 1, there were $\frac{6}{5}$ times the number of passengers at stop 2 so at the first stop 108 passengers got on the tube.

**Question 13: E**

Some students born in winter like English, art and music

**A – incorrect** – we are not given enough information to tell whether some students born in spring like both biology and maths.

**B – incorrect** – we don't know what the students born in spring think about art.

**C – incorrect** – as we don't know what the students born in winter think about biology.

**D – incorrect** – it is possible that some of the students born in winter who like are may also like biology, we are not specifically told that all students born in winter dislike biology.

**E – correct** – all students born in winter like music and some like art. We are told specifically that everyone likes English. Some students born in winter like English, art and music, so, statement E is correct!

| Subject | TIME OF BIRTH | | |
|---|---|---|---|
| | SPRING | AUTUMN | WINTER |
| English | Everyone likes | Everyone likes | Everyone likes |
| Biology | Some like | No one likes | |
| Art | | Everyone likes | Some like |
| Music | | | Everyone likes |
| Maths | Some like | | |

**Question 14: A**

The main conclusion is option **A** - that some works of modern art no longer constitute art. **B** is not an assumption made by the author as the main conclusion does not rely on all modern art being ugly to be valid. **C** is not an assumption because the argument does not rely on artists studying for decades to produce pieces of work that constitute art. This point is simply used to support the main argument. Options **D** and **E** are stated in the argument so are not assumptions.

**Question 15: E**

Reducing the price of the sunglasses by 10% is equivalent to multiplying the price by 0.9. The price of the sunglasses is successively reduced by 10% three times and so the price on Monday is $0.9^3$ the price of the sunglasses on Friday. $0.9^3$ is equal to 0.729 and so the price of the sunglasses on Monday is 72.9% of the price of the sunglasses on Friday.

**Question 16: C**

It is probably quickest to just use the values given in the options A – E!

**A – incorrect** – 277 – 27 = 250
**B – incorrect** – 527 – 52 = 475
**C – correct** – 627 – 62 = **565**
**D – incorrect** – 667 – 66 = 601
**E – incorrect** – 6277 – 667 = 5650

**Question 17: E**

Look at the flat cube net and note the shapes that are adjacent to each other. Sides that are joining on the net will be beside each other on the formed cube. Work through to deduce option E can be formed from the cube net shown.

**Question 18: E**

The H shape is comprised of 12 squares. The shape's area of 588 can be divided by 12 to give 49, which is the area of each individual square. The square root of 49 is 7 and so the side length of each individual square is 7cm. The perimeter of the shape is comprised of 26 sides and the length of each side is 7 so the perimeter of the shape is 182cm.

**Question 19: B**

The main conclusion is that EnergyFirst is expected to expand its customer base at a rate exceeding its competitors in the ensuing months. **A** does not directly contradict the main argument. It demonstrates a flaw in the argument in that it ignores the fact that other companies may be stronger in other areas and attract customers by other means. However, it does not serve to weaken the main argument. **C** does not contradict the main conclusion; EnergyFirst could still expand its customer base at the fastest rate even if there is not much competition between energy companies. **D** would not weaken the argument as it refers to the rate of new customer intake rather than the number of new customers attracted. **E**, if true, would strengthen the argument because it suggests that visual advertising would attract new customers. **B** would weaken the main argument because if it were true then investing the most money in advertising would not serve to attract the most customers.

**Question 20: A**

Option **B** points out a flaw in the argument, which attributes the healthier circulatory system of vegetarians to diet, but ignores other potential contributory factors to a healthy circulatory system such as exercise. **C** is not an assumption: the health benefits of a vegetarian and omnivorous diet are not discussed; rather the argument is centred on the negative health ramifications. **D** is stated in the argument so is not an assumption and option **E** is a counter argument, not an assumption. Option **A** is required to support the main conclusion but is not stated in the argument so is an assumption made in the argument.

**Question 21: A**

First, calculate the number of hours spent flying and waiting. It takes 24 hours in total from Auckland to London, 11.5 hours from London to Calgary and 8 hours from Calgary to Boston. In total this amounts to 43.5 hours of flying and waiting. Boston is 16 hours behind Auckland and so when Sam arrives in Boston it will be 27.5 hours ahead of 10am. The time in Boston will therefore be 13:30 pm.

## Question 22: B

This question requires you to find the lowest common multiple. This is the product of the highest power in each prime factor category.

$18 = 3^2 \times 2$

$33 = 3 \times 11$

$27 = 3^3$

Therefore, $3^3$, 11 and 2 need to be multiplied together which equals 594 seconds between simultaneous flashes. 5 minutes or 300 seconds needs to be subtracted from 594 in order to find the length of time until the next flash. The time that they will next flash simultaneously is 294 seconds.

## Question 23: C

Option **A** may explain why young drivers are involved in more accidents but does not need to be true for the main conclusion to hold. **B** would weaken the argument if true as drivers that spend more time driving will have a greater chance of being involved in accidents regardless of age. **D** is not an assumption, but if true may weaken the argument as it attributes the accidents to unsafe cars rather than unsafe driving. **E** is irrelevant to the main conclusion: it does not matter whether the young drivers are male or female; arguably steps should still be taken to reduce the number of accidents. Option **C** represents an assumption that is not stated in the argument but is required to support the main conclusion.

## Question 24: B

**B**- If the advice was appropriate, regardless of vested interests, it would still stand. **A**- It is explicitly stated this is only a possibility. **C**- Is irrelevant to the conclusion. **D**- Vested interests not misjudging the virus is the issue. **E**- is irrelevant.

## Question 25: C

**A**-1 posits fewer rats than 3. **B**- For 1 there are potentially fewer rats than for 4. **D**-There could be more rats than people for 2, and more people than rats for 4. **E**- 3 there may be more rats than people, but for 4 there are not. **C**- 2 and 3 are equivalent.

## Question 26: A

**B** cannot be inferred from the passage. Although **C** and **D** could be argued, they are not argued for in the text. **E** is wrong; although the impact on the elderly is noted but it is not argued that they should be prioritized over work. **A** is the conclusion of all the arguments in the paragraph.

## Question 27: E

**E** undermines the argument competition should prevent more information becoming public. **A**- The passage is about development of new drugs. **B** and **C** could be deduced from the text alone. **D** does not influence the effects of competition between drug companies.

## Question 28: C

**C** is the conclusion of all the arguments in the paragraph. **B** and **D** are arguments not conclusions. **E** is not mentioned in the text. **A** is wrong since changing the character of older buildings is mentioned but is not what the argument is about.

## Question 29: C

**C** is the conclusion of the arguments presented. **A** is not argued in the text. **B** is not the central conclusion. **D** is stated as a belief only. **E** is implied but is not the conclusion.

## Question 30: B

A.  True, but not far-reaching enough.

B.  Correct answer. Sugar does indeed have an addictive potential as it causes the release of endorphins and the health concerns are well known.  This characteristic makes it like alcohol and smoking, and potentially suitable for similar policies.

C.  True, but similar to option A) and thus too limited.

D.  Potentially true, but also too limited.

## Question 31: B

**B** is **correct** – the main conclusion is that we should not wait for proof of climate change.

**A** and **D** are both reasons to **support** the main conclusion, but they are not the main conclusion.

**C** is an **analogy**, rather than a conclusion.

**E** is a **counter-argument** to the main conclusion.

## Question 32: D

**D** is the closest parallel, as it focuses on the benefits to both the individual and society. **A** doesn't address the question of pay in sufficient detail, **B** is a possible extension of the argument, but not a parallel. **C** is almost right, but is too focused on the advantage to employers. **E** is also close, but doesn't include the educational element.

### END OF SECTION

## SECTION 2

### Question 1: E

**1 – incorrect** – lipid molecules contain carbon, as they have a backbone of carbon. Thus, they are part of the carbon cycle.

**2 – incorrect** – plasmids are composed of DNA or RNA. DNA and RNA both contain carbon, hence plasmids are part of the carbon cycle.

**3 – incorrect** – proteins contain carbon, thus these proteins are a part of the carbon cycle.

Note that this question asks which is **not** involved in the carbon cycle – always read the question carefully!

Remember, during the carbon cycle, carbon is incorporate into complex molecules in organisms! Thus, these complex molecules are a part of the carbon cycle.

### Question 2: C

Statement 1 is true. High temperatures and pH extremes cause a permanent alteration to the highly specific shape of the active site so that the substrate can no longer bind, and the enzyme no longer works.
Statement 2 is false. Amylase is produced in the salivary glands, pancreas, and small intestine.
Statement 3 is true.
Statement 4 is false. Bile is stored in the gall bladder, but it does travel down the bile duct to neutralise hydrochloric acid found in the stomach.

### Question 3: C

The combining of food with bile and digestive enzymes occurs in the duodenum of the small intestine. In the ileum of the small intestine, the digested food is absorbed into the blood and lymph. The digested food then progresses into the large intestine. In the colon, water is reabsorbed. Faeces are then stored in the rectum and leave the alimentary canal via the anus.

### Question 4: C

Statement 1 is true.
Statement 2 is true. For example, the drug curare, a South American plant toxin which is used in arrow poison, stops the nerve impulse from crossing the synapse and causes paralysis and can stop breathing.
Statement 3 is false. The sheath provides insulation for the nerve axon and increases the speed of impulse transmission via saltatory conduction.
Statement 4 is false. The peripheral nervous system includes motor and sensory neurons carrying impulses between receptors, effectors, and the central nervous system. The CNS consists of the spinal cord and the brain.
Statement 5 is true. A reflex arc travels from sensory neuron to relay neuron to motor neuron and is an innate mechanism designed to keep the animal safe. For example, it allows a person to quickly draw their hand away from a flame.

### Question 5: C

Statement 1 is true.

Statement 2 is false. The transition metals are both malleable and ductile, they conduct heat and electricity and they form positive ions when reacted with non-metals.

Statement 3 is true. Thermal decomposition is a reaction whereby a substance breaks down into two or more other substances due to heat. When a transition metal carbonate is heated, metal oxide and carbon dioxide are produced. The carbon dioxide can be collected and will turn limewater cloudy.

An example of this reaction is: $CuCO_3 \rightarrow CuO + CO_2$

Statement 4 is false. Transition metal hydroxides are insoluble in water.

Statement 5 is true.

## Question 6: E

There are 9 Sulphur atoms on the left so there must be 9 on the right. Therefore, the values of B and C must add to make 9. This can be written as an equation: B+C=9

It is now useful to try to balance the Oxygen atoms: 4A+36 = 10+4B+4C+14

Simplify to give: 12 = 4B+4C-4A

Equation 1 can now be substituted into equation 2 to give: 12 = (4x9)-4A

24 = 4A

A = 6

There are 6 Potassium atoms on the left. This means that there must also be 6 potassium atoms on the right, so B must by 3. As shown in equation 1, B and C add to make 9 so C must be 6.

**5** $PhCH_3$ + **6** $KMnO_4$ + **9** $H_2SO_4$ = **5** PhCOOH + **3** $K_2SO_4$ + **6** $MnSO_4$ + **14** $H_2O$

## Question 7: B

Statement 1 is true. Males have one X chromosome so if the allele is present they will be affected. Females have two X chromosomes so both need to be affected to be red-green colour blind as the condition is recessive

Statement 2 is true because according to the Punnett square below half of the children will have the homozygous recessive tt genotype and so will be non-rollers.

|   | T | t |
|---|---|---|
| t | Tt | tt |
| t | Tt | tt |

Statement 3 is true because all of the male children will inherit an X chromosome from the mother which will carry the colour-blind allele.

## Question 8: B

Start by multiplying each term by $ax$ to give: $a(y+x)=x^2+a^2$

Expand the brackets: $ay+ax=x^2+a^2$

Subtract $ax$ from both sides: $ay=x^2+a^2-ax$

Lastly, divide the both sides by a to get: $y = \frac{x^2+a^2-ax}{a}$

## Question 9: A

This question requires the use of the equation: $C = \frac{n}{v}$ where C= concentration, n= moles and v=volume

Convert 25cm³ into litres to get 0.025 litres and plug the values for concentration and volume into the equation to get the number of moles:   $0.1 = \frac{n}{0.025}$ so n=0.0025

This question also requires the use of the equation: $n = \frac{m}{Mr}$   where m=mass, n=moles and Mr= molecular mass

The molecular mass is the sum of one calcium and two chlorine atoms which is equal to 111gmol⁻¹.

Inserting the molecular mass and number of moles into the above equation can be used to calculate the mass of calcium chloride: $m = 0.0025 \; x \; 111 = 0.28g$

## Question 10: C

Solve as simultaneous equations

Start by substituting x = $\frac{y}{3}$ into equation B.

This gives y = $\frac{18}{y} - 7$

Multiply every term by y to give:

0=y² +7y – 18

Factorise this quadratic to give:

0=(y+9)(y-2)

Where the graphs meet, y is equal to 2 and 9. Then y=3x so the graphs meet when x = 6 and x = 27

## Question 11: D

Statement 1 is false because the pulmonary artery carries deoxygenated blood from the right ventricle to the lungs.

Statement 2 is true. This property of the aorta allows it to carry blood at high pressure and is why it pulsates.

Statement 3 is false because the mitral valve, otherwise known as the bicuspid valve, is between the left atrium and left ventricle.

Statement 4 is true.

## Question 12: D

The Ar of Carbon is 12, Hydrogen is 1 and Oxygen is 16. Therefore, 12g of carbon is 1 mole of carbon; 2g of H is 2 moles of hydrogen and 16g of O is 1 mole of oxygen. The empirical formula is therefore $CH_2O$. The molecular weight is 30 g.mol⁻¹, which goes into 120 g.mol⁻¹ exactly 4 times. The empirical formula must therefore be multiplied by 4 to obtain the molecular formula so the molecular formula is $C_4H_8O_4$.

## Question 13: B

To win one game, Rupert must win one squash game and one tennis game. In order to calculate the probability one winning one game, it is necessary to add the probability of winning one tennis game and losing one squash game to the probability of losing one tennis game and winning one squash game. The following calculation must be performed: $(\frac{3}{4} x \frac{2}{3}) + (\frac{1}{4} x \frac{1}{3}) = \frac{7}{12}$

## Question 14: C

The numbers can all be written as a fraction over 36:

$0.\dot{3}$ is the same as $\frac{12}{36}$

$\frac{11}{18}$ is the same as $\frac{22}{36}$

$0.25$ is the same as $\frac{9}{36}$

$0.75$ is the same as $\frac{27}{36}$

$\frac{62}{72}$ is the same as $\frac{31}{36}$

$\frac{7}{7}$ is the same as $\frac{36}{36}$

Ordering them from lowest to highest gives: $\frac{7}{36}$ ; $0.25$; $0.\dot{3}$ ; $\frac{11}{18}$ ; $0.75$; $\frac{62}{72}$ ; $\frac{7}{7}$

Therefore, the median value is $\frac{11}{18}$

## Question 15: E

This question requires use of the equation: Percentage yield $= \frac{actual\ yeild\ (g)}{predicted\ yield\ (g)}$ x 100.

If all of the benzene was converted to product (100 percent yield) then 20.5g of nitrobenzene would be produced:

$13g\ C_6H_6 \times \frac{1\ mol\ C6H6}{78g\ C6H6} \times \frac{123g\ C6H5NO2}{1\ mol\ C6H5NO2} = 20.5g\ C_6H_5NO_2$

However, only 16.4g are actually produced. Using the equation, we can now calculate the percentage yield:

$\frac{16.4g}{20.5g}$ x 100 = 80% yield.

## Question 16: C

Statement 1 is true.

Statement 2 is false because infrared has a longer wavelength than visible light.

Statement 3 is true.

Statement 4 is false because gamma radiation and not infrared radiation is used to sterilise food and to kill cancer cells.

Statement 5 is true because darker skins contain a higher amount of melanin pigment, which absorbs UV light.

## Question 17: B

This question requires the use of the equation:
p=mv where p=momentum, m=mass and v=velocity.

The total momentum before the collision is equal to the sum of the momentum of carriage 1 (12000 x 5) and carriage 2 (8000 x 0), which is 60,000 kg ms$^{-1}$. Momentum is conserved before and after the collision so the total momentum after the event also equal 60,000 kg ms$^{-1}$. The carriages now move together so the combined mass is 20,000kg. Using the equation again, the total momentum (60,000 kg ms$^{-1}$) divided by the total mass (20,000 kg) gives the velocity of the train carriages after the crash, which is equal to 3 ms$^{-1}$.

## Question 18: C

**Statement 1** is **false**. In a nuclear reactor, all uranium nuclei split to release energy and three neutrons. An explosion could occur if all the neutrons were absorbed by further uranium nuclei as the reaction would escalate out of control. Control rods that are made of boron absorb some of the neutrons and control the chain reaction.

**Statement 2** is **false**. Nuclear fusion occurs when a deuterium and tritium nucleus are forced together. The nuclei both carry a positive charge and consequently, very high temperatures and pressures are required to overcome the electrostatic repulsion. These temperatures and pressures are expensive and hard to repeat and so fusion is not currently suitable as a source of energy.

**Statement 3** is **true**. Alpha particles are composed of 2 protons and 2 neutrons which leave the nucleus of the radioactive element during alpha decay. It has an Ar of 4 and is the equivalent of a helium nucleus.

**Statement 4** is **true**. During beta decay, a neutron transforms into a proton and an electron. The proton remains in the nucleus, whereas the electron is emitted and is referred to as a beta particle. The carbon-14 nucleus now has one more proton and one less neutron, so the atomic number increases by 1 and the atomic mass number remains the same.

**Statement 5** is **false**. Beta particles are more ionising than gamma rays and less ionising than alpha particles.

## Question 19: E

Firstly, deal with the term in the brackets: $3^3 = 27$

$(x^{½})^3 = x^{1.5}$

$(3x^{½})^3 = 27x^{1.5}$

Next, divide by $3x^2$: $\frac{27}{3} = 9$

$\frac{x^{1.5}}{x^2} = x^{-0.5} = \frac{1}{\sqrt{x}}$

Answer = $\frac{9}{\sqrt{x}}$

## Question 20: E

Statement 1 is true.

Statement 2 is true. Decomposers in the soil break down urea and the bodies of dead organisms and this results in the production of ammonia in the soil.

Statement 3 is true.

Statement 4 is true.

## Question 21: A

Write $\frac{\sqrt{20}-2}{\sqrt{5}+3}$ in the form $p\sqrt{5} + q$

Firstly, multiply the term by $\frac{\sqrt{5}-3}{\sqrt{5}-3}$ (ie 1) and write $\sqrt{20}$ as $2\sqrt{5}$

This gives: $\frac{10-6\sqrt{5}-2\sqrt{5}+6}{5-9}$

This simplifies to: $\frac{16-8\sqrt{5}}{-4}$

This simplifies to: $2\sqrt{5} - 4$

Therefore p = 2 and q = -4

## Question 22: E

The question is asking for which of the statements are *false*.

Statement 1 is true.

Statement 2 is true.

Statement 3 is false. Ionic compounds do conduct electricity when dissolved in water or when melted because the ions can move and carry current. On the other hand, solid ionic compounds do not conduct electricity.

Statement 4 is true. Alloys contain different sized atoms, making it harder for the layers to slide over each other.

## Question 23: A

The equation for a circle, with centre at the origin and radius r is $x^2 + y^2 = r^2$

The equation of this circle is therefore $x^2 + y^2 = 25$

Solve the problem using simultaneous equations or by drawing the line onto the graph.

$x^2 + (3x - 5)^2 = 25$

This simplifies to $10x^2 - 30x = 0$

$10x(x - 3) = 0$

So, $x = 3$ or $x = 0$ where the two graphs intersect

## Question 24: C

Statement 1 is false. Heat energy is transferred from hotter to colder places by convection.

Statement 2 is true.

Statement 3 is true. Radiation can travel through a vacuum like space.

Statement 4 is false. Shiny surfaces are poor at reflecting and absorbing infrared radiation and dull surfaces are good at absorbing and reflecting infrared radiation.

## Question 25: C

Statement 1 is true.

Statement 2 is false. The melting and boiling points increase as you go down the group.

Statement 3 is true.

Statement 4 is false. Chloride is more reactive than bromine, so no displacement reaction occurs.

Statement 5 is true.

## Question 26: C

ABC and DBE are similar triangles because all of the angles are equal.

Therefore: $\frac{BE}{BC} = \frac{DE}{AC}$

This is the case because the side lengths of the small and large triangles are in proportion to each other. Substitute the side lengths into the expression:

$\frac{4}{6} = \frac{DE}{9}$

DE=6cm

## Question 27: E

This question requires the use of the equation:

$v^2 = u^2 + 2ah$   where v=final velocity, u=initial velocity, a=acceleration and h=height

From the information provided in the question, we know that v=0ms$^{-1}$, u=40ms$^{-1}$ and a=-10ms$^{-2}$. Inserting these values into the equation gives:

0=1600 + 2(-10h)

The maximum height reached is therefore 80m. **END OF SECTION**

# SECTION 3

*'The NHS should not treat obese patients'*

**Explain what this statement means. Argue to the contrary. To what extent do you agree with the statement?**

The statement argues that free health care should not be given to patients with a BMI of 30 or more. This essay will consider both perspectives before arriving at a conclusion.

There are several arguments to support the treatment of obesity by the NHS. The first is that it is in accordance with the definition of a disease; namely that is reduces life expectancy, negatively impacts normal body function and can be induced by genetic factors. Obesity often has a genetic basis, for example the melanocortin-4 receptor polymorphism and leptin receptor deficiency, which shift the homeostatic balance towards weight gain and are associated with hyperphagia and obesity. Obesity can also be a major feature of certain syndromes such as Prader-Willi syndrome, Bardet-Biedl syndrome and Cohen syndrome. If obesity is either classified as a disease or is an unavoidable ramification of certain syndromes, then surely it should be treated by the NHS just the same as any other disease.

Moreover, if the NHS refuses to treat obese patients, it will become difficult to decide where to draw the line. Should smokers or people who drink alcohol also be denied free health treatment and how many cigarettes or units per week should qualify? Should all obese people be denied free health treatment or just in cases where it is not an unavoidable secondary result of certain syndromes? Obesity is often a consequence of mental illnesses such as depression and it may be hard to differentiate cause from effect.

On the other hand, obesity in certain cases could be considered as a self-induced condition rather than an actual illness. Individuals arguably exercise a degree of free will and are responsible for the number of calories that they consume and the amount of exercise that they do. There is an argument that obesity is driven by structural changes in the environment and is a mass phenomenon influenced by advertising and propaganda. Perhaps societal changes in the outlook towards healthy living are required to address the obesity problem.

Many NHS organisations already ration surgery for overweight patients and will not for example pay for joint or hip replacements for patients with a BMI of over 30. Surely NHS funds and taxpayers' money is better spent on people who make an effort to maintain a good level of health, for instance patients who are subject to largely unpreventable and serious diseases such as certain cancers.

I would suggest that each case should be considered on an individual basis and that obesity treatments should be included on the NHS where they may act to significantly improve the patient's life in the longer term.

*'We should all become vegetarian'*

**Explain what this statement means. Argue to the contrary, that we should not all become vegetarian. To what extent do you agree with this statement?**

This statement is saying that everyone should stop eating meat. This essay will consider both perspectives before arriving at a conclusion.

Some animals are raised in poor living conditions. Circumstances can be cramped and due to growth rate maximisation, animals can develop serious joint problems. Pig tails are cut, chickens have their toenails and beaks clipped and cows are dehorned without painkillers. The slaughter process can also be stressful and inhumane. Halal meat is not stunned before the jugular vein is slit and death is not instantaneous. It could be considered unethical to kill animals for food in this way when vegetarian options are available. Moreover, if farmers grew crops in place of livestock, this would generate more food and potentially alleviate world hunger.

Farming meat also has environmental implications. The overgrazing of livestock entails significant deforestation, which destroys natural habitats and endangers wild species. Enteric fermentation generates huge greenhouse gas emissions and ammonia and hydrogen sulphide leach poisonous nitrate into the water.

A vegetarian diet also has notable health benefits. Diets high in animal protein can cause excretion of calcium, oxalate and uric acid, which contribute to the development of kidney stones and gallstones. Vegetarians absorb more calcium: meat has a high renal acid content which the body neutralises with calcium leached from bones, which can weaken them. A diet rich in legumes, nuts and soy proteins can improve glycaemic control in diabetics. Moreover, growing crops instead of farming livestock can reduce antibiotic use and minimise the development of resistance.

However, there are advantages to eating meat. Meat contains healthy saturated fats that enrich the function of the immune and nervous system. Meat is the best source of vitamin B12 required for nervous and digestive system function and is a better source of iron than vegetables (the body absorbs 15-35% of heme iron found in meat compared to only 2-20% of the non-heme iron found in vegetable sources). Most plants do not contain sufficient levels of essential amino acids.

Moreover, a vegetarian diet can actually have negative environmental consequences. For example, some herbicides utilised on genetically modified crops are toxic to wild plants and animals are often killed during harvest. Eating meat could be considered as natural rather than cruel or unethical. Moreover, the problem of world hunger could partly be attributed to economics and distribution as opposed to insufficient amounts of food.

I would argue that it is ethically acceptable to eat meat so long as it is raised in a satisfactory way. It provides important nutrients, especially for growing children. However, it would be better if we reduced the amount of meat we eat in order to reduce the environmental impact of enteric fermentation and deforestation.

*'Certain vaccines should be mandatory'*

## Explain what this statement means. Argue to the contrary. To what extent do you agree with the statement?

Vaccines are antigenic substances derived from the infectious microorganism itself that provide immunity against a disease. The statement argues that some vaccines should be compulsory. This essay will consider both perspectives before arriving at a conclusion.

Vaccines can protect the individuals that receive them against terrible debilitating diseases. Moreover, vaccines can also protect others in the population. If a certain proportion of the population are protected, herd immunity can be achieved. This means that people who cannot be vaccinated, for instance if they are immunocompromised or undergoing chemotherapy, will not contract the disease. Vaccines can also protect later generations. For instance, mothers vaccinated against rubella reduce the chance of their unborn children acquiring birth defects such as loss of vision, heart defects, cataracts and mental disabilities. Some vaccines have completely eradicated diseases for example the last case of Smallpox occurred in Somalia in 1977. Rinderpest, a disease of cattle, has also been eradicated and the instance of Polio has been substantially reduced.

Although many vaccines are available on the NHS and are funded by the taxpayer, they ultimately cost less to administer than the expense involved in time off work to care for a sick child, long term disability care and medical costs.

Nonetheless, vaccines sometime have serious and occasionally fatal consequences. About one in a million children are at risk of anaphylactic shock. The rotavirus vaccination can result in a type of bowel blockage known as intussusception; and the DPT and MMR vaccines have been associated with seizures, coma and permanent brain damage. Some physicians have raised concerns over the ingredients used in vaccinations. For example, thimerosal has been linked to autism, aluminium taken in excess can cause neurological harm and formaldehyde is a carcinogen that can result in coma, convulsions and death.

It could also be argued that the decision to be vaccinated should constitute a personal medical decision and individuals should be allowed to exert freedom of choice. There are also religious objections to vaccinations. For example, the Amish object to vaccines and mandatory vaccinations. The Catholic Church is also opposed to the ingredients of certain vaccinations. For example, the MMR vaccine is cultivated in cells derived from two foetuses aborted in the 1960s.

However, the chance of serious side effects is incredibly small and furthermore the ingredients in vaccines are safe in the tiny amounts used: the exposure of children to aluminium is higher in breast milk than it is in vaccines. The FDA (food and drug administration) requires vaccines to be tested for up to 10 years before they are licensed and even after licensing, they continue to be monitored. In my view, the wider benefits of vaccines outweigh the minimal risk of poor side effects. In addition, it could be argued that personal decisions should be restricted when they affect the health of others. Therefore, I am supportive of certain vaccinations being mandatory.

'Compassion is the most important quality of a healthcare professional'

**Explain what this statement means. Argue to the contrary. To what extent do you agree with the statement?**

The statement argues that in careers involved in caring for the sick, kindness and empathy for the patients is the most important professional attribute. I will provide reasons for why this might be the case, whilst also discussing the importance of a sound scientific knowledge. I will then decide which quality I believe to be the most important.

A lack of compassion shown by staff working in care homes and hospitals could be held partly responsible for inexcusable cases of patient neglect. For example, care home members have been mocked and tortured and in hospitals, patients have been left surrounded in their own urine and forced to drink water from flower vases. Arguably this neglect has arisen from a lack of care and compassion from the healthcare professionals. However, at the same time it must partly be attributed to understaffing, lack of resources and training. Moreover, it is difficult to assess someone's level of compassion and it is uncertain whether this is something that can actually be taught.

A greater level of compassion would lead to better diagnoses. A large aspect of healthcare involves listening and communicating to patients. If a doctor has more empathy, patients are more likely to trust their doctor and disclose more personal information. An empathetic manner has also been shown to reduce patient anxiety and lead to faster patient recovery.

On the other hand, too much empathy could actually hamper healthcare professionals. Doctors and other health workers often require a degree of objectivity in order to make optimal decisions that may go against the patient's wishes. A level of detachment would also help professionals to remain calm in stressful clinical situations. Clearly, it is desirable for doctors and other healthcare professionals to have a detailed and comprehensive medical knowledge contributing to faster diagnoses, more skilled treatments and faster recoveries.

I would argue that scientific knowledge is the most important quality of a doctor especially because it is a necessity in order to practice medicine. However, compassion is also a highly important quality in a healthcare worker and is what separates an adequate doctor or nurse from an exceptional one.

**END OF PAPER**

# FINAL ADVICE

### Arrive well rested, well fed and well hydrated

The BMAT is an intense test, so make sure you're ready for it. Unlike the UCAT, you'll have to sit this at a fixed time (normally at 9AM). Thus, ensure you get a good night's sleep before the exam (there is little point cramming) and don't miss breakfast. If you're taking water into the exam then make sure you've been to the toilet before so you don't have to leave during the exam. Make sure you're well rested and fed in order to be at your best!

### Move on

If you're struggling, move on. Every question has equal weighting and there is no negative marking. In the time it takes to answer one hard question, you could gain three times the marks by answering several easier ones. Be smart to score maximum points- especially in section two where some questions are far easier than others.

### Make Notes on your Essay

Some universities may ask you questions on your BMAT essay at the interview. Sometimes you may have the interview as late as March which means that you **MUST** make short notes on the essay title and your main arguments after the essay. This is especially important if you're applying to UCL and Cambridge where the essay is discussed more frequently.

### Afterword

Remember that the route to a high score is your approach and practice. Don't fall into the trap that "*you can't prepare for the BMAT*"– this could not be further from the truth. With knowledge of the test, some useful time-saving techniques and plenty of practice you can dramatically boost your score.

Work hard, never give up and do yourself justice.
Good Luck!

# WHAT'S NEXT?

Preparing for the BMAT is just **one step** on your path to medical school.

To make the most of your preparation, we would strongly recommend that you ensure you perform at your very best in your **interviews** as well.

Don't worry though, we have you covered. Medical interviews can be unpredictable, and are *always* tough, but UniAdmissions is the UK's best medical admissions company for a reason, and our expertise is key to mastering your interviews.

The Ultimate Medical School Interview Guide is your next step – take control of your application, and your future, here and save up to 50%: https://amzn.to/3NJoJWl

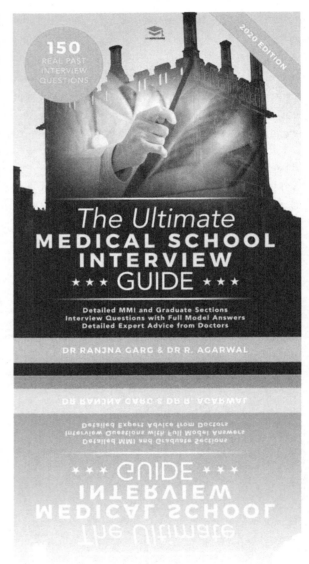

# ACKNOWLEDGEMENTS

I would like to thank Rohan and the UniAdmissions Tutors for all their hard work and advice in compiling this book, and both my parents and Meg for their continued unwavering support.

*Matthew*

# ABOUT US

UniAdmissions currently publishes over 85 titles across a range of subject areas – covering specialised admissions tests, examination techniques, personal statement guides, plus everything else you need to improve your chances of getting on to competitive university courses such as medicine and law, as well as into universities such as Oxford and Cambridge.

This company was founded in 2013 by Dr Rohan Agarwal and Dr David Salt, both Cambridge medical graduates with several years of tutoring experience. Since then, every year, hundreds of applicants and schools work with us on our programmes. Through the programmes we offer, we deliver expert tuition, exclusive course places, online courses, best-selling textbooks and much more.

With a team of over 1,000 Oxbridge tutors and a proven track record, UniAdmissions have quickly become the UK's number one admissions company.

Visit and engage with us at:
Website (UniAdmissions): www.uniadmissions.co.uk
Facebook: www.facebook.com/uniadmissionsuk

# YOUR FREE BOOK

Thanks for purchasing this Ultimate Book. Readers like you have the power to make or break a book — hopefully you found this one useful and informative. *UniAdmissions* would love to hear about your experiences with this book. As thanks for your time we'll send you another ebook from our Ultimate Guide series absolutely <u>FREE</u>!

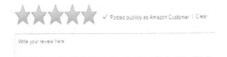

## How to Redeem Your Free Ebook

1) Find the book you have on your Amazon purchase history or your email receipt to help find the book on Amazon.

2) On the product page at the Customer Reviews area, click 'Write a customer review'. Write your review and post it! Copy the review page or take a screen shot of the review you have left.

3) Head over to www.uniadmissions.co.uk/free-book and select your chosen free ebook!

Your ebook will then be emailed to you — it's as simple as that!
Alternatively, you can buy all the titles at

<u>www.uniadmissions.co.uk</u>

Printed in Great Britain
by Amazon

83857909R00244